Recent Progress in Steroids Research

Recent Progress in Steroids Research

Editor: Dwyane Mason

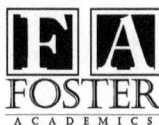

FA FOSTER
ACADEMICS

www.fosteracademics.com

www.fosteracademics.com

FOSTER
ACADEMICS

Cataloging-in-Publication Data

Recent progress in steroids research / edited by Dwyane Mason.
    p. cm.
Includes bibliographical references and index.
ISBN 978-1-63242-827-1
1. Steroids. 2. Steroids--Research. 3. Steroid drugs. I. Mason, Dwyane.
RM297.S74 R43 2019
615.36--dc23

Foster Academics,
118-35 Queens Blvd., Suite 400,
Forest Hills, NY 11375, USA

ISBN 978-1-63242-827-1 (Hardback)

Contents

Preface

Every book is initially just a concept; it takes months of research and hard work to give it the final shape in which the readers receive it. In its early stages, this book also went through rigorous reviewing. The notable contributions made by experts from across the globe were first molded into patterned chapters and then arranged in a sensibly sequential manner to bring out the best results.

The core structure of a steroid comprises of seventeen carbon atoms, bonded in four fused rings. These include one five-member cyclopentane ring, and three six-member cyclohexane rings. Steroids are biologically active organic compounds which have four rings arranged in a specific molecular configuration. These are found in several animals, fungi and plants. They are usually formed in the cells from the sterols lanosterol or cycloartenol. Steroids can be modified by slight changes to the ring structure. Gonane is the simplest steroid, which is the fundamental nucleus of all steroids. It consists of the fusion of a phenanthrene ring with a cyclopentane ring. This book brings forth some of the most innovative concepts and elucidates the unexplored aspects of steroids. It is a valuable compilation of topics, ranging from the basic to the most complex advancements in the research of steroids. The book is appropriate for students seeking detailed information in this area as well as for experts.

It has been my immense pleasure to be a part of this project and to contribute my years of learning in such a meaningful form. I would like to take this opportunity to thank all the people who have been associated with the completion of this book at any step.

Editor

Effects of Intramuscular or Bioadhesive Buccal Testosterone Treatment on Antioxidant Systems in Secondary Hypogonadism

Mancini A[1]*, Raimondo S[1], Di Segni C[1], Persano M[1], Cammarano M[1], Pontecorvi A[1], Festa R[2], Tiano L[3], Silvestrini A[4] and Meucci E[4]

[1]Department of Medical Sciences, Division of Endocrinology, The Catholic University School of Medicine, Rome, Italy
[2]Department of Clinical and Molecular Sciences, Polytechnic University of Marche, Ancona, Italy
[3]Institute of Biochemistry, Polytechnic University of the Marche, Ancona, Italy
[4]Institute of Biochemistry and Clinical Biochemistry, Catholic University of the Sacred Heart, Rome, Italy

Abstract

From cross-sectional studies in healthy men, lower plasma total testosterone levels seem to be associated with hyperinsulinemia, decreased glucose tolerance, and a higher level of cardiovascular risk factors. Despite in vitro and in vivo experiments suggest a key role of testosterone in modulating antioxidant systems in different tissues, few data are reported in humans. Extending our previous results, we show that treatment with testosterone, both in intramuscular or bioadhesive buccal formulations, increase plasma levels of Coenzyme Q10, lipophilic antioxidant, and total antioxidant capacity, measured with colorimetric method, in patients with secondary hypogonadism. Hypogonadism could represent a condition of oxidative stress, in turn related with augmented cardiovascular risk in such patients.

Keywords: Hypogonadism; Hyperinsulinemia; Testosterone

Introduction

From cross-sectional studies in healthy men, lower plasma total testosterone (T) levels seem to be associated with hyperinsulinemia, decreased glucose tolerance, and a higher level of cardiovascular risk factors [1-4]. A relatively low blood concentration of testosterone in the older men may have adverse effects, promoting atherosclerosis, and explain the higher incidence of coronary heart disease in the male [5]. Therefore, male hypogonadism can be associated to metabolic syndrome and increased cardiovascular risk [6]. Oxidative stress (OS), due to an imbalance between reactive oxygen species (ROS) and antioxidant defense, is a possible mechanism involved both in complications of metabolic syndrome and male infertility [7]. It has already been recognized that seminal Total Antioxidant Capacity (TAC, which reflects non enzymatic antioxidants) significantly correlates with FSH, LH, free-T3 (fT3), but not with testosterone [8]. In previous works we have demonstrated alterations of plasma coenzyme Q10 (CoQ10, lipidic antioxidant, also endowed with bioenergetic properties) in pituitary diseases, such as acromegaly or secondary hypothyroidism: in particular, a significant inverse correlation between plasmatic values of CoQ10 and thyroid hormones, fT3 and free-T4 (fT4), was observed; in patients with acromegaly, plasmatic value of CoQ10 was low [7]. Moreover, a relationship between sex hormones and plasmatic TAC was already observed. Finally, we have demonstrated that Testosterone treatment induced a significant change both in CoQ10 level and LAG in secondary hypogonadism [9].

To further investigate the role of gonadal steroids in the regulation of systemic antioxidants, we have determined blood plasma CoQ10 and TAC in a group of post-surgical hypogonadal patients, before and after treatment with two different testosterone formulations.

Materials and Methods

20 patients, aged 20-70 yrs, were studied at 6-12 months after trans-sphenoidal operation for pituitary tumors (prolactinomas or non secreting tumors of the hypothalamus-pituitary region). All were hypopituitaric, but exhibited a normalization of thyroidal and adrenal hormone values with replacement therapy (50-100 mcg of L-thyroxine daily and 20-30 mg of hydrocortisone daily). Replacement therapy for hypogonadism was performed, randomly assigning the patients to two groups: testosterone enantate (250 mg i.e. every 3 weeks, group A, n=15) bioadhesive buccal testosterone (30 mg/daily, group B, n=5). 10 normal subjects, aged 30-55 yrs, were studied as control group.

Main outcome measures

CoQ10 levels were measured by a well recognized HPLC (high-performance liquid chromatography) method [10]. The method is based on oxidation of CoQ10 in the sample by treating it with para-benzoquinone followed by extraction with 1-propanol and direct injection into the HPLC apparatus. Preoxidation of the sample ensures quantification of total CoQ10 by U.V. detection. This method achieves a linear detector response for peak area measurements over the concentration range of 0.05-3.47 μM. Diode array analysis of the peak was consistent with CoQ10 spectrum. Supplementation of the samples with known amounts of CoQ10 yielded a quantitative recovery of 96–98.5%; the method showed a level of quantitation of 1.23 nmol per HPLC injection (200 μl of propanol extract containing 33.3 μl of plasma). A good correlation was found with a reference electrochemical detection method ($r = 0.99$, $p<0.0001$). Within run precision showed a CV% of 1.6 for samples approaching normal values (1.02 μM). Day-to-day precision was also close to 2%. Moreover, CoQ10 values were related to plasma cholesterol concentration, measured by a cholesterol oxidase enzymatic test.

Total Antioxidant Capacity (TAC) was evaluated, with a modification of the method developed by Rice-Evans and Miller [11], as previously described [12]. The method is based on the antioxidants inhibition of the absorbance of the radical cation

---

*Corresponding author: Mancini A, Department of Medical Sciences, Division of Endocrinology, The Catholic University School of Medicine, Rome, Italy, E-mail: me4224@mclink.it

2,2¹-azinobis (3-ethylbenzothiazoline-6 sulphonate) (ABTS·⁺) formed by interaction between ABTS (150 μM) and ferryl myoglobin radical species, generated by activation of meta myoglobin (2.5 μM) with H_2O_2 (75 μM). Aliquots of the frozen plasma were thawed at room temperature and 10 μl of the samples were tested immediately. The manual procedure was used with only minor modifications, i.e., temperature at 37°C to be in more physiological conditions and each sample assayed alone to carefully control timing and temperature. The reaction was started directly in cuvette through H_2O_2 addition after 1 min equilibration of all other reagents (temperature control by a thermocouple probe, model 1408 K thermocouple, Digitron Instrumentation Ltd, Scunthorpe, United kingdom) and followed for 10 min under continuous stirring, monitoring at 734 nm, typical of the spectroscopically detectable ABTS·⁺. The presence of chain-breaking antioxidants induces a lag time (the Lag phase) in the accumulation of ABTS·⁺ whose duration is proportional to the concentration of this type of antioxidants. Antioxidant capacity afforded by chain-breaking antioxidants is expressed as length of Lag phase (sec). Trolox, a water-soluble tocopherol analog, was used as a reference standard and assayed in all experiments to control the system. Absorbance was measured with a Hewlett-Packard 8450A UV/Vis spectrophotometer (Palo Alto, CA) equipped with a cuvette stirring apparatus and a constant temperature cell holder. Measurements of pH were made with a PHM84 Research pH meter (Radiometer, Copenhagen, Denmark,); the electrode response was corrected for temperature. Unless stated differently, experiments were repeated two to three times; qualitatively similar results were obtained with individual values varying<8%.

In the Lag mode, the assay mainly measures nonprotein and nonenzymatic antioxidants that are primarily extracellular chain breaking antioxidants, such as ascorbate, urate and glutathione [12].

Statistics

Distribution of data was estimated by the test of Kolmogorov-Smirnov. Since the data were not distributed normally, the comparison among groups was made using Mann-Whitney U test; the comparison in the same patients, before and after therapy was performed using Wilcoxon-Runk Sum test. Linear correlation analysis was also employed. The Software Arcus Quickstat (Software Publishing Biomedical version 1.2) was used for this statistic analysis.

Results

Hypogonadal patients, considered as a whole group, showed lower values of antioxidant systems than control subjects. The figure 1 shows mean ± SEM CoQ10 values, significantly lower in hypogonadal patients (0.66 ± 0.07 vs 0.93 ± 0.11 μg/ml respectively, p<0.05). The figure 2 shows mean ± SEM TAC values, expressed as LAG (71 ± 5.5 vs 76 ± 9.91 sec), with a trend toward lower levels in hypogonadal patients.

Testosterone treatment induced a change both in CoQ10 level (0.81 ± 0.43 in group A; 0.67 ± 0.03 μg in group B) and LAG (78.33 ± 4.53 sec in group A and 80 ± 4.03 sec in group B) (Table 1).

CoQ10 and LAG values significantly correlated (r=0, 7; p<0.001), when CoQ10 was corrected for cholesterol values (Figure 3), suggesting an inter-relationship between different antioxidants.

Discussion

Low testosterone levels may predict increased cardiovascular risk in men [13]. Moreover, treatment with exogenous testosterone improved arterial vasodilation [14] and lipid profile [15] in patients

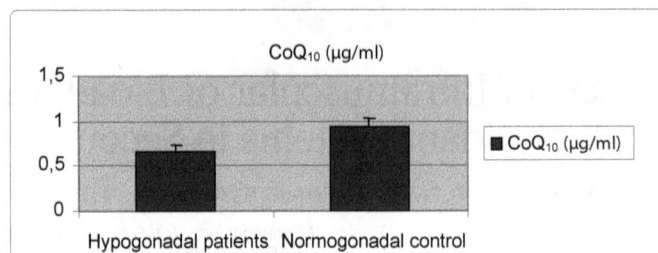

Figure 1: Mean (± SEM) CoQ10 values in patients with secondary hypogonadism and normal controls.

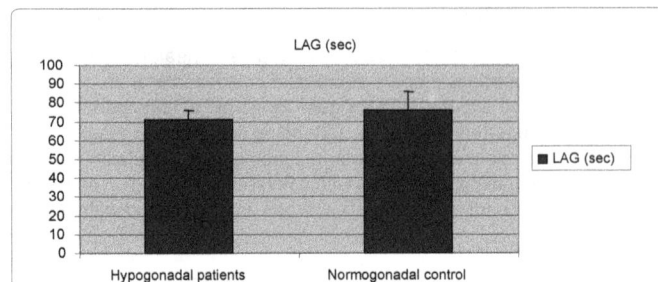

Figure 2: Mean (± SEM) Total antioxidant capacity values, expressed as LAG, in patients with secondary hypogonadism and normal controls.

	Group A		Group B	
	Pretreatment	Post treatment Pre	Pretreatment	Post treatment
CoQ10 (μg/ml)	0.65 ± 0.21	0.81 ± 0.43	0.43 ± 0.06	0.67 ± 0.03
LAG (sec)	56.66 ± 4.08	78.33 ± 4.53	56 ± 8.16	80 ± 4.03

Table 1: Mean ± SEM CoQ10 and LAG values, before and after treatment, in the two groups of patients, treated with different testosterone formulations.

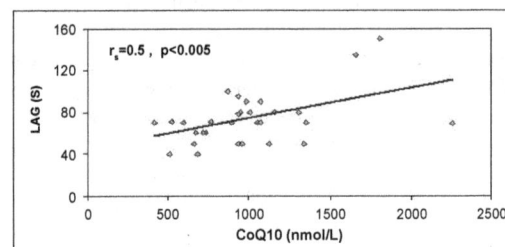

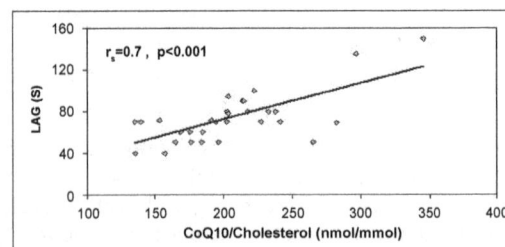

Figure 3: Graphical representation of simple regression analysis, plotting CoQ10 values (upper panel) or CoQ10/cholesterol values (lower panel) and LAG values in our patients.

with cardiovascular disease. In particular, testosterone induced a decrease of serum triglycerides, LDL cholesterol and an increase in HDL cholesterol.

Oxidative stress could be a mechanism involved in progression of cardiovascular disease, in part for the oxidation of LDL-cholesterol [16], and in part for the activation of neutrophils, that contribute to ROS production through NADPH oxidase activation and release of myeloperoxidase, with a vicious circle inducing more toxic oxidant species. This mechanism can be counteracted by testosterone [17].

The role of androgens in the regulation of antioxidant systems is not fully understood. No significant effects of androgens were reported on antioxidant enzymes in erythrocytes [18]; conflicting results have also been reported about regulation of nitric oxide (NO) synthesis in immune system [19]; however antioxidant properties of testosterone in human neutrophils have been recently demonstrated, as indicated by suppression of superoxide anion and thiobarbituric acid-reactive substances (TBARS) levels, increase of NO levels, glutathione reductase activity and thiol groups; so testosterone administration at physiological concentrations had a greater antioxidant potential than higher concentrations [20].

Oxidative stress is claimed as responsible for toxicity and apoptosis of cardiomyocites induced by doxorubicin; in AR (androgen receptor)-KO mice mitochondrial damage induced by the drug, with following ROS generation, is aggravated and the effect again counteracted by the system androgen-AR [21]. Castration induced an elevated prooxidant state in LV of adult Wistar rats, with a significant decrease of Superoxide Dismutase (SOD), Glutathione peroxidase (GPX), catalase (CAT), Glutathione Reductase (GR), and a trend toward lower levels of glutathione (GSH) and protein thiols, and an increase in lipid peroxidation and higher nitrotyrosine concentrations. The reestablishment of physiological T levels by androgen replacement resulted in a further decrease in the antioxidant defence [22].

Direct action at endothelial levels has been demonstrated [23]. Moreover testosterone attenuated expression of vascular cell adhesion molecule-1 by conversion to estradiol by aromatase [24]. Both in vitro and in vivo experiments also indicate direct testosterone effects on NO synthesis, and on tissue plasminogen activactor (t-PA) and plasminogen activator inhibitor-I (PAI-I) expression. However differential effects are exerted by physiological or supraphysiological T doses.

Testosterone can have protective effects against oxidative stress in many other tissues and systems. OS causes β-cell apoptosis in streptozotocin-diabetic mice [25]; testosterone has been shown to exert a cytoprotective action in gonadectomized rats, inducing an increase in catalase and Cu/Zn SOD; however this effect was sex-specific, inducible only in male rats, treated with testosterone, but not in female rats or male rats treated with estradiol or progesterone [26]. Another important site of action is central nervous system (CNS): testosterone protects cerebellar granule cells from oxidative stress-induced cell death by receptor-mediated mechanism [27], through an increase in catalase activity. Differential effects of glucocorticoid and gonadal steroids on glutathione levels were exerted in neuronal and glial cells: models of neuronal hippocampal cells (HT22) and glioma cells (C6) were tested and testosterone effects were also observed in long-term experiments [28]. The same group also showed increase in catalase activity after both short- and long-term incubation with gonadal steroids [29]. Testosterone was able to protect from OS and cell damage in the striatum, induced by ovariectomy (via caspase-3) and further increased by administration of 3-nitropropionic acid [30]. These studies are of fundamental importance for the investigation of neurodegenerative disorders, since OS has been implicated in the development of Alzheimer's disease, Parkinson disease and amyotrophic lateral sclerosis [31].

As genital apparatus is concerned, different studies have been performed on testis and prostate. Hypoxia exposure initiates low serum testosterone levels that could be attributed to down-regulated androgen biosynthesizing genes, such as StAR (steroidogenic acute regulatory protein) and 3-β-HSD (hydroxysteroid dehydrogenase) in the testis, associated with OS and increase in chaperones of endoplasmic reticulum, modulated by a reduction in calcium influx (ER stress) [32]. A protective effect was demonstrated for low dose testosterone supplementation in TM3 cell line (obtained by mouse and characterized by the presence of AR): significantly reduced ROS generation, lipid peroxide contents and hypoxia induction-factor (HIF)-1α stabilization and activation were found with 100-nmol l^{-1} testosterone treatment; a 1.58-fold increase in StAR expression was found in 50- nmol l^{-1}; however there was a 1.72-fold increase in ROS generation in the 500- nmol l^{-1}, compared with the 100- nmol l^{-1} testosterone treatment [33].

Finally, androgens could exert an important role in the regulation of redox state in the prostate. It has been demonstrated that castration induced a discrete OS in the acinar epithelium of rat ventral prostate (VP), as evidenced from marked increases in 8-hydroxy-2'-deoxyguanosine and 4-hydroxynonenal protein adduct in the regressing epithelium [34]. Castration induced a dramatic increase of three ROS-generating NAD(P)H oxidases (Nox1, gp91phox and Nox4), a significant reduction of key ROS-detoxifying enzymes (SOD 2, GPX 1, thioredoxin, peroxiredoxin 5); catalase, glutathione reductase, γ-glutamyl trasnpeptidase, and glutathione synthetase levels remained unchanged. Testosterone replacement partially reduced OS in VP epithelia of castrated animals, however without restoring a fully normal pattern: it partially reduced expression of Noxs, but restored expression of SOD 2, GPX 1, thioredoxin, peroxiredoxin 5; moreover it induced a compensatory increase in expression of catalase, glutathione reductase, γ-glutamyl trasnpeptidase, and glutathione synthetase in the regenerating VP [35].

The present results, extending our previous data [9], confirm that hypogonadal patients present lower levels of antioxidant defence and therefore are more vulnerable to oxidative damage than normal eugonadal controls. The levels of CoQ10 were significantly lower, while TAC exhibited a trend toward lower levels.

TAC, as previously described [7], is a measurement of the non-enzymatic antioxidants that are primarily extracellular (ascorbate, urates, albumin, tocopherol and glutathione). They are "chain-breaking" molecules able to block the propagation chain of lipid peroxidation and to prevent the amplification of radical generation and the subsequent biochemical damage. Differently by enzymes, they are consumed at the moment in which they act and this fact could explain the reduction in their levels in biological fluids producing ROS (for example, the high levels of ROS and a low TAC in the seminal fluid of infertile males suggests oxidative stress is associated to a variety of etiologies of male infertility) [36]. The dosage of TAC is considered a better index of the total antioxidant status of a biological sample than the measurement of one or more specific antioxidant, that could not carefully reflect the combined effect of the various antioxidants and their "collaboration" during the oxidative stress. CoQ10 is a key component of the mitochondrial oxidative phosphorylation chain as link between flavoproteins and cytochromes in inner mitochondrial membrane. It has also many other functions, first of all a powerful antioxidant activity, and new roles in different cellular functions are coming out in last times, because this molecule can participate in oxido-reductive reactions not only in mitochondria, but also in lysosomial, in Golgi apparatus and plasmatic membranes [37], even contributing to membrane fluidity. Moreover CoQ10 can take part in many aspects of the oxido-reductive control of the cellular signalling origin and transmission; in fact the autooxidation of semi-quinon, formed in various membranes during the electronic transportation, can be a primary source for the H2O2 generation, which activates some transcription factors, as NFkB, to induce gene expression [38].

We observed a significant direct correlation between CoQ10 and TAC in our patients, suggesting an important CoQ10 contribution to TAC and an inter-relationship between the different antioxidants. The greater impact on CoQ10 could be attributed to its lipophilic nature and the alterations of lipidic pattern in hypogonadal patients. There is a relationship between low concentrations of plasma CoQ10 and coronary disease, even if this correlation is not so strong to be considered a casual relation [39]. Ubiquinol/ubiquinone ratio is considered an oxidative stress marker in coronary disease and LDL/CoQ10 ratio is an index of coronary risk factor [40]. Therefore our data underline, according to the protective role of ubiquinone in cardiovascular disease, a mechanism underlying the cardiovascular risk of hypogonadal patients.

Testosterone administration induced a significant increase in both parameters, independently from pharmacological route of adimistration, reinforcing the concept of a positive influence of testosterone *per se* on antioxidant systems.

In conclusion, the role of androgens in modulating the balance between ROS generation and antioxidant defences is very complex and related the different models investigated, time and dose of administration, different metabolic pathways of testosterone itself. Very few data are reported in vivo in humans. Our data allow to affirm that CoQ10 and TAC are significantly lower in secondary hypogonadic patients and that testosterone treatment exerts a positive effect on such values. Hypogonadism could represent a condition of oxidative stress, in turn related with augmented cardiovascular risk in such patients.

References

1. Kaufman JM, Vermeulen A (2005) The decline of androgen levels in elderly men and its clinical and therapeutic implications. Endocr Rev 26: 833-876.

2. Matsumoto AM (2002) Andropause: clinical implications of the decline in serum testosterone levels with aging in men. J Gerontol A Biol Sci Med Sci 57: M76-99.

3. Rodriguez A, Muller DC, Metter EJ, Maggio M, Harman SM, et al. (2007) Aging, androgens, and the metabolic syndrome in a longitudinal study of aging. J Clin Endocrinol Metab 92: 3568-3572.

4. Vermeulen A (2001) Androgen replacement therapy in the aging male--a critical evaluation. J Clin Endocrinol Metab 86: 2380-2390.

5. Camacho EM, Huhtaniemi IT, O'Neill TW, Finn JD, Pye SR, et al. (2013) Age-associated changes in hypothalamic-pituitary-testicular function in middle-aged and older men are modified by weight change and lifestyle factors: longitudinal results from the European Male Ageing Study. Eur J Endocrinol 168: 445-455.

6. Wu FC, von Eckardstein A (2003) Androgens and coronary artery disease. Endocr Rev 24: 183-217.

7. Mancini A, Festa R, Di Donna V, Leone E, Littarru GP, et al. (2010) Hormones and antioxidant systems: role of pituitary and pituitary-dependent axes. J Endocrinol Invest 33: 422-433.

8. Mancini A, Festa R, Silvestrini A, Nicolotti N, Di Donna V, et al. (2009) Hormonal regulation of total antioxidant capacity in seminal plasma. J Androl 30: 534-540.

9. Mancini A, Leone E, Festa R, Grande G, Silvestrini A, et al. (2008) Effects of testosterone on antioxidant systems in male secondary hypogonadism. J Androl 29: 622-629.

10. Littarru GP, Tiano L (2005) Clinical aspects of coenzyme Q10: an update. Curr Opin Clin Nutr Metab Care 8: 641-646.

11. Rice-Evans C, Miller NJ (1994) Total antioxidant status in plasma and body fluids. Methods Enzymol 234: 279-293.

12. Meucci E, Milardi D, Mordente A, Martorana GE, Giacchi E, et al. (2003) Total antioxidant capacity in patients with varicoceles. Fertil Steril 79 Suppl 3: 1577-1583.

13. Svartberg J, von Mühlen D, Mathiesen E, Joakimsen O, Bønaa KH, et al. (2006) Low testosterone levels are associated with carotid atherosclerosis in men. J Intern Med 259: 576-582.

14. Webb CM, McNeill JG, Hayward CS, de Zeigler D, Collins P (1999) Effects of testosterone on coronary vasomotor regulation in men with coronary heart disease. Circulation 100: 1690-1696.

15. Wu S, Weng X (1992) Therapeutic effect of andriol on serum lipids and apolipoproteins in elderly male coronary heart disease patients. Chin Med Sci J 7: 137-141.

16. Griendling KK, Sorescu D, Ushio-Fukai M (2000) NAD(P)H oxidase: role in cardiovascular biology and disease. Circ Res 86: 494-501.

17. Békési G, Kakucs R, Várbíró S, Rácz K, Sprintz D, et al. (2000) In vitro effects of different steroid hormones on superoxide anion production of human neutrophil granulocytes. Steroids 65: 889-894.

18. Massafra C, Gioia D, De Felice C, Picciolini E, De Leo V, et al. (2000) Effects of estrogens and androgens on erythrocyte antioxidant superoxide dismutase, catalase and glutathione peroxidase activities during the menstrual cycle. J Endocrinol 167: 447-452.

19. Friedl R, Brunner M, Moeslinger T, Spieckermann PG (2000) Testosterone inhibits expression of inducible nitric oxide synthase in murine macrophages. Life Sci 68: 417-429.

20. Marin DP, Bolin AP, dos Santos Rde C, Curi R, Otton R (2010) Testosterone suppresses oxidative stress in human neutrophils. Cell Biochem Funct 28: 394-402.

21. Ikeda Y, Aihara K, Akaike M, Sato T, Ishikawa K, et al. (2010) Androgen receptor counteracts Doxorubicin-induced cardiotoxicity in male mice. Mol Endocrinol 24: 1338-1348.

22. Kłapcińska B, Jagsz S, Sadowska-Krepa E, Górski J, Kempa K et al. (2008) Effects of castration and testosterone replacement on the antioxidant defense system in rat left ventricle. J Physiol Sci 58: 173-177.

23. Campelo AE, Cutini PH, Massheimer VL (2012) Testosterone modulates platelet aggregation and endothelial cell growth through nitric oxide pathway. J Endocrinol 213: 77-87.

24. Mukherjee TK, Dinh H, Chaudhuri G, Nathan L (2002) Testosterone attenuates expression of vascular cell adhesion molecule-1 by conversion to estradiol by aromatase in endothelial cells: implications in atherosclerosis. Proc Natl Acad Sci U S A 99: 4055-4060.

25. O'Brien BA, Harmon BV, Cameron DP, Allan DJ (1996) Beta-cell apoptosis is responsible for the development of IDDM in the multiple low-dose streptozotocin model. J Pathol 178: 176-181.

26. Palomar-Morales M, Morimoto S, Mendoza-Rodríguez CA, Cerbón MA (2010) The protective effect of testosterone on streptozotocin-induced apoptosis in beta cells is sex specific. Pancreas 39: 193-200.

27. Ahlbom E, Prins GS, Ceccatelli S (2001) Testosterone protects cerebellar granule cells from oxidative stress-induced cell death through a receptor mediated mechanism. Brain Res 892: 255-262.

28. Schmidt AJ, Krieg J-, Vedder H (2002) Differential effects of glucocorticoids and gonadal steroids on glutathione levels in neuronal and glial cell systems. J Neurosci Res 67: 544-550.

29. Schmidt AJ, Krieg JC, Vedder H (2005) Effects of steroid hormones on catalase activity in neuronal and glial cell systems. Eur Neuropsychopharmacol 15: 177-183.

30. Túnez I, Feijóo M, Collado JA, Medina FJ, Peña J, et al. (2007) Effect of testosterone on oxidative stress and cell damage induced by 3-nitropropionic acid in striatum of ovariectomized rats. Life Sci 80: 1221-1227.

31. Barron AM, Fuller SJ, Verdile G, Martins RN (2006) Reproductive hormones modulate oxidative stress in Alzheimer's disease. Antioxid Redox Signal 8: 2047-2059.

32. Liu GL, Yu F, Dai DZ, Zhang GL, Zhang C, et al. (2012) Endoplasmic reticulum

stress mediating downregulated StAR and 3-beta-HSD and low plasma testosterone caused by hypoxia is attenuated by CPU86017-RS and nifedipine. J Biomed Sci 19: 4.

33. Hwang TI, Liao TL, Lin JF, Lin YC, Lee SY, et al. (2011) Low-dose testosterone treatment decreases oxidative damage in TM3 Leydig cells. Asian J Androl 13: 432-437.

34. Kohen R, Nyska A (2002) Oxidation of biological systems: oxidative stress phenomena, antioxidants, redox reactions, and methods for their quantification. Toxicol Pathol 30: 620-650.

35. Tam NN, Gao Y, Leung YK, Ho SM (2003) Androgenic regulation of oxidative stress in the rat prostate: involvement of NAD(P)H oxidases and antioxidant defense machinery during prostatic involution and regrowth. Am J Pathol 163: 2513-2522.

36. Lewis SE, Boyle PM, McKinney KA, Young IS, Thompson W (1995) Total antioxidant capacity of seminal plasma is different in fertile and infertile men. Fertil Steril 64: 868-870.

37. Crane FL (2001) Biochemical functions of coenzyme Q10. J Am Coll Nutr 20: 591-598.

38. Kaltschmidt B, Sparna T, Kaltschmidt C (1999) Activation of NF-kappa B by reactive oxygen intermediates in the nervous system. Antioxid Redox Signal 1: 129-144.

39. Yalcin A, Kilinc E, Sagcan A, Kultursay H (2004) Coenzyme Q10 concentrations in coronary artery disease. Clin Biochem 37: 706-709.

40. Tomasetti M, Alleva R, Solenghi MD, Littarru GP (1999) Distribution of antioxidants among blood components and lipoproteins: significance of lipids/CoQ10 ratio as a possible marker of increased risk for atherosclerosis. Biofactors 9: 231-240.

2

Myeloperoxidase Anti-neutrophil Cytoplasmic Antibody Glomerulosclerosis Associated with Pulmonary Disorders

Toru Sanai*, Takako Hirakawa, Toru Mizumasa, and Hideyuki Koga

Department of Internal Medicine and Clinical Research Institute, National Kyushu Medical Center, 1-8-1 Jigyohama, Chuo-ku, Fukuoka-city, 810-8563 Fukuoka, Japan

Abstract

Seven patients presented a specific renal lesion of rapidly progressive glomerulonephritis with myeloperoxidase anti-neutrophil cytoplasmic antibody. Rapidly progressive glomerulonephritis with myeloperoxidase anti-neutrophil cytoplasmic antibody can be associated with pulmonary hemorrhage and/or pulmonary interstitial fibrosis. The patients included three men and four women with a mean age of 62.4 years. All courses of renal lesions revealed rapidly progressive glomerulonephritis and the serum creatinine levels were 7.1 ± 3.9 mg/dl and the myeloperoxidase anti-neutrophil cytoplasmic antibody was 473 ± 471 EU before treatments. Steroid therapy was administered to all patients, immunosupressive agent to four and hemodialysis in six cases. Four patients experienced a pulmonary hemorrhage and died, but all of three patients with pulmonary interstitial fibrosis survived. All of four cases died due to an infection in pulmonary hemorrhage. Although three patients with pulmonary interstitial fibrosis were survived, pulmonary hemorrhage indicated a poor prognosis. Pulmonary infection may be fetal in pulmonary hemorrhage, but pulmonary infection was a few in pulmonary interstitial fibrosis.

Keywords: Infection; Myeloperoxidase anti-neutrophil cytoplasmic antibody; Pulmonary Hemorrhage; Pulmonary interstitial fibrosis; Rapidly progressive glomerulonephritis; Steroid

Introduction

Many patients experience rapidly progressive glomerulonephritis (RPGN) with myeloperoxidase anti-neutrophil cytoplasmic antibody (MPO-ANCA) [1,2]. As RPGN with MPO-ANCA can be associated with Pulmonary Hemorrhage (PH) and/or pulmonary interstitial fibrosis (PIF), which are often fatal [3,4]. Cough, chest pain, and shortness of breath may be present and chest radiographic features consist of patchy, bilateral airspace opacities caused by alveolar hemorrhage in PIF [4]. Seven patients with renal lesions characteristic of RPGN with MPO-ANCA experienced pulmonary disorders in this study.

Cases and Methods

This study of seven patients suffering from RPGN with MPO-ANCA was performed at the Department of Internal Medicine, National Kyushu Medical Center over an approximate 5-year period. A renal biopsy was performed in 2 of 7 cases (cases 1 and 4) and case 4 was undergoing regular hemodialysis. All of the patients were suffering from RPGN and pulmonary disorders.

Table 1 show that all seven patients were diagnosed with RPGN with MPO-ANCA. The patients included three men and four women with a mean age of 62.4 years (47-72 year old). All of the renal lesions were characteristic of RPGN and the serum creatinine levels were 7.1 ± 3.9 [means ± SD] mg/dl and the MPO-ANCA was 474 ± 471 EU before treatments. Four of the patients experienced PH and died, but three patients with PIF thereafter recovered.

Case	Age/Sex (Year old)	Original Disease	Course Kidney	OB/Before Tx Cr (mg/dl)	MPO-ANCA (EU)	ABG PO2 (mmHg)	Dx of lung
1	64 M	CrGN	RPGN	3+/4.3	22	70 (room air)	PH
2	47F	CrGN	RPGN	3+/12.8	108	88 (room air)	PH
3	72M	CrGN	RPGN	3+/4.5	924	56 (mask 10 l/min)	PH
4	57F	CrGN	RPGN, rHD	anuria/6.5	100	34 (nasal 3 l/min)	PH (4 times)
5	65F	RA, AA, MPA	CRF→MPA RPGN	3+/5.0	1000	83 (room air)	PIF
6	66F	MPA	RPGN	-/3.8	136	93 (room air)	PIF
7	66M	MPA	RPGN	±/12.6	126	102 (room air)	PIF

Table 1: Patient profiles of MPO-ANCA glomerulonephritis. Tx=treatment, ABG=arterial blood gas analysis on the admission, Dx=diagnosis,OB=urinary occult blood, Cr=creatinine, CrGN=crescent glomerulonephritis, MPA=microscopic polyangiitis, RA=rheumatic arthritis, AA=secondary amyloidosis, RPGN=rapidly progressive glomerulonephritis, rHD=regular hemodialysis, CRF=chronic renal failure, PH=pulmonary hemorrhage, and PIF=pulmonary interstitial pneumonia.

*Corresponding author: Toru Sanai, MD, The Division of nephrology, Fukumitsu Hospital, 4-10-1 Kashiihama Higashi-ku, Fukuoka-city, 813-0016 Fukuoka, Japan, E-mail: sunny@fukumitsu-hospital.jp

Seven patients of RPGN with MPO-ANCA and pulmonary disorders clinicopathologically examined. Table 2 shows that steroids (pulse in six cases and oral in one case) were administered to all of patients, a immunosuppressive agent (cyclophosphamide) to four patients and hemodialysis in six patients (endotoxin absorption therapy was added in case 2 and plasma exchange in case 3). Cyclophosphamide pulse and corticosteroid pulse therapy was used in case 5. Among the four

patients who died from PH (all were founded by autopsy), pneumonia and disseminated intravascular coagulation were observed in case 1, fungus, cytomegalovirus infection, pneumonia, disseminate, intravascular coagulation and sepsis in cases 2 and 4 and pneumonia (haemophilus influenza) in case 3 (Title 3). Antibiotics were used in case 1-4, but were not used in case 5-7.

Case	Steroid	Immunosupression	Hemdialysis	Other Therapy
1	pulse	-	-	-
2	pulse	+	+	endotoxin absorption
3	pulse	+	+	plasma exchange
4	pulse	+	+	-
5	pulse, oral	-	+	-
6	pulse	+	+	-
7	oral	-	+ (hemodialysis off)	-

Table 2: Treatment of MPO-ANCA glomerulosclerosis.

The serum MPO-ANCA levels remained at 48 ± 92 EU after treatments. There was no correlation between the MPO-ANCA titers and the pulmonary disorders. Although the risk of PH was high, all three patients with PIF were recovered. Pulmonary infection was a few in pulmonary interstitial fibrosis (Table 3). The autopsies of three patients

revealed vasculitis in only one case. The patients were observed for a mean of 32.9 months (0-72 months). Cases 5 and 6 were undergoing maintenance hemodialysis. CRP was negative in PIF, IgG lower than 600 mg/dl in case 4, neutrophil lower than 500 /mm3 in none, and lymphocyte lower than 500/ mm3 in cases 2, 3, 4 and 7 (Title 3).

Case	Association	CRP (mg/dl)	WBC/N/L (X102/mm3)	IgG (mg/dl)	Prognosis
1	pn, DIC	29.64	81/67/10	2862	died
2	fungus, CMV, pn, DIC, sepsis	48.27	177/162/0.9	850	died
3	pn (hemo.inf)	27.17	204/189/4	1294	died
4	fungus, CMV, pn, DIC, sepsis	32.8	16/10/0.3	481	died
5	-	< 0.3	82/62/13	783	alive
6	-	< 0.3	70/38/9	748	alive
7	-	< 0.3	85/64/2	1975	alive

Table 3: Association and Course of MPO-ANCA glomerulosclerosis pn=pneumonia, DIC=disseminat intravascular couagulation, CMV=cytomegarovirus, hemo.inf=hemofirusu infuensa, CRP=C-reactive protein, WBC=white blood cell, N=neutrophil, and L=lymphocyte. Neutrophil and leukocyte; cases 1-4 at the time of death and cases 5-7 at the time on discharge.

Discussion

These seven patients were all thought to have a specific renal lesion known as RPGN with MPO-ANCA. As RPGN with MPO-ANCA can be associated with PH and PIF, four of the patients died from PH and clinicopathologically examined.

The acute management of systemic vasculitis may also require intensive immunosuppressive therapy [3]. However, immunosuppressive therapy can be associated with fungus, cytomegalovirus infection, pneumonia, sepsis and the patients may die due to an infection in PH.On the other hands, PIF and chronic MPO- ANCA glomerulonephritis may require the treatment of infection [5]. Especially, it is necessary that we take preventive drugs such as pentamidine, amphotericin B and itraconazole.

Three of the seven cases with cytoplasmic (C)-ANCA experienced an extensive intra-alveolar hemorrhage while four of the seven patients had perinuclear (P)-ANCA. PIF was detected in two of four cases with C-ANCA vs. three of four cases with P-ANCA. In contrast, the fatal

cases include 3 of the 4 patients with C-ANCA vs. one of the five patients with P-ANCA. Therefore, P-ANCA was associated with a poor prognosis [6].

The mortally rate is higher in patients that experience a hemorrhage in Goodpasture's syndrome (56%) than those who do not (18.4%) [7]. On the other hands, five of six patients with PIF died [4]. Furthermore, three of the four patients with PIF were fatal [2]. PIF has not been commonly appreciated as an accompanying of microscopic polyangitis [8]. However, the involvement of the respiratory system is a very common and important aspect of ANCA associated systemic vasculitis [9,10]. Moreover, PIF may be an early manifestation of the disease, antedating the diagnosis of microscopic polyangititis by two or more years and is associated with a poor prognosis [4]. In the present study, all of the three patients with PIF survived.

Conclusion

RPGN with MPO-ANCA was observed in patients associated with PH and/or PIF. Steroid therapy was administered to all patients. Four of all the patients died due to the PH but those with PIF survived. Pulmonary infection was fetal in PH, but pulmonary infection was a few in PIF.

Acknowledgement

We thank Dr. M. Nakayama at the Department of Internal Medicine, National Kyushu Medical Center.

References

1. Nachman PH, Jennette JC, Falk RJ (2008) Primary glomerular disease. In: Brenner BM (ed.), The Kidney, 8th ed. Philadelphia, W.B. Sauders 987-1066.

2. Hiromura K, Nojima Y, Kitanhara T (2000) Four cases of anti- myeloperoxidase antibody-related rapidly progressive glomerulonephritis during the course of idiopathic pulmonary fibrosis. Clin Nephrol 53: 384-389.

3. Elsharkawy AM, Perrin F, Farmer CK, Abbs IC, Muir P, et al. (2004) Symptomatic cytomegalovirus infection complicating treatment of acute systemic vasculitis. Clin Nephrol 62: 319-326.

4. Eschum GM, Mink SN, Sharma S (2003) Pulmonary interstitial fibrosis as a presenting manifestation in perinuclear antineutrophilic cytoplasmic antibody micrscopic polyangitis. Chest 123: 297-301.

5. Kamesh L, Harper L (2002) Savage COS. ANCA-positive vasculitis. J Am Soc Nephrol 13: 1953-1960.

6. Gal AA, Salinas FF, Staton GW Jr (1994) The clinical and pathological spectrum of antineutrophil cytoplasmic autoantibody-related pulmonary disease. A comparison between perinuclear and cytoplasmic antineutrophil cytoplasmic autoantibodies. Arch Pathol Lab Med 118: 1209-1214.

7. Nagashima T, Ubara Y, Tagami T (2002) Anti-glomerular basement membrane antibody disease: a case report and a review of Japanese patients with and without alveolar hemorrhage. Clin Exp Nephrol 6: 49-59.

8. Souid M, Terki NH, Nochy D (2001) Myeloperoxidase anti-neutrophil cytoplasmic antibody (MPO-ANCA)-related rapidly progressive glomerulonephritis (RPGN) and pulmonary fibrosis (PF) with dissociated evolution. Clin Npehrol 55: 337-338.

9. Manganelli P, Fietta P, Carotti M, Pesci A, Salaffi F (2006) Respiratory system involvement in systemic vasculitides. Clin Exp Rheumatol 24: S48-59.

10. Jennette JC, Falk RJ, Andrassy K, Bacon PA, Churg J, et al. (1994) Nomenclature of systemic vasculitides. Proposal of an international consensus conference. Arthritis Rheum 37: 187-192.

Protective Effect of Taurine on Thiopurine-Induced Testicular Atrophy in Male Albino Rats

Basma K Ramadan[1], Mona F Schaalan[2]* and Eman S Mahmoud[3]

[1]Department of Physiology, Faculty of Medicine for Girls (Cairo), Al-Azhar University, Egypt
[2]Department of Clinical Pharmacy, Faculty of Pharmacy, Misr International University, Cairo, Egypt
[3]Department of Histology, Faculty of Medicine for Girls (Cairo), Al-Azhar, University, Egypt

Abstract

Background: Though the use of Azapress (Azathioprine) in cancers and autoimmune diseases has proved therapeutic effectiveness in numerous prospective clinical trials, some cases of testicular toxicity has been reported, that were referred to the evolved oxidative stress and inflammatory milieu. Taurine (TAU) is an amino acid found abundantly in brain, heart, and reproductive organ cells and with reported antioxidant and anti-inflammatory benefits.

Objective: The aim of the work was to investigate the protective effects of Taurine against Azapress-induced testicular dysfunction in male albino rats and unravel the contributing mechanisms.

Material and methods: Forty adult male albino rats were allocated into four equal groups; (i) normal control rats (Control group), (ii) Azapress group (AZP, 1mg/day for four weeks); (iii) Taurine group(Tau; 100 mg/kg bw/day for 6 weeks), (iv) Taurine and AZP group).

Results: AZP caused alterations in sperm parameters, increased DNA damage, and sex hormones disturbance. Moreover, significant decreased levels of superoxide dismutase (SOD) and catalase (CAT) activities, and upregulated levels of the pro-inflammatory cytokines, tumor necrosis factor-alpha (TNF-α) and interleukin-1beta (IL-1β), as well as apoptotic markers; Bcl2 and caspase-9 expression it were evident in the testicular tissues. In contrast, taurine pretreatment significantly alleviated these toxic effects that were further evidenced histologically.

Conclusion: Our data suggest that oxidative stress and inflammation are involved in AZP-induced destruction in the male reproductive system and that co-administration of taurine exerts a protective effect against AZP-induced male reproductive testicular atrophy. This could open new horizon to its usage as an add-on complementary approach to chemotherapy supportive care.

Keywords: Taurine; Testicular atrophy; Azapress; Bcl2, Caspase-9; DNA fragmentation; IL-1β

Introduction

Thiopurines were first described in the 1950s by Gertrude Elion and George Hitchings and comprised three chemical structures: 6-thioguanine (6-TG), mercaptopurine (MP) and azathioprine [1]. The latter is an immunomodulatory drug, available as Azapress® and Imuran® in the market and often used to treat inflammatory bowel disease, autoimmune disorders, prevent rejection of transplanted organs and acts as an anticancer drug [2]. It acts via multifaceted pathways; it inhibits purine metabolism leading to DNA damage [3], its anti-inflammatory effect is mainly mediated via inhibition of the small GTPase Rac1, leading to apoptosis of activated T-lymphocytes, whereas high chemotherapeutic dosages in oncological treatment are associated with inhibition of DNA synthesis [4]. Upon its administration, it is rapidly converted into several toxic and non-toxic metabolic compounds, including the active 6-mercaptopurine (6-MP) which is formed through a conjugation reaction with glutathione (GSH) and leads to the depletion of GSH) [5]. This conversion can occur spontaneously or by enzymatic conversion through glutathione S-transferase, leading to surge of reactive oxygen species (ROS). 6-MP is metabolized by xanthine oxidase (XO) to thiouric acid, a reaction that is also known to create ROS [6]. The major reported adverse effect of thiopurines is immune suppression, with consequent lowering of infection-fighting white blood cells, hence increasing the vulnerability to infection [7].

The aforementioned antimetabolic drugs interfere with the availability of precursors of purine nucleotides by competing with them in the synthesis of DNA or RNA. Despite their effectiveness, these drugs may cause drug-induced toxicity with increased risk of death, even when used in standard doses [8]. One of these major drug–related disorders is developing testicular atrophy and infertility with a possible contributing mechanism of the genetic polymorphisms of thiopurine methyltransferase (TPMT) enzyme, which is responsible for thiopurine metabolism. Population studies have shown that patients with low enzymatic activity have a high risk for severe potentially fatal toxicities [9]. The common side effect of azathioprine treatment in both animal and human is bone marrow depression and lymphocyte depletion, which are anticipated findings for immunosuppressive drugs. However, its active metabolite, 6-mercaptopurine (6- MP) inflicts damage on rapidly dividing cells, such as bone marrow, intestinal epithelium and the reproductive organs in adults [10,11].

Amino acids have been recognized as important signaling mediators in different cellular functions. Taurine is a sulfur-containing

*Corresponding author: Mona F Schaalan, Department of Biochemistry Faculty of Pharmacy, Misr International University, Cairo, Egypt,
E-mail: mona.schaalan@miuegypt.edu.eg

amino acid, which does not contribute to protein synthesis, and is traditionally considered as an inert molecule without any reactive groups. Besides the well-known conjugation with bile acids, taurine has a number of other physiological functions such as intracellular osmolyte for volume regulation and some antioxidant properties [12,13]. It can be obtained either exogenously through dietary source as poultry, beef, pork, seafood, and processed meats or endogenously through biosynthesis from methionine and cysteine precursors. Both sources are important to maintain the physiologic levels of taurine, and either can help to compensate the other in cases of deficiency. Moreover, it has been found in variable amounts in the liver, muscle, kidney, pancreas, spleen, small intestine, lungs and in the male and female reproductive organs. Its supplementation has been proposed to have beneficial effects in the treatment of epilepsy, heart failure and cystic fibrosis [14]. It has also been reported that taurine can be biosynthesized by male reproductive organs [15]. It has been localized to Leydig cells of the testes, the cellular source of testosterone in males, as well as the cremaster muscle, efferent ducts, and peritubular myoid cells surrounding seminiferous tubules. Taurine has been detected in the testes of humans and has been identified as the major free amino acid of sperm cells and seminal fluid [16].

It has become increasingly apparent that oxidative stress plays a major role in a broad range of human diseases and in many diseases including the destruction of male rat reproductive system. Taurine, by virtue of its antioxidant activity, has been shown to play a crucial role as a cytoprotectant and in the attenuation of apoptosis [17]. There is a growing consensus that oxidative stress is linked to mitochondrial dysfunction and that the beneficial effects of taurine are due to its antioxidant properties [18], added to its ability to improve mitochondrial function by stabilizing the electron transport chain and inhibiting the generation of reactive oxygen species [19]. Levels of taurine in spermatozoa are correlated with sperm quality, presumably by protecting against lipid peroxidation through taurine's antioxidant effects, as well as through the spermatozoa maturation by facilitating the capacitation, motility, and the acrosomal reaction of the sperm [20,21].

To the best of our knowledge, there was no previous focus on the effect of taurine supplementation on AZP induced testicular atrophy in a rat model. Accordingly, this study aimed to evaluate the effect of AZP on the testicular functions and unravel the possible protective effects of TAU combination with AZP to alleviate such adverse effects.

Material and Methods

Material

- Commercial chow diet (balanced diet), containing 67% carbohydrates, 10% fat, and 23% protein as the energy sources (overall calories: 3.6 kcal/g), was purchased from El Gomhorya company (Cairo, Egypt).

- Azapress® (AZP): manufactured by EXCELLA Gmbh and Co. Feucht, Germany.

- Taurine (TAU): 2-amino ethane sulfonic acid was supplied by GALL Pharma, Austria- Pharmaceuticals.

Methods

Experimental design: Forty adult male albino rats, 7-8-weeks old, weighing 130-150 g were purchased from the Nile Pharmaceuticals Company, Cairo, Egypt. They were housed in laboratory standard cages ($25 \times 30 \times 30$ cm) 5 rats/cage, under specific pathogen-free conditions in facilities maintained at 21-24°C with a 40-60% relative humidity and 12 hr light/dark cycle. All animals have free access to chow diet and water *ad libitum*. They were acclimated for one week prior to initiation of the experiment in the laboratory of Physiology, Faculty of Medicine Al-Azhar University. All Animal Care Committee procedures were approved. The principles of laboratory animal care were followed, as well as specific national laws were applicable.

The rats were divided into 4 equal groups (10 rats each)

- **Group I (Control):** Rats were served as control group. They received normal balanced chow and saline orally by gastric gavage tube for 10 weeks.

- **Group II (TAU):** Rats received TAU daily at a dose of 100 mg/kg b/w, orally. It was freshly prepared by dissolving it in 0.9% saline for 6 weeks according to Abd El-Twab et al. [22].

- **Group III (AZP):** Rats received normal diet for six weeks, and then they were treated with AZP dissolved in distilled water and given orally by gastric gavage in a dose of 1mg/day, for four weeks [11].

- **Group IV (TAU/AZP):** Rats received TAU daily at a dose of 100 mg/kg b/w, orally and then were given AZP by the same dose and duration as AZP group.

Serum and tissue collection: At the end of the experiment, after overnight fasting, blood samples were collected from retro-orbital venous plexus by capillary tubes under light phenobarbitone anesthesia. The blood was then centrifuged at 3000 rpm for 15 minute for serum collection. Serum was separated in aliquots in Eppendorf tubes and stored frozen at -80°C until analysis for detection of sex hormone activities. Finally the animals were decapitated and both testes were removed, the right one was used for preparation of the homogenate to be used for determination of DNA fragmentation, oxidative stress marker activities, pro-inflammatory cytokines, and gene expression for caspase 9 and Bcl2 in the testis. The left was rapidly immersed in Bouin's fixative for 24 hr for histology and immunohistochemistry.

Sperm count: The two fresh cauda epididymis were used to study sperm abnormalities including, sperm motility, epididymal count and vitality. They were hold in 4 ml of saline solution (0.9% NaCl); by squeezing process, the sperms became free in the saline solution. A haemocytometer slide was used for sperm counting; the sperms were counted in four squares at 40 magnifications. The motility assessment was expressed as percentage motile forms. The epididymal filtrate was then mixed in equal volume with eosin-nigrosin stain and a smear made of it was used for epididymal sperm vitality [23]. The caudal epididymal sperm reserve was determined using standard hemocytome tric method [24].

Tissue preparation of the homogenate: The right testis was washed in ice-cold saline and kept in 1 ml physiological saline (0.9% NaCl). The testes were sliced into small pieces, and then homogenized in 1 ml physiological saline. The homogenates were centrifuged at 20,000 xg for 30 min at 4°C. The supernatants were collected and stored at −20°C until DNA, SOD, CAT, TNF-α and IL-1β assay were conducted.

Biochemical Analysis

Sex hormone assay

Serum levels of testosterone, Luteinizing hormone (LH) and Follicle stimulating hormone (FSH), were estimated using enzyme-linked immunosorbent assay (ELISA) kits (Diagnostic System Laboratories Inc., USA), according to the manufacturer's instruction.

Superoxide dismutase (SOD) activity

SOD activity in testicular cells was estimated following the method described by Kono (1978) [25]. SOD was generated by the oxidation of hydroxylamine hydrochloride. The reduction of nitroblue tetrazolium to blue formAZPn mediated by superoxide anions was measured at 560 nm under aerobic conditions. Addition of SOD inhibited the reduction of nitroblue tetrazolium and the extent of inhibition was taken as a measure of enzyme activity.

Testicular catalase (CAT) activity

CAT activity was estimated following the method described by Aebi [26]. Briefly, 0.5 mL of the post-mitochondrial supernatant was mixed with 50 mM phosphate buffer (pH 7.0) and 20 mM H_2O2. The estimation was done using spectrophotometer following the decrease in absorbance at 240 nm.

Testicular tumor necrosis factor alpha (TNF-α) and interleukin-1B (IL-1B) level

Proinflammatory cytokines including TNF-α and IL-1β levels in testicular cells were assessed and quantified (pg/mg protein) by using ELISA technique (R and D systems, USA).The DNA fragmentation was determined according to the chemical method of Collins et al. [27]. After tissue homogenization, centrifugation and precipitation of DNA was done by addition of 1 ml TTE solution and vortexing vigorously to allow the release of fragmented DNA. DNA was hydrolyzed by adding 160μl of 5% TCA to each pellet and heating 15 minutes at 90˚C in a heating block. Colorimetrical quantitation on staining with diphenylamine (DPA) was assessed at a wave length 600 nm against blank reagent and the values are given as % fragmented DNA.

Protein extraction and Western Blotting for Bcl2

Testis was homogenized in RIPA buffer supplemented with protease inhibitors using the liquid nitrogen grinding, followed by incubation on ice for 10 min. The samples were centrifuged thoroughly to obtain protein supernatants. The protein concentrations were determined using a BCA Protein Assay Kit (Pierce). Twenty mg protein for each sample was resolved on 12% Bis-Tris or 4-12% gradient Bis/Tris gels (Life Technologies) and then transferred to PVDF membranes (Millipore). After blocking in 10% skim milk, the immunoblotting membrane was probed with indicated antibodies and visualized by ECL kit (Pierce). Lastly, images of indicated protein bands were recorded on the BioMax film (Kodak), and quantification was conducted by using Image J software (Bio-Rad). Antibodies used in this study were diluted as anti-Bcl2 (1:500, Santa Cruz Biotechnology).

Determination of caspase-9 enzymatic activity

The activity of caspase-9 was measured by Caspase-Glo-9 assay kit according to the manufacturer's instructions (Promega).

Histopathological Analysis

Light microscopic examination

After removal of the left testis, it was weighed and rapidly immersed in Bouin's fixative for 24 hr. Then, washed in several changes of 70% ethanol, dehydrated, cleared and embedded in paraffin [28]. The tissue was sectioned at 5 μm thick, mounted and stained with Hematoxylin and Eosin (H and E) for studying the general structure, Masson's Trichrome stain for staining the collagen fibers [29], and Periodic Acid-Schiff reaction (PAS) for demonstration of mucopolysaccharides [30].

Immunohistochemical study

BCL2 the immunohistochemical technique was used to evaluate the protein expression of BCL2 in the testes of the different experimental groups. BCL2 is an oncoprotein that inhibits the programmed cell death (apoptosis) [31]. Positively charged paraffin sections were deparaffinized in xylene and rehydrated using ascending grades of alcohol. The process of antigen retrieval was performed in 10 mM sodium citrate buffer. Endogenous peroxidase activity was blocked using 0.03% hydrogen peroxide for 5 min. at room temperature. Tissue sections were washed gently with phosphate buffered saline (PBS) and then incubated with anti-apoptotic protein BCL2 (1:50) biotinylated primary antibodies for 15 min. Sections were gently washed with the buffer and kept in a buffer bath in a humid chamber. A sufficient amount of streptavidin biotin peroxidase was then added and incubated for 15 min. Diaminobenzidine-substrate chromagen (DAB) was added to the sections and incubated for 7 min., followed by washing and counterstaining with hematoxylin for 5 sec [32,33].

Histomorphometrical analysis

For the estimation of spermatogenesis in testicular tissue, different indices were used. In 20 randomly selected round and nearly round seminiferous tubules, the seminiferous tubule diameter (STD), the epithelial height (EH) the tubular differentiation index (TDI), the repopulation index (RI) and the spermiogenesis index (SPI) were measured for each testis in H and E stained sections. In addition, optical density of PAS and Masson's trichome stained sections respectively, were measured too. To determine TDI, the number of seminiferous tubules that have more than three layers of germinal cells derived from type A of spermatogonia was calculated. To find out RI, the ratio of active spermatogonia (having lightly stained nuclei) to inactive spermatogonia (with darkly stained nuclei) was calculated and to determine the SPI, the ratio of the number of seminiferous tubules with spermatozoids versus empty tubules was calculated according to Movahed et al. [34]. A lica Qwin 500 LTD image was used to count the apoptotic cells in 10 high power fields (HPF) and optical density of BCL2 in all groups.

Statistical analysis

All the data were expressed as mean ± standard error (SEM). Statistical analysis was performed using one-way analysis of variance (ANOVA) followed by Bonferroni post hoc multiple comparison test using the program Statistical Package for the Social Sciences (SPSS). The values of $P<0.05$ were considered significant.

Results

Effect of AZP and TAU on rat's body and testis weights, levels of serum testosterone, LH and FSH (Table 1)

Since there was no difference between control group receiving TAU and control group, only those for control are utilized in the current study for statistical comparison. As illustrated in Table 1, there was a significant decrease in the body and testis weights in AZP treated group (8.7%, 22.4%, respectively), when compared to control group. TAU treatment successfully normalized the body and testis weights when compared to AZP treated group, as illustrated in Table 1. Moreover, AZP had a negative effect on the steroidogenic hormones, reflected as significant decrease in the serum levels of testosterone (41.74%), LH (71.6%) and FSH (52.4%), when compared to control group. Upon TAU treatment, the aforementioned altered levels were mitigated to reach nearly the normal levels.

Groups / Parameters	Group I (Control)	Group II (TAU)	Group III (AZP)	Group IV (TAU/AZP)
body weight (g)	285 ± 2.5	289 ± 2.9	260[a] ± 1.59	275[a,b] ± 4.3
Testicular weight (g)	1.25 ± 0.5	1.85 ± 0.4	0.97[a] ± 0.3	1.19[b] ± 0.7
Testosterone (ng/ml)	5.15 ± 0.35	4.8 ± 0.5	3.02[a] ± 0.54	4.97[b] ± 0.15
Luteinizing hormone (LH) (mIU/ml)	3.01 ± 0.33	3.2 ± 0.5	0.85[a] ± 0.45	2.95[b] ± 0.45
Follicle stimulating hormone (FSH) (mIU/ml)	4.1 ± 0.25	4.3 ± 0.4	1.95[a] ± 0.51	3.98[b] ± 0.33

Data were expressed as Mean ± SEM and analyzed using one-way ANOVA followed by Bonferroni post hoc multiple comparison test (n=10). Difference between groups was considered statistically significant when $P \leq 0.05$. (a) Significant values versus group control, (b) Significant values versus AZP group.

Table 1: Effects of TUA, AZP, and their combination on the body and testicular weights, serum testosterone (ng/ml), Luteinizing hormone (LH) (mIU/ml) and Follicle stimulating hormone (FSH) (mIU/ml).

Group / Parameters	Group I (Control)	Group II (TAU)	Group III (AZP)	Group IV (TAU/AZP)
TNF-α (pg/mg protein)	31.95 ± 2.2	33.8 ± 2.5	70.65[a] ± 4.6	40.05[a,b] ± 2.1
IL-1β (pg/mg protein)	34.05 ± 1.5	35.2 ± 1.7	61.15[a] ± 3.1	39.52[a,b] ± 1.3
SOD (U/mg protein)	1.8 ± 0.1	1.92 ± 0.2	0.9[a] ± 1.35	1.5[b] ± 2.95
CAT (U/mg protein)	6.1 ± 1.2	6.7 ± 1	3.5[a] ± 2.55	5.9[b] ± 4.45

Data were expressed as Mean ± SEM and analyzed using one-way ANOVA followed by Bonferroni post hoc multiple comparison test (n=10). Difference between groups was considered statistically significant when $P \leq 0.05$.
(a) Significant values versus group control,
(b) Significant values versus AZP group.

Table 2: Effects of TUA, AZP, and their combination on testicular levels of TNF-α (pg/mg protein), IL-1β (pg/mg protein), Superoxide dismutase (SOD) (U/mg protein), and Catalase (CAT) (U/mg protein) in experimental groups.

Groups / Parameters	Group I (Control)	Group II (TAU)	Group III (AZP)	Group IV (TAU/AZP)
Sperm Motility (%)	90.45 ± 5.01	88.5 ± 4.5	51.59[a] ± 1.59	86.13[b] ± 4.32
Caudal epididymal sperm count (10^6/ml)	95.01 ± 2.15	92.3 ± 2.2	30.75[a] ± 2.66	89.99[b] ± 3.65
Sperm vitality (Live: Death ratio)	14.15 ± 1.02	13.8 ± 1.3	5.95[a] ± 0.65	13.01[b] ± 1.25

Data were expressed as Mean ± SEM. and analyzed using one-way ANOVA followed by Bonferroni post hoc multiple comparison test (n=10). Difference between groups was considered statistically significant when $P \leq 0.05$.
(a) Significant values versus group control,
(b) Significant values versus AZP group.

Table 3: Effects of TUA, AZP, and their combination on percentage of sperm motility, epididymal count (10^6/ml) and sperm vitality (Live: Death ratio).

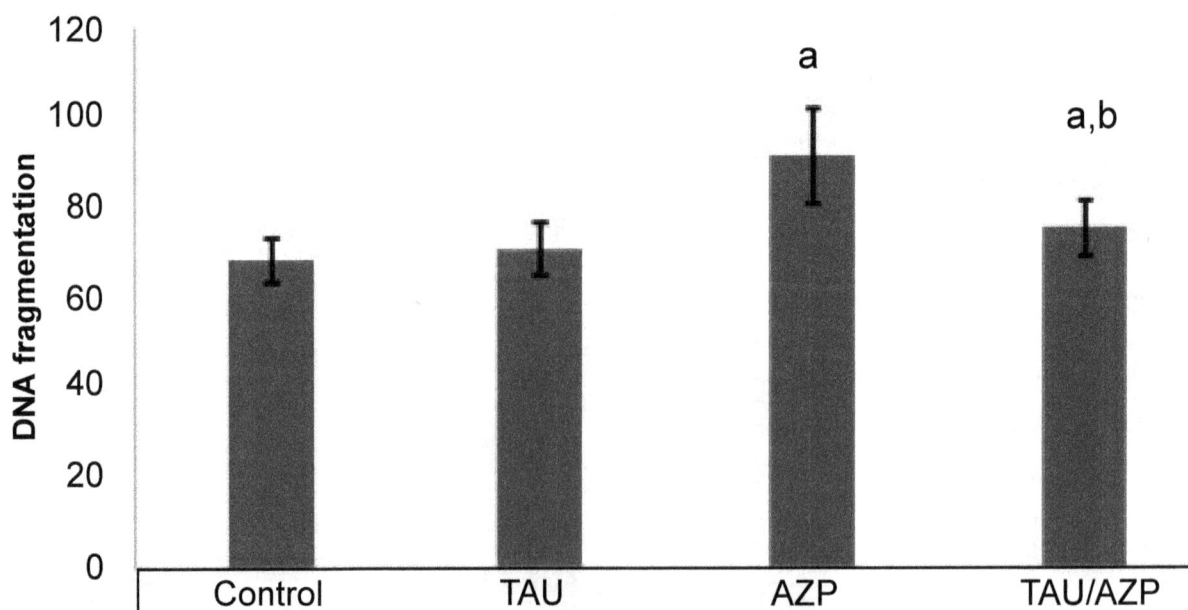

Figure 1: The percentage of DNA fragmentation in different groups. Data were presented as means ± SEM (n=10), (a) Significant difference from control; (b) Significant difference from AZA group; all at $P<0.05$.

Effect of AZP and TAU on rats' testicular pro-inflammatory cytokines TNF-α and IL-1β and antioxidant enzymes, SOD and CAT (Table 2)

The testicular levels of pro-inflammatory cytokines including TNF-α and IL-1β were significantly increased in AZP supplemented rats (2.2,1.8 folds, respectively), compared to the control animals. TAU supplementation for six weeks ameliorated successfully the elevated cytokine levels, when compared to AZP treated rats, data presented in (Table 2). AZP supplementation for four weeks induced a robust oxidative stress, reflected by significant reduction of testicular activities of CAT and SOD (42.6, 50%, respectively), when compared to normal rats. TAU supplementation for six weeks significantly increased their level when compared to AZP supplemented group.

Effect of AZP and TAU on rat's epididymal sperm count, motility and viability (Live:Death ratio) on AZP treated rats (Table 3)

Significant reduction of sperm motility (42.9%), caudal epididymal sperm count (67.6%) and vitality (57.8%) were observed in AZP treated

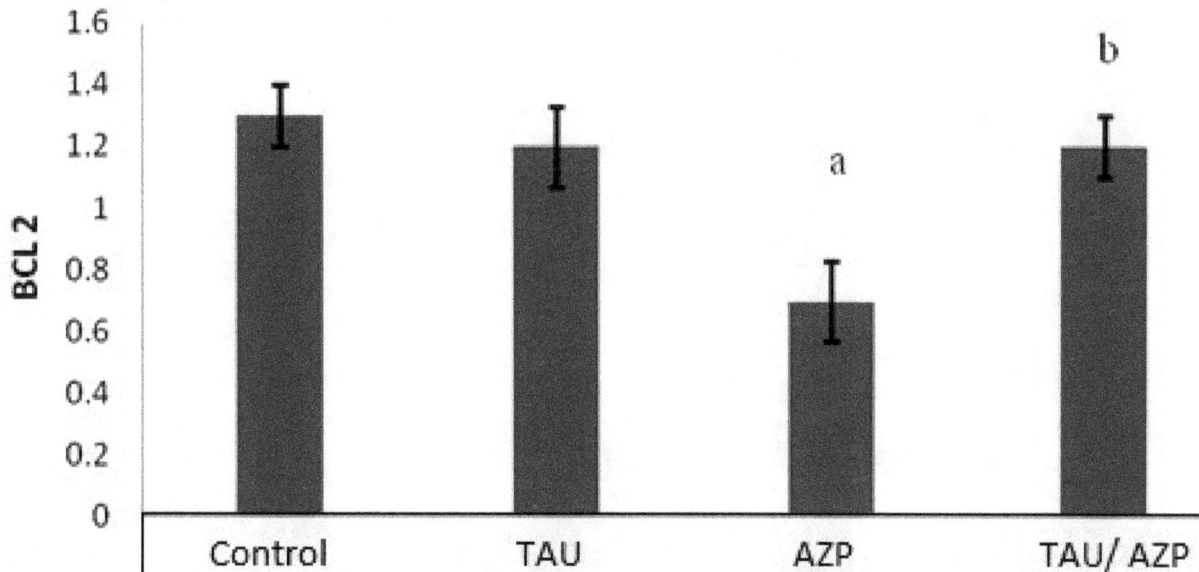

Figure 2: Transcriptional expression of BCL2 measured by real-time qPCR. Data were presented as means ± SEM (n=10), (a) Significant difference from control; (b) Significant difference from AZA group; all at P<0.05.

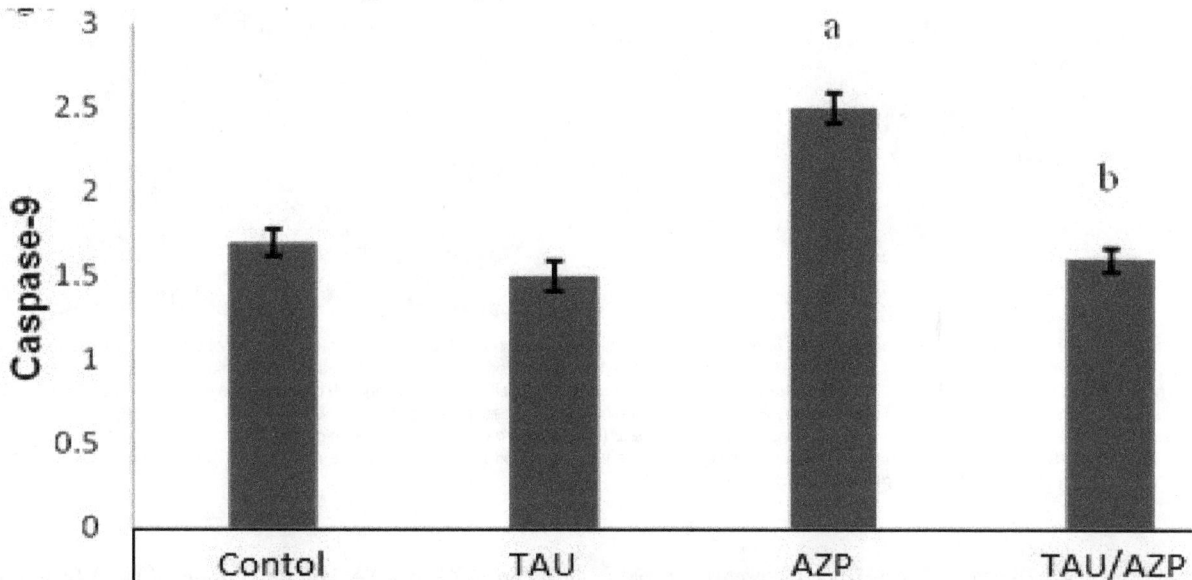

Figure 3: Transcriptional expression of Caspase 9 measured by real-time qPCR. Data were expressed as means ± SEM (n=10), (a) Significant difference from control; (b) Significant difference from AZA group; all at P<0.05.

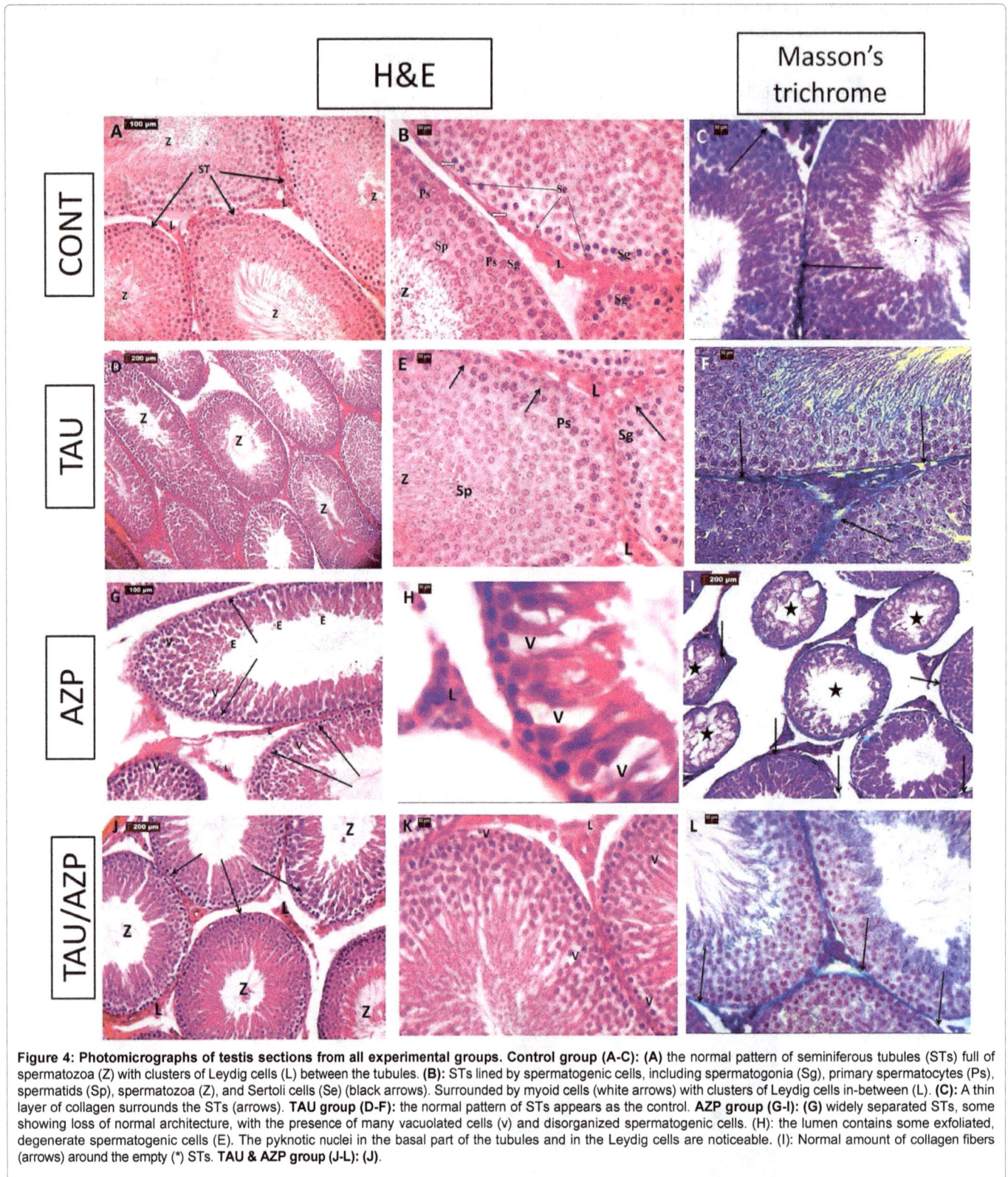

Figure 4: Photomicrographs of testis sections from all experimental groups. Control group (A-C): (A) the normal pattern of seminiferous tubules (STs) full of spermatozoa (Z) with clusters of Leydig cells (L) between the tubules. **(B):** STs lined by spermatogenic cells, including spermatogonia (Sg), primary spermatocytes (Ps), spermatids (Sp), spermatozoa (Z), and Sertoli cells (Se) (black arrows). Surrounded by myoid cells (white arrows) with clusters of Leydig cells in-between (L). **(C):** A thin layer of collagen surrounds the STs (arrows). **TAU group (D-F):** the normal pattern of STs appears as the control. **AZP group (G-I): (G)** widely separated STs, some showing loss of normal architecture, with the presence of many vacuolated cells (v) and disorganized spermatogenic cells. **(H):** the lumen contains some exfoliated, degenerate spermatogenic cells (E). The pyknotic nuclei in the basal part of the tubules and in the Leydig cells are noticeable. **(I):** Normal amount of collagen fibers (arrows) around the empty (*) STs. **TAU & AZP group (J-L): (J).**

rats when compared with control rats. These reductions were improved by TAU treatment to reach nearly the normal levels on comparison to AZP treated rats, data highlighted in Table 3.

Effect of AZP and TAU on percentage of DNA fragmentation, caspase-9 and Bcl2 expression

A significant increase in the DNA fragmentation was noticed after

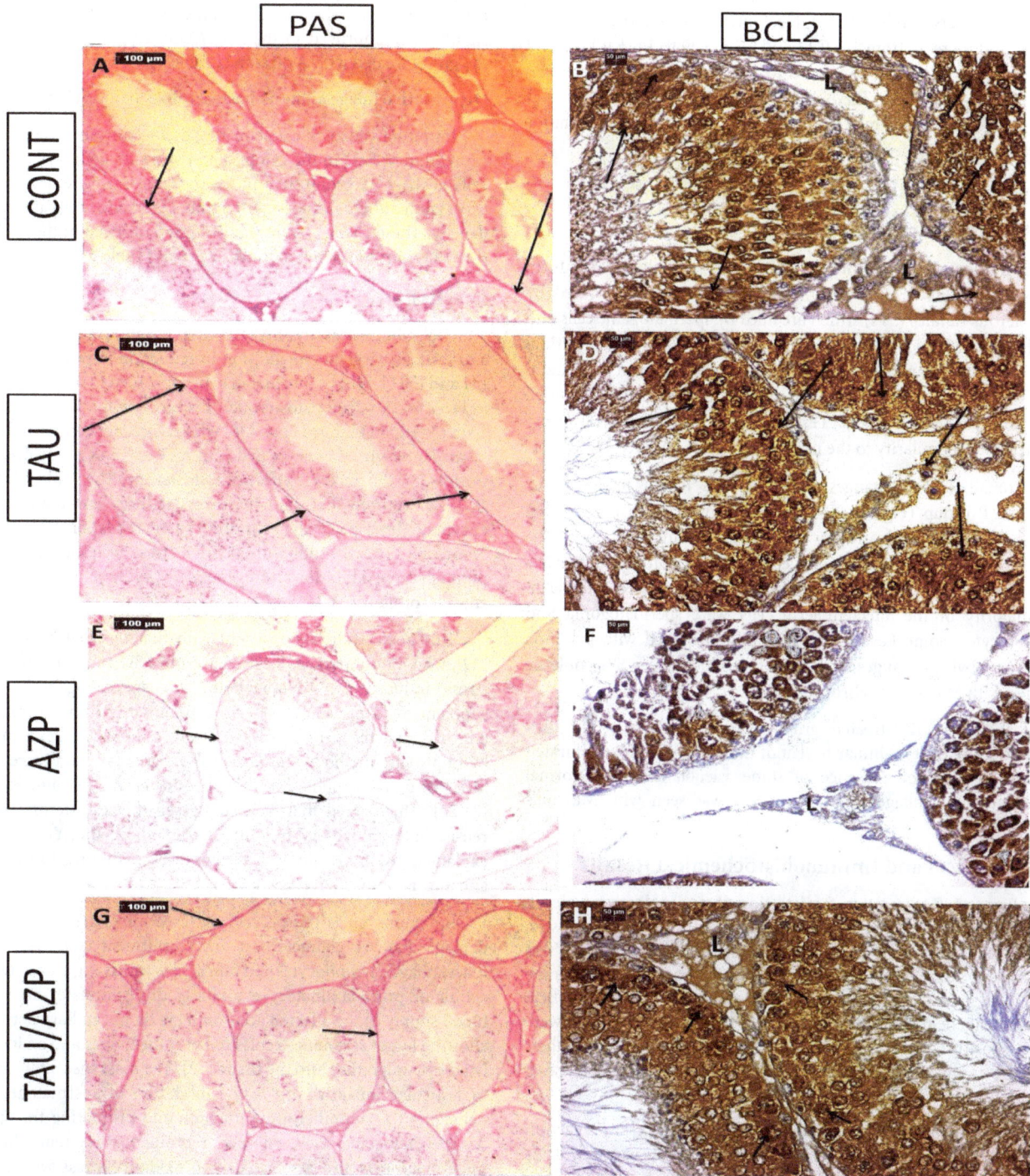

Figure 5: PAS reaction of the basement membrane of seminiferous tubules and Bcl2 immunohistochemistry in the different groups. Control group (A&B): **(A)** the normal pattern of PAS-positive reaction of the basement membrane of STs (arrows). **(B):** Most of the spermatogenic and Leydig cells show a strong Bcl2-positive reaction (arrows). **TAU group (C&D):** similar results as the control are noticed. **AZP group (E&F): (E)** a weak PAS reaction in the basement membrane of STs (arrows). **(F):** Only some spermatogenic cells have a weak Bcl2-positive reaction (arrows), and Bcl2 was negative in Leydig cells (L). **TAU & AZP group (G&H): (G)** nearly normal pattern of PAS-positive reaction of the basement membrane of STs (arrows). **(H):** Most of the basal spermatogenic cells have equivocally positive BCL2 staining (arrows), with weakly positive staining of Leydig cells (L).

AZP treatment from 70.55 ± 6 to 91.27 ± 10.5. Administration of TAU prior to AZP administration decreased the latter level significantly to 68.19 ± 4.8, when compared to AZP treated group (Figure 1). The overall activity of Bcl2 (Figure 2) and caspase-9 (Figure 3) in the homogenates of AZP treated rats' testes were significantly reduced from 1.7 ± 0.07 and 1.3 ± 0.08 to 1 ± 0.13 and 0.7 ± 0.09, respectively when compared to the control rats. While TAU supplementation for six weeks revealed a significant increase from 1 ± 0.13 and 0.7 ± 0.09 to 1.6 ± 0.1 and 1.2 ± 0.07, respectively when compared to AZP treated rats. Collectively, these results showed that the Bcl2-capase-9 pathway was activated in the testis of AZP treated rats, which is corrected by TAU treatment for six weeks.

Histological Results

Light microscopic examination

Light microscopic examination of sections of adult rat testis from the control group (Figure 4A-C) showed that testis is formed by seminiferous tubules (STs) which are lined by spermatogenic cells and Sertoli cells. Leydig (interstitial) cells were present in the interstitial space between STs and surrounded by blood vessels as seen by H and E stain. In Masson's trichrome stained sections the STs were surrounded with, thin collagenous fibers. Testicular sections in the TAU group revealed a high similarity to the normal ST pattern (Figure 4D-4F).

Histopathological changes were observed in the testis of rats in the AZP group (Figure 4G-I), including widening of interstitial spaces, disruption and atrophy of the STs, disorganization of the spermatogonia, few spermatogenic cells and spermatozoa, numerous cells with pyknotic nuclei and eosinophilic or vacuolated cytoplasm. The majority of the affected germ cells were spermatogonia and spermatocytes. Some Leydig cells appeared atrophied with pyknotic nuclei. No obvious changes in collagen fibers in-between STs could be detected with Masson's trichrome stain.

In the TAU/AZP-treated group (Figure 4J-4L) the histology appeared more or less similar to that of the control, with ameliorated changes, in spite of presence of some vacuolated cells. Normal condensation of collagen in-between STs was seen with Masson's trichrome stain.

Histochemical and Immunohistochemical Results

In Figure 5, PAS reaction for detection of mucopolysaccharides in the basement membrane of the STs and Bcl2 immunohistochemistry, which is an oncoprotein that inhibits apoptosis, was used to assess the different groups. In the control group, the basement membrane of the STs gave a strong positive PAS reaction (Figure 5A). Bcl2 immunohistochemistry revealed that most of spermatogonia were strongly positive, with the appearance of dark brown granules in their cytoplasm (Figure 5B) Examination of testis from the TAU-treated groups gave similar results too (Figures 5C and 5D).

Conversely, in the AZP group (Figure 5E) a weak PAS reaction was observed in the basement membranes of STs. There were few Bcl2-positive cells; these positive cells were situated on the basal side, while the remaining cells had many vacuoles and were negative for Bcl2 (Figure 5F). A strong positive PAS reaction was detected in the TAU / AZP group, similar to that in the control group (Figure 5G) and most of the basal spermatogenic cells have equivalent positive BCL2 staining with weakly positive staining of Leydig cells (Figure 5H).

Histomorphometrical results

Significant decreases in the seminiferous tubule diameter (STD), epithelial height (EH), tubular differentiation index (TDI), repopulation index (RI), spermiogenesis index (SPI) and PAS density in the AZP

group were noted. While a non-significant increase in the collagen fiber area percentage was observed in the AZP group compared to the control group in Masson's trichrome staining. These changes were significantly improved in the TAU/AZP-treated group compared to the group treated with AZP alone (Table 4).

Quantitative image analysis-based evaluation of BCL2

Immunohistochemical stain revealed significant decreases in the expression of Bcl2 in the cytoplasm of spermatogenic cells and Sertoli cells in the AZP group than in the other groups. The decrease in the expression of Bcl2 includes both number of stained cells and its optical density. These changes were significantly improved in the TAU/AZP-treated group compared to the AZP group (Table 5).

Discussion

Oral administration of AZP caused a significant decrease in body and testicular weights in addition to reduction in serum testosterone, LH and FSH levels; events that may be attributed to the oxidative stress induced by this drug testosterone. This agrees with the results of Sachin et al. [35] and Onanuga et al. [36] who noticed a decrease in body and testicular weight of mice treated with AZP and was rationalized by the decrease of the anabolic effect of testosterone. The study of Bairyk et al. [37], reported that oxidative stress reduced enzymatic and non-enzymatic level in Leydig cells and caused reduction of testosterone. Therefore, the AZP-induced oxidative stress in testicular tissue may rationalize the inhibition androgenesis by Leydig cells at the level of the anterior pituitary [38].

This postulation is consistent with that revealed by Duan et al. [39], who found marked decline in serum FSH and LH with oxidative stress induced by 4-Nonylphenol on spermatogenesis. Taurine supplementation, which is a free β-amino acid with remarkable antioxidant activity, for 6 weeks improved these changes significantly by improving the body and testicular weights [40] and increasing the levels of gonadotrophic hormones; testosterone, LH and FSH levels [21,22]. They stated that TAU increased the testosterone hormone release both in vivo and in vitro. On the other hand, Yang et al. [41], explained this increase in testosterone levels to the anti-oxidative stress and anti-apoptotic effects of TAU.

Inflammation is the process of responding to injury and tissue damage that is characterized by recruitment and activation of macrophages, lymphocytes and other cells, which trigger a coordinated action of proinflammatory cytokines. This stimulates an increased blood supply to the affected area, an increase in capillary permeability allowing larger serum molecules to enter the tissues and an increase in leukocyte migration into the tissue [42]. The most susceptible response to testicular inflammation is the inhibition of spermatogenesis, by damaging the seminiferous epithelium and promoting the apoptosis of spermatogenic cells in the reproductive system. Moreover, inflammation is also associated with oxidative stress which impairs sperm function [43]. This crosstalk between inflammation and spermatogenesis is evidenced by the current histological results. Thereby, we suggest a direct association between AZP supplementation and testicular inflammation evidenced by elevated testicular IL1-ß and TNF-α. This agrees with the study of Ramonda et al. [44], who reported an increase of TNF–α level in semen associated with reduced sperm count, motility and morphology. These disturbances were successfully ameliorated by Taurine, as evidenced by the study of Ahmed [45], who attributed these corrective effects to anti-inflammatory, antiapoptotic (intrinsic apoptotic pathway) and steroidegenic effects of TAU.

Parameters	Group I	Group II	Group III	Group IV
	(Control)	(TAU)	(AZP)	(TAU & AZP)
STD(μm)	230.35 ± 10.1	232.14 ± 15.01	210.88[a] ± 8.09	224.45 ± 9.43[b]
EH(μm)	41.645 ± 2.12	43.132 ± 3.12	29.865[a] ± 1.82	36.665[a,b] ± 2.76
TDI %	91 ± 6.87	94 ± 5.57	47[a] ± 2.34	60[a,b] ± 5.54
RI %	82.74 ± 4.421	83.29 ± 6.457	75.34[a] ± 5.81	79.45[b] ± 5.12
SPI %	90.89 ± 4.12	91.37 ± 4.49	53.5[a] ± 4.43	65.24[b] ± 4.31
Collagen fiber area %	5.262 ± 0.35	5.345 ± 0.53	5.96[a] ± 1.33	6.13[b] ± 2.21
PAS density	0.354 ± 0.01	0.432 ± 0.05	0.23[a] ± 0.11	0.32[b] ± 0.012

Data were expressed as Mean ± SEM and analyzed using one-way ANOVA followed by Bonferroni post hoc multiple comparison test (n=10). Difference between groups was considered statistically significant when P ≤ 0.05.

(a) Significant values versus group control,

(b) Significant values versus AZP group.

STD: Diameters of seminiferous tubules ; EH: Epithelial height , TDI: Tubular differentiation index ; RI: Repopulation index; SPI: Spermiogenesis index; PAS: Periodic acid Schiff reaction

Table 4: Effects of TUA, AZP, and their combination on spermatogenesis indices in the seminiferous tubules.

Groups	Group I	Group II	Group III	Group IV
Parameters	(Control)	(TAU)	(AZP)	(TAU & AZP)
Apoptotic index (ratio of apoptotic cells to normal cells)	0.078 ± 0.015	0.075 ± 0.013	1.1[a] ± 0.12	0.6[b] ± 0.05
BCL2 optical density	137 ± 16	140 ± 8	48[a] ± 6.5	110[b] ± 9

Data were expressed as Mean ± SEM and analyzed using one-way ANOVA followed by Bonferroni post hoc multiple comparison test (n=10). Difference between groups was considered statistically significant when P ≤ 0.05.   (a) Significant values versus group control,

(b) Significant values versus AZP group

Table 5: Effects of TAU, AZP, and their combination on the Bcl2 expression in the cytoplasm of spermatogenic and sertoli cells.

Any inflammatory damage on the male genital tract leads to the increased generation of reactive oxygen species (ROS). Oxidative stress arises when excess free radicals exceed the antioxidant defence of the male reproductive tract, thereby damaging male reproductive tract. Superoxide, hydroxyl and hydrogen hydroxide radicals are the major ROS present in seminal plasma [46]. Various oxidants can damage cells by starting chemical chain reactions such as lipid peroxidation, or by oxidizing DNA or proteins [47], mutations that are major causes of cancer, and can be reversed by DNA repair mechanism [48]. AZP is one of these oxidants that caused a marked DNA fragmentation of the testicular tissue in rats of the present study.

AZP treatment for four weeks in the present study induced testicular inflammation and hence significant reduction of SOD and CAT levels; this decrease was corrected by pre-treatment of TAU for 6 weeks. Sperm quality and quantity are critical factors to the male fertility [49]. There is a positive correlation between abnormal and immature sperms with oxidative stress [50]. Consistent with these findings [51], reported that ROS promoted apoptosis which may lead to a decrease in sperm viability and density. In the present study, we demonstrated that the percentage of abnormal sperms was significantly increased in the AZP group as well as an increase in the percentage of immature, immotile and dead sperms associated with decreased in the levels of SOD and CAT in testicular tissues [52].

TAU was also reported to have the ability to scavenge reactive oxygen species (ROS) and attenuate lipid peroxidation and, consequently, stabilizes biological membranes [53]. The anti-inflammatory action of TAU, evidenced in the current study, confirms previous findings of [54], who demonstrated the effective role of TAU as an anti-inflammatory supplement when given to alleviate the inflammation induced in the kidney by chronic ethanol ingestion.

The potent antioxidant properties of TAU are additionally associated with increased antioxidant enzyme activity, SOD, catalase and GSH which are the key cellular antioxidant enzymes. The antioxidant effects attributed to TAU may be associated with its sulfur moiety, and the modulation of GSH and GSH levels by TAU is critical in the cellular defence against oxidative stress. Consistent with the antioxidant properties of taurine observed in the present study [55], also found protective role of TAU on hepatocytes subjected to iron-overload as a way of oxidative stress.

In the present study, treatment by AZP for four weeks induced activation of caspase-9 (an upstream protease of caspase-3 and downstream effectors of the Bcl2 mitochondrial apoptosis pathway) which indicates an increase in the apoptotic activity in the testicular tissue. Bcl2 is a prosurvival multidomain protein that regulates apoptosis by preventing the release of proapoptogenic factors from the mitochondria (e.g., cytochrome c) and subsequent caspase activation. In our study the anti-apoptotic protein BCL2 level was significantly reduced with AZP treatment. This dysregulation of the fine-tuned apoptotic pathway is considered one of the mechanisms of AZP-induced injury of the testicular function which might be the reason for decreased sperm viability and mobility. In alignment with our findings [56], documented an increase in the activity of Bcl2/Caspase-9 apoptosis pathway in the testis of mice subjected to apoptotic inducers.

The protective role of TAU is highlightened in the adjustment of caspase-9 activity and Bcl2 level towards the control values in order to properly control the proliferation and differentiation of germ cells during spermatogenesis. This anti-apoptotic effect of TAU was also demonstrated by Takatani et al. [57], who suggested that Taurine inhibits apoptosis by preventing formation of the Apaf-1/caspase-9 apoptosome. In addition, Zulli et al. [58] reported an anti-apoptotic effect of taurine, results that encourage the usage of Tau as a dietary supplement.

A sensitive and indispensable method for revealing disturbances in spermatogenesis is histopathological examination [59]. Our histological results revealed widening of the interstitial spaces, disruption and atrophy of many seminiferous tubules with scanty spermatogenic cells and spermatozoa in AZP group. These results agree with those of Akinlolu [60] and Padmanabhan, et al. [61], while cytoplasmic vacuolations was further reported by Karawya and El-Nahas [62]. The current study noticed a decrease in the diameters of the seminiferous tubules which was proved by the morphometrical studies and agrees with the results of Shrestha et al. and Khayatnouri et al. [63,64]. Many cells appeared shrieked with pyknotic nuclei and deeply acidophilic cytoplasm, which may indicate apoptosis. Sun et al. [65], reported that early injury of the cells occurred mainly in the form of apoptotic cells and cellular apoptosis are associated with the release of cytochrome c and others apoptosis-promoting substances. Kumar et al. [66], described pyknosis as irreversible condensation of chromatin in the nucleus of a cell necrosis, while Kroemer et al. [67], referred pyknosis to apoptosis.

AZP induced reproductive disorders was confirmed by histomorphometrical, as it significantly decreased in the diameter and epithelial height of the seminiferous tubules due to cell loss from the epithelium and epithelial sloughing in some tubules in addition to Leydig cells atrophy. Moreover, the results of this study demonstrated a decrease in RI, TDI and SPI. As testosterone supports spermatogenesis, sperm maturation and sexual function, thus any disruption in testosterone biosynthesis can adversely affects male fertility [68]. In another study of El-Sharaky et al. [69], the use of a Leydig cell toxicant resulted in decrease of testosterone level in rats, resulting in increased germ cell apoptosis. In addition, testosterone can affect Sertoli cells function and germinal cell degeneration; thus, dislocation could take place due Sertoli cells dysfunction and decreased testosterone level, the latter enhance premature detachment of epithelial cells [70,71]. Atrophy of Leydig cells can be responsible for the reduction in serum testosterone level. Therefore, the changes in the seminiferous tubules, observed in the current histopathological findings, may be a result of hormonal effect and not a consequence of a direct effect.

Considering the fact that the normal spermatogenesis is directly associated with reduction of oxidative stress and increasing endocrine activity by Leydig and Sertoli cells, TAU proved to protect spermatogenesis and decrease tubular atrophy. This may be partly by down-regulating oxidative stress enzymes and as well by improving testosterone biosynthesis. These results were confirmed by the histopathological finding that showed a remarkably higher seminiferous tubules diameter as well as germinal epithelium height in the testes in the TAU and AZP group, compared to AZP group. Taurine not only improved the morphological and histomorphometrical damage, but also the apoptotic cells number and morphology, which confirms Taurine's ability to decrease the toxic effects of AZP. Previous studies reported that Tau treatment prevented significantly the morphological damage, and the amount of apoptotic cells through suppressing the increased oxidative stress in diabetes-induced testicular dysfunction in the rat [72], through its antioxidant effect [73,74].

Conclusion

Conclusively, the present study suggests that AZP plays a destructive impact on reproductive system functions in male rats, while TAU supplementation has beneficial effects on the induced inflammation, testicular function and apoptosis. Taurine's benefit in reducing the oxidative stress and inflammatory response, hence testicular hypofunction, induced by AZP treatment, would encourage its supplementation as an add-on therapy when the use of AZP is mandatory. This could open new horizon to its usage as an adjunctive, complementary approach to chemotherapy supportive care.

References

1. Meijer B, Seinen ML, Leijte NN, Mulder CJ, van Bodegraven AA, et al. (2016) Clinical value of mercaptopurine after failing azathioprine therapy in patients with inflammatory bowel disease. Ther Drug Monit 38: 463-470.

2. La Duke KE, Ehling S, Cullen JM, Bäumer W (2015) Effects of azathioprine, 6-mercaptopurine, and 6-thioguanine on canine primary hepatocytes. Am J Vet Res 76: 649- 655.

3. Barbara S (2010) Inflammatory bowel disease and male fertility. LIJ Health System 516:734-850.

4. de Boer NK, van Bodegraven AA, Jharap B, de Graaf P, Mulder CJ (2007) Drug insight: Pharmacology and toxicity of thiopurine therapy in patients with IBD. Nat Clin Pract Gastroenterol Hepato 4: 686-694.

5. van Asseldonk DP, Sanderson J, de Boer NK, Sparrow MP, Lémann M, et al. (2011) Difficulties and possibilities with thiopurine therapy in inflammatory bowel disease--proceedings of the first thiopurine task force meeting. Dig Liver Dis 43: 270-276.

6. Lee AU, Farrell GC (2001) Mechanism of azathioprine-induced injury to hepatocytes: Roles of glutathione depletion and mitochondrial injury. J Hepatol 35: 756-764.

7. Weersma RK, Peters FTM, Oostenbrug LE, van den Berg AP, van Haastert M, et al. (2004) Increased incidence of azathioprine induced pancreatitis in Crohn's disease compared with other diseases. Alimentary Pharmacology & Therapeutics. 20: 843-850.

8. Al-Judaibi B, Schwarz UI, Huda N, Dresser GK, Gregor JC, et al. (2016) Genetic predictors of azathioprine toxicity and clinical response in patients with inflammatory bowel disease. J Popul Ther Clin Pharmacol 23: e26-36.

9. Lee MN, Kang B, Choi SY, Kim MJ, Woo SY et al. (2015) Impact of genetic polymorphisms on 6-thioguanine nucleotide levels and toxicity in pediatric patients with IBD treated with azathioprine. Inflamm Bowel Dis 21: 2897-2908.

10. Polifka J, Friedman JM (2002) Azathioprine and 6-Mercaptopurine. Tratology 65: 240-261.

11. Bendre SV, Shaddock JG, Patton RE, Dobrovolsky VN, Albertini RJ et al. (2007) Effect of chronic Azathioprine treatment on germ-line transmission of Hprt in mice. Environmental and Molecular mutagenesis 48: 744-753.

12. Bouckenooghe T, Remacle C, Reusens B (2006) Is taurine a functional nutrient? Curr Opin Clin Nutr Metab Care 9: 728-733.

13. El Mesallamy HO, El-Demerdash E, Hammad LN El Magdoub HM (2010) Effect of taurine supplementation on hyperhomocysteinemia and markers of oxidative stress in high fructose diet induced insulin resistance. Diabetology & Metabolic Syndrome 2:46-56.

14. Caine JJ, Geracioti TD (2016) Taurine, energy drinks, and neuroendocrine effects. Cleve Clin J Med 83: 895-904.

15. Li JH, Ling YQ, Fan JJ, Zhang XP, Cui S (2006) Expression of cysteine sulfinate decarboxylase (CSD) in male reproductive organs of mice. Histochem. and Cell Biology 125:607-613.

16. Aaronson DS, Iman R, Walsh TJ, Kurhanewicz J, Turek PJ (2010) A novel application of 1H magnetic resonance spectroscopy: Non-invasive identification of spermatogenesis in men with non-obstructive azoospermia. Hum Reprod 25: 847-852.

17. Das J, Sil PC (2012) Taurine ameliorates alloxan-induced diabetic renal injury, oxidative stress-related signaling pathways and apoptosis in rats. Amino Acids 43:1509-1523.

18. Marcinkiewicz J, Kontny E (2012) Taurine and inflammatory diseases. Amino Acids 46:7-20.

19. Jong CJ, Azuma J, Schaffer S (2012) Mechanism underlying the antioxidant activity of taurine: Prevention of mitochondrial oxidant production. Amino Acids 42: 2223-2232.

20. Das J, Ghosh J, Manna P, Sinha M, Sil PC (2009) Taurine protects rat testes against NaAsO (2)-induced oxidative stress and apoptosis via mitochondrial dependent and independent pathways. Toxicol. Lett 187:201-210.

21. Yang J, Wu G, Feng Y, Lv Q, Lin S, et al. (2010) Effects of taurine on male reproduction in rats of different ages. J Biomed Sci 17: S9.

22. Abd El-Twab SM, Mohamed HM, Mahmoud AM (2016) Taurine and pioglitazone attenuate diabetes-induced testicular damage by abrogation of oxidative stress and up-regulation of the pituitary-gonadal axis. Can J Physiol Pharmacol 94: 651-661.

23. Lasley JF, Easely GT, McKenzie FF (1944) Staining method for the differentiation of live and dead spermatozoa. Anat Rec 82: 167-174.

24. Amann RP, Almquist JO (1961) Reproductive capacity of dairy bulls. I. Technique for direct measurement of gonadal and extra-gonadal sperm reserves. J. Dairy Sci. 44:1537-1543.

25. Kono Y (1978) Generation of superoxide radical during autoxidation of hydroxylamine and an assay for superoxide dismutase. Arch Biochem Biophys 186:189-95.

26. Aebi H (1974) Catalase In Methods in enzymatic analysis. Volume 2, New York, USA.

27. Collins JA, Schandl CA, Young KK, Vesely J, Willingham MC (1997) Major DNA fragmentation is a late event in apoptosis. J Histochem Cytochem 45: 923-934.

28. Carson F (1992) Histotechnology A self-instructional text (1st edn.) American Society of Clinical Pathology (ASCP) press. pp:19-29.

29. Drury RA, Wallington EA (1980) Carlton's histological technique (5th edn.) Oxford University press, New York, London.

30. Bancroft JD, Stevens A (1996) Theory and practice of histological techniques. (4th edn.) Churchill Livingstone, New York, London.

31. Ozen OA, Kus MA, Kus I, Kus I, Alkoc OA, et al. (2008) Protective effect of melatonin against formaldehyde induced oxidative damage and apoptosis in rat testes: An immunohistochemical and biochemical study. Systems Biology in reproductive medicine. 54:169-176.

32. Agnieszk P, Zbigniew B, Marcin W, Justynian V (2005) Ultrastrucural and immunohistochemical evaluation of apoptosis in foetal rat liver after adriamycin administration. Bull Vet Inst Pulawy 49: 475-448.

33. Zhou XH, Han YL, Yang HM et al. (2007) Effects of SSTF on the expression of apoptosis-associated gene BCL2 and Bax by cardiomyocytes induced by H2O2 Guangdong. Med J 28: 1590-1591.

34. Movahed E, Nejati V, Sadrkhanlou R, Ahmadi A (2013) Toxic effect of acyclovir on testicular tissue in rats. Iran J Reprod Med 11: 111-118.

35. Bendre SV, Shaddock JG, Patton RE, Dobrovolsky VN, Albertini RJ, et al. (2005) Lymphocyte Hprt mutant frequency and sperm toxicity in C57BL/6 mice treated chronically with Azathioprine. Mutation Research 578: 1-14.

36. Onanuga IO, Ibrahim RB, Amin A, Omotoso GO (2014) Testicular alteration in over dosage of azazthioprine:A histological and histochemical study in Wistar rats. African Journal of Cellular Pathology 2: 83-88.

37. Bairyk L, Kumar G, Rao Y (2009) Effect of acyclovir on the sperm parameters of albino mice. Indian J Physiol Pharmacol. 53: 327-333.

38. Millsop JW, Heller MM, Eliason MJ, Murase JE (2013) Dermatological medication effects on male fertility. Dermatol Ther 26: 337-346.

39. Duan P, Hu C, Butler HJ, Quan C, Chen W et al. (2017) 4-Nonylphenol induces disruption of spermatogenesis associated with oxidative stress-related apoptosis by targeting p53-Bcl2/Bax-Fas/FasL signaling. Environ Toxicol 32: 739-753.

40. Tsounapi P, Honda M, Dimitriadis F, Shimizu S, Hikita K et al. (2016) Post-fertilization effect of bilateral primary testicular damage induced by unilateral cryptorchidism in the rat model. Andrology. Mar 4: 297-305.

41. Yang J, Zong X, Wu G, Lin S, Feng Y, et al. (2015) Taurine increases testicular function in aged rats by inhibiting oxidative stress and apoptosis. Amino Acids 47:1549-1558.

42. Hedger MP (2011) Immunophysiology and pathology of inflammation in the testis and epididymis. J Androl 32: 625-640.

43. Imamoğlu M, Bülbül SS, Kaklikkaya N, Sarihan H (2012) Oxidative, inflammatory and immunologic status in children with undescended testes. Pediatr Int 54: 816-829.

44. Ramonda R, Foresta C, Ortolan A, Bertoldo A, Oliviero F et al.(2014) Influence of tumor necrosis factor α inhibitors on testicular function and semen in spondyloarthritis patients. Fertil Steril 101: 359-365.

45. Ahmed MA (2015) Amelioration of nandrolone decanoate-induced testicular and sperm toxicity in rats by taurine: Effects on steroidogenesis, redox and inflammatory cascades, and intrinsic apoptotic pathway. Toxicol Appl Pharmacol. 282 : 285-296.

46. Moazamian R, Polhemus A, Connaughton H, Fraser B, Whiting S et al.(2015) Oxidative stress and human spermatozoa: Diagnostic and functional significance of aldehydes generated as a result of lipid peroxidation. Mol Hum Reprod 21: 502-515.

47. Akinloye O, Abbiyesuku FM, Oguntibeju OO, Arowojolu AO, Truter EJ (2011) The impact of blood and seminal plasma zinc and copper concentrations on spermogram and hormonal changes in infertile Nigerian men. Reprod Biol 11: 83-98.

48. Tian H, Gao Z, Li H, Zhang B, Wang G et al. (2015) DNA damage response--a double-edged sword in cancer prevention and cancer therapy.Cancer Lett 358: 8-16.

49. Stanislavov R, Rohdewald P (2014) Sperm quality in men is improved by supplementation with a combination of L-arginine, L-citrulline, roburins and Pycnogenol. Minerva. Urol. Nefrol 66: 217-23.

50. Türk G, Sönmez M, Ceribaşi AO, Yüce A, Ateşşahin A (2010) Attenuation of cyclosporine A-induced testicular and spermatozoal damages associated with oxidative stress by ellagic acid. Int Immunopharmacol 10:177-82.

51. Park HJ, Choi YJ, Lee JH, Nam MJ (2017) Naringenin causes ASK1-induced apoptosis via reactive oxygen species in human pancreatic cancer cells. Food Chem Toxicol 99: 1-8.

52. Ghyasi R, Sepehri G, Mohammadi M, Badalzadeh R, Ghyasi A (2012) Effect of mebudipine on oxidative stress and lipid peroxidation in myocardial ischemic-reperfusion injury in male rat. J Res Med Sci 17: 1150–1155.

53. Jang HJ, Kim SJ (2013) Taurine exerts anti-osteoclastogenesis activity via inhibiting ROS generation, JNK phosphorylation and COX-2 expression in RAW264.7 cells. J Recept Signal Transduct Res 33: 387-391.

54. Latchoumycandane C, Nagy LE, McIntyre TM (2015) Myeloperoxidase formation of PAF receptor ligands induces PAF receptor-dependent kidney injury during ethanol consumption. Free Radic Biol Med 86: 179-90.

55. Zhang Z, Liu D, Yi B, Liao Z, Tang L, et al. (2014) Taurine supplementation reduces oxidative stress and protects the liver in an iron-overload murine model. Mol Med Rep 10: 2255-2262.

56. Xu W, Guo G, Li J, Ding Z, Sheng J, et al. (2016) Activation of Bcl2-Caspase-9 Apoptosis Pathway in the Testis of Asthmatic Mice. PLoS ONE 11: e0149353.

57. Takatani T, Takahashi K, Uozumi Y, Shikata E, Yamamoto Y, et al. (2004) Taurine inhibits apoptosis by preventing formation of the Apaf-1/caspase-9 apoptosome. Am J Physiol 287: C 949-953.

58. Zulli A, Lau E, Wijaya B, Jin X, Sutarga K, et al. (2009) High dietary taurine reduces apoptosis and atherosclerosis in the left main coronary artery association with reduced CCAAT/enhancer binding protein homologous protein and total plasma homocysteine but not lipidemia. Hypertension 53: 1017-1022.

59. Biró K, Barna-Vetró I, Pécsi T, Szabó E, Winkler G, et al. (2003) Evaluation of spermatological parameters in ochratoxin A--challenged boars. Theriogenology 60: 199-207.

60. Padmanabhan S, Tripathiathi DN, Vikram A, Ramarao, Jena GB (2009) Methotrexate-induced cytotoxicity and genotoxicity in germ cells of mice: intervention of folic and folinic acid. Mutat Res 673: 43-52.

61. Nouri HS, Azarmi Y, Movahedin M (2009) Effect of growth hormone on testicular dysfunction induced by methotrexate in rats. Andrologia 41: 105-110.

62. Karawya FD, El-Nahas AF (2006) The protective effect of vitamin C on Azathioprine induced seminiferous tubular structural changes and cytogenetic toxicity in albino rats. Cancer Ther 125-134.

63. Shrestha S, Dhungel S, Saxena AK, Bhattacharya S, Maskey D (2007) Effect of methotrexate (MTX) administration on spermatogenesis: An experimental study on animal model. Nepal Med Coll J 9: 230-233.

64. Khayatnouri M, Safavi SE, Safarmashaei S, Mikailpourardabili, Babazadeh BD (2011) Effect of saffron on histomorphometric changes of testicular tissue in rat. Am J Anim Vet Sci 6: 153-159.

65. Sun K, Liu Z, Sun Q (2004) Role of mitochondria in cell apoptosis during hepatic ischemia and protective effect of ischemic post conditioning. World J Gastroenterol 10: 1934-1938.

66. Kumar SG, Narayana K, Bairy KL, D'Souza UJ, Samuel VP, et al. (2006) Dacarbazine induces genotoxic and cytotoxic germ cell damage with

concomitant decrease in testosterone and increase in lactate dehydrogenase concentration in the testis. Mutat Res 607: 240-252.

67. Kroemer G, Galluzzi L, Vandenabede P (2009) Classification of Cell death: Recommendation of The Nomenclature committee on Cell death. Cell Death Diffen 16: 3-11.

68. Benzoni E, Minervini F, Giannoccaro A, Fornelli F, Vigo D, et al. (2008) Influence of in vitro exposure to mycotoxin zearalenone and its derivatives on swine sperm quality. Reprod Toxicol 25: 461-467.

69. El-Sharaky AS, Newairy AA, Elguindy NM, Elwafa AA (2010) Spermatotoxicity, biochemical changes and histological alteration induced by gossypol in testicular and hepatic tissues of male rats. Food Chem Toxicol 48: 3354-3361.

70. Najafi G, Razi M, Hoshyar A, Shahmohamadloo S, Feyzi S (2010) The effect of chronic exposure with imidacloprid insecticide on fertility in mature male rats. Int J Fertil Steril 4: 9-16.

71. Tsounapi P, Saito M, Dimitriadis F, Koukos S, Shimizu S, et al. (2012) Antioxidant treatment with edaravone or taurine ameliorates diabetes-induced testicular dysfunction in the rat. Mol Cell Biochem 369: 195-204.

72. Kang IS, Kim C (2013) Taurine chloramine administered in vivo increases NRF2-regulated antioxidant enzyme expression in murine peritoneal macrophages. Adv Exp Med Biol 775: 259-267.

73. Kim W, Kim HU, Lee HN, Kim SH, Kim C, et al. (2015) Taurine Chloramine Stimulates Efferocytosis Through Upregulation of Nrf2-Mediated Heme Oxygenase-1 Expression in Murine Macrophages: Possible Involvement of Carbon Monoxide. Antioxid Redox Signal 23: 163-177.

74. Kim C, Cha YN (2014) Taurine chloramine produced from taurine under inflammation provides anti-inflammatory and cytoprotective effects. Amino Acids 46: 89-100.

4

The Best Use of Systemic Corticosteroids in the Intensive Care Units

Mohammad S Abdallah[1*], **Ahmad F Madi**[2] **and Muhammad A Rana**[2]

[1]*Critical Care Clinical Pharmacist at King Saud Medical City Riyadh, Saudi Arabia*
[2]*ICU consultant at King Saud Medical City Riyadh, Saudi Arabia*

Abstract

Corticosteroids are one of the most common medications that are used in the intensive care units (ICUs); corticosteroids are used for a variety of indications, including septic shock, acute respiratory distress syndrome (ARDS), bacterial meningitis, tuberculous meningitis, lupus nephritis, severe chronic obstructive pulmonary disease (COPD) exacerbations and many others.

Corticosteroids are associated with many severe side effects that affect morbidity and mortality of the patients like increased risk of infections, glucose intolerance, hypokalemia, sodium retention, edema, hypertension, myopathy etc. In order to make the best use of these medications and to minimize the unwanted side effects we should follow some particular protocol. Please keep in our mind that there is controversy about dosing and tapering of steroids, so effort has been made to include the best available evidence.

This review discusses mainly the most common indications of corticosteroids in ICU, dosing of corticosteroids in those indications and how to taper corticosteroids according to the best evidence that recommends their use.

Literature search was done using Medline, BMJ, Uptodate, Chochrane database, Google scholar and the best evidence based guidelines in which steroids are recommended to treat ICU related disorders. Sex hormones are not discussed in this review since its use is rare in the intensive care units.

Keywords: Corticosteroids; Tapering; Steroids; Withdrawal symptoms; Intensive care

Abbreviations

ACTH: Adrenocorticotropic Hormone; ARDS: Acute Respiratory Distress Syndrome; COPD: Chronic Obstructive Pulmonary Disease; CSF: *Cerebrospinal Fluid*; ETT: *Endotracheal Tube;* ICU: Intensive Care Unit; IPF: Idiopathic Pulmonary Fibrosis; IV: Intravenous; NIH: National Institutes of Health; PEFR: Peak Expiratory Flow Rate; PO: per os; SLE: *Systemic Lupus Erythematosus*; TB: Tuberculous.

Introduction

Corticosteroids are molecules produced by the adrenal cortex (the outer part of the adrenal gland), Corticosteroids are classified to either glucocorticoids that are produced in response to stress and have important effects on intermediary metabolism and immune function or mineralocorticoids that maintain the balance of salt and water within the body. The major glucocorticoid in humans is cortisol which its release is mainly controlled by adrenocorticotropic hormone (ACTH) and the most important mineralocorticoid is aldosterone which its release is mainly controlled by angiotensin [1]. These medications (glucocorticoids and mineralocorticoids are associated with severe side effects that sometimes cause their discontinuation in many patients.

We observed many times that we are not using these medications properly in patients by using wrong doses of steroids, using inappropriate tapering regimens and sometimes by using steroids for indications that literature does not support their use in such indications. To avoid the recurrence of medication errors and side effects that are associated with corticosteroids we wrote this review that can be used by health care providers who are working in different Intensive Care Units. This review discusses mainly the most common indications of corticosteroids in ICU, dosing of corticosteroids in those indications and how to taper corticosteroids according to the best evidence that recommends their use (Tables 1 and 2).

Compound	Anti-inflammatory of potency	Na retaining potency	Duration of action	Equivalent dose
Cortisol	1	1	S	20
Cortisone	0.8	0.8	S	25
Dexamethasone	25	0	L	0.75
Prednisone	4	0.8	I	5

*Corresponding author: Abdallah Mohammad S, Critical Care Clinical Pharmacist at King Saud Medical City Riyadh, Saudi Arabia, E-mail: mohasulmoha@yahoo.com

Prednisolone	4	0.8	I	5
Methyprednisolone	5	0.5	I	4
Triamcinolone	5	0	L	4
Betamethasone	25	0	L	0.75

Equivalent doses apply only to oral or intravenous preparations-S Short (8-12 Hrs), L- Long (36-72 Hrs), and I Intermediate (12-36 Hrs).Prednisone and prednisolone are potent glucocorticoids and weak mineralocorticoids. Methylprednisolone and dexamethasone have no mineralocorticoid effect. NOTE: Glucocorticoid doses which provide a mineralocorticoid effect that is approximately equivalent to 0.1 mg fludrocortisone are: prednisone or prednisolone 50 mg, or hydrocortisone 20 mg. Equivalent dose shown is for oral or IV administration. Relative potency for intra-articular or intramuscular administration may vary considerably. Data for cortisol, endogenous corticosteroid hormone, are included for comparison with synthetic preparations listed. Fludri cortisone is not used for an anti-inflammatory effect its minaralo corticoid activity is 125 and its antiinflamatory activity is 10. Prednisone itself is biologically inactive, but it is rapidly converted to the active form prednisolone. However, patients with severe liver disease may have difficulty converting prednisone to prednisolone; in such patients, it is possible that one might not get the same effect from prednisone as from prednisolone. In addition, certain drug interactions can affect the metabolism and bioavailability of prednisone. As an example, phenytoin, barbiturates or rifampin, attenuate the biological effects of glucocorticoids.

Table 1: Comparison of various corticosteroids.

Indication of corticosteroids*	Dosing regimen and tapering §
1) Septic shock	Hydrocortisone at a dose of 200 mg per day as continuous infusion. Should be tapered when vasopressors are no longer required
2) Airway edema	Dexamethasone is 0.5-2 mg/kg divided over 4-6 hrs started 24 hours before extubation and continued for 24 hours after extubation
3) Spinal cord injury	Methylprednisolone should be initiated within eight hours of injury using an initial bolus of 30 mg/kg by IV for 15 minutes followed 45 minutes later by a continuous infusion of 5.4 mg/kg/hour for 23 hours
4) ARDS	loading dose of 1 mg/kg of methyl prsnisolone followed by an infusion of 1 mg/kg/d from day 1 to day 14, then 0.5 mg/kg/d from day 15 to day 21, then 0.25 mg/kg/d from day 22 to day 25, and finally 0.125 mg/kg/d from day 26 to day 28. In the study if the patient was extubated between days 1 and 14, the patient was advanced to day 15 of drug therapy and tapered according to schedule
5) Bacterial meningitis	Dexamethasone 0.15 mg/kg q6 h for 2–4 days with the first dose administered 10–20 min before, or at least concomitant with, the first dose of antimicrobial therapy
6) Tuberculous (TB) meningitis	Patients with grade II or III disease should receive intravenous treatment of dexamethasone for four weeks (0.4 mg per kilogram per day for the first week, 0.3 mg per kilogram per day for the second week, 0.2 mg per kilogram per day for the third week, and 0.1 mg per kilogram per day for the fourth week) and then oral treatment for four weeks, starting at a total of 4 mg per day and decreasing by 1 mg each week Patients with grade I disease should receive lower dose of intravenous dexamethasone therapy with shorter duration of two weeks (0.3 mg per kilogram per day for the first week and 0.2 mg per kilogram per day for the second week) and then four weeks of oral therapy (0.1 mg per kilogram per day for the third week, then a total of 3 mg per day, decreasing by 1 mg each week)
7) Pneumocystis jirovecii pneumonia	Prednisone 40 mg q 12 hrs per os (PO) for 5 days followed by 40 mg q24 hrs PO for 5 days and then 20 mg q24 hrs PO for 11 days
8) Lupus Nephritis	IV pulse methylprednisolone of 1 gram per day for 3 days monthly for 6 months, with 0.5-1.5 mg of oral prednisone per kilogram between pulses
9) COPD exacerbations	Methyl prednisiolone succinate IV 125 mg every 6 hours for 3 days then 60 mg daily for 4 days then 40 mg daily for 4 days then 20 mg daily for 4 days.
10) Asthma exacerbations	120 to 180 mg/day of prednisone, prednisolone, or methylprednisolone in 3 or 4 divided doses for 48 hours and then 60 to 80 mg/day until peak expiratory flow rate (PEFR) reaches 70% of predicted
11) Brain edema.	Dexamethasone with initial dose of 10 mg intravenously or orally, followed by 4 mg every 6 hours
12) Anaphylaxis	Prednisone 1 mg/kg up to 50 mg orally or hydrocortisone 1.5-3 mg/kg IV
13) Pulmonary fibrosis	Corticosteroids should be tapered within 2 to 3 weeks. This can be done by decreasing the dose by 50% every 4 days Methyl prednisiolone pulse therapy (1000 mg/day for 3 days, 500 mg/day for 2 days, 250 mg/day for 2 days, 125 mg/day for 2 days, and 80 mg/day for 2 days), followed by oral prednisolone (1 mg per kilogram per day, reduced by about 20% each week)

14) Thyroid storm	Hydrocortisone 300 mg intravenous loading followed by 100 mg every 8 hours
15) Myxedema	Intravenous hydrocortisone should be given at a dosage of 100 mg every eight hours
16) Brain dead patients that are candidates for organ donation	Methylprednisolone 15 mg/kg IV every 24 hours

* Many other indications of corticosteroids are not covered like autoimmune hemolytic anemia, prevention and treatment of rejection of transplanted organs, hypercalcemia and many others because their incidence in the ICUs is rare.
§ There is controversy about dosing and tapering of steroids, so effort has been made to include the best available evidence.

The Most Common Indications of Corticosteroids in ICU

Septic shock

A plenty of data is available in the literature about using and dosing of corticosteroids in septic shock. In this review we included the recommendation of the latest Surviving Sepsis Campaign guideline that was published in Feb.2013. The guideline recommended not using intravenous hydrocortisone to treat adult septic shock patients if adequate fluid resuscitation and vasopressor therapy are able to restore hemodynamic stability. If this case is not achievable, the intravenous hydrocortisone alone at a dose of 200 mg per day as continuous infusion is suggested, repetitive bolus application of hydrocortisone leads to a significant increase in blood glucose; this peak effect was not detectable during continuous infusion [2]. Other recommendations about corticosteroids that were included in the aforementioned guideline were not using the Adrenocorticotropic hormone(ACTH) stimulation test to identify adults with septic shock who should receive hydrocortisone, not using corticosteroids for the treatment of sepsis in the absence of shock and corticosteroids should be tapered when vasopressors are no longer required [2].

Airway edema

Laryngeal edema is one of the most common complications in ICU that can cause stridor, dyspnoea and reintubation. These complications, especially reintubation, can result in many adverse outcomes, including longer hospital stay, higher costs and increased mortality. Risk factors of laryngeal edema and the development of postextubation stridor include older age, female gender, low Glasgow Coma Scale score, excessive endotracheal tube (ETT) size, elevated Acute Physiologic and Chronic Health Evaluation II score and a prolonged intubation period (more than 36 hrs) [3].

Corticosteroids (mainly dexamethasone and methylprednisolone) were shown to be effective in decreasing the incidence of postextubation stridor in adult patients at high risk to develop airway obstruction [3].

The dose of dexamethasone is 0.5-2 mg/kg divided over 4-6 hrs started 24 hours before extubation and continued for 24 hours after extubation [4]. Current evidence also suggests that prophylactic intravenous (IV) methylprednisolone therapy (20-40 mg every 4-6 h) should be considered 12-24 hours prior to a planned extubation in patients at high-risk for postextubation laryngeal edema [5].

Usually laryngeal edema occurs within eight hours after extubation, that's why the administration of steroids immediately after extubation might be too late. The benefit of steroids before selected extubation is assumed to be due to protection against or treating mucosal edema in the glottic region caused by pressure or irritation from the endotracheal tube [6].

Spinal cord injury

A phase three randomized trial proved the efficacy of methylprednisolone sodium succinate in enhancing sustained neurologic recovery after spinal cord injury [7]. Methylprednisolone should be initiated within eight hours of injury using an initial bolus of 30 mg/kg by IV for 15 minutes followed 45 minutes later by a continuous infusion of 5.4 mg/kg/hour for 23 hours. If the maintenance therapy is extended for 48 hours, further improvement in motor function recovery has been shown to occur. This is evident when the initial bolus dose could only be administered three to eight hours after the trauma.

ARDS

Corticosteroids were studied to prevent and to treat early and late ARDS. While using corticosteroids in preventing ARDS showed higher mortality and rate of ARDS development, there is a mixed data about its role in treating early ARDS. These drugs have no benefits in late stage of ARDS and are associated with bad outcomes [8].

Since the direction of the systemic inflammatory response is established in the early stage of ARDS, we suggest to use low-dose methylprednisolone (1 mg/kg/d) tested in early ARDS (within 72 h of diagnosis) since it was tested and was shown to down regulate systemic inflammation and lead to earlier resolution of pulmonary organ dysfunction and a reduction in duration of mechanical ventilation and ICU stay according to a randomized controlled trial that was done by Meduri [9].

The regimen that was used in the aforementioned study is the beginning of administration of a loading dose of 1 mg/kg of methyl prsnisolone followed by an infusion of 1 mg/kg/d from day 1 to day 14, then 0.5 mg/kg/d from day 15 to day 21, then 0.25 mg/kg/d from day 22 to day 25, and finally 0.125 mg/kg/d from day 26 to day 28. In the study if the patient was extubated between days 1 and 14, the patient was advanced to day 15 of drug therapy and tapered according to schedule [9].

Bacterial meningitis

Corticosteroids reduce brain edema, intracranial hypertension and meningeal inflammation in experimental models of bacterial meningitis. It is also proven to be associated with reduced mortality and lower frequency of hearing loss and neuropsychological sequelae in adult patients [10].

However, there is a concern about impaired antibiotics penetration as a consequence of dexamethasone therapy [11].

Dexamethasone (0.15 mg/kg q6 h for 2–4 days with the first dose administered 10–20 min before, or at least concomitant with, the first dose of antimicrobial therapy) in adults with suspected or proven pneumococcal meningitis [10]. Dexamethasone should only be continued if the cerebrospinal fluid (CSF) Gram stain reveals gram- positive diplococci, or if blood or CSF cultures are positive for S. pneumonia [10].

Adjunctive dexamethasone should not be given to adult patients who have already received antimicrobial therapy [10].

Delayed treatment is not beneficial as dexamethasone does not reverse existing brain edema or intracranial hypertension in later stages of meningitis [11].

Tuberculous meningitis

As in bacterial meningitis corticosteroids are also effective in reducing the risk of death or disabling residual neurological deficit. However, corticosteroids in TB meningitis are used for prolonged period (6 to 8 weeks) rather than 2 to 4 days (as in bacterial meningitis), so all patients with TB meningitis receive adjunctive corticosteroids regardless of disease severity at presentation [12]. Dexamethasone and prednisolone were mainly given for TB meningitis with variable dosing regimens and there is no data from controlled trials comparing different corticosteroid regimens [13].

There is insufficient evidence to recommend routine adjunctive corticosteroids for all patients with tuberculomas without meningitis, or with spinal cord tuberculosis. However, they may be helpful in those patients whose symptoms are not controlled, or are worsening, on anti-tuberculosis therapy, or who have acute spinal cord compression secondary to vertebral tuberculosis [12].

Patients with grade II or III disease should receive intravenous treatment of dexamethasone for four weeks (0.4 mg per kilogram per day for the first week, 0.3 mg per kilogram per day for the second week, 0.2 mg per kilogram per day for the third week, and 0.1 mg per kilogram per day for the fourth week) and then oral treatment for four weeks, starting at a total of 4 mg per day and decreasing by 1 mg each week [12].

Patients with grade I disease should receive lower dose of intravenous dexamethasone therapy with shorter duration of two weeks (0.3 mg per kilogram per day for the first week and 0.2 mg per kilogram per day for the second week) and then four weeks of oral therapy (0.1 mg per kilogram per day for the third week, then a total of 3 mg per day, decreasing by 1 mg each week) [12].

Corticosteroids are not recommended in other forms of Tuberculosis except in tuberculous pericarditis where some evidence suggests its use in this indication [14].

Pneumocystis jirovecii pneumonia

Corticosteroids are used as adjunctive initial therapy only in patients with HIV infection who have severe P jirovecii pneumonia as defined by an arterial-alveolar O2 gradient that exceeds 35 mm Hg or a room air arterial oxygen pressure of less than 70 mm Hg or. In patients without HIV infection adjunctive steroids are not recommended [15].

During antimicrobial therapy microbial degradation and clearance may result in further inflammation that can exacerbate a severe inflammatory response that includes the production of cytokines and other inflammatory markers and cells to dying organisms in the lungs that often worsens after therapy is begun. Adjunctive steroids can blunt this inflammatory response that result in lung tissue damage [15]. Consequently, this will lead to good outcomes by improving survival, decreasing episodes of respiratory decompensation and decreasing the need for mechanical ventilation.

Prednisone 40 mg q 12 hrs per os (PO) for 5 days followed by 40 mg q24 hrs PO for 5 days and then 20 mg q24 hrs PO for 11 days [15].

Methylprednisolone at 75% of the respective prednisolone dose should be administered if intravenous therapy is necessary [15].

Lupus Nephritis

Corticosteroid therapy is a major component in therapeutic regimens for systemic lupus erythematosus (SLE). It is known to suppress the clinical expression of disease and is considered by many to be a major factor in the improved survival and prognosis. Although most clinical trials of corticosteroid therapy in SLE patients have been conducted in patients with severe lupus nephritis, the evidence suggests that they are also effective in the treatment of severe and life threatening cases of, pneumonitis, polyserositis, vasculitis, thrombocytopenia, CNS disease and other clinical manifestations [16].

The IV pulse methylprednisolone is used for life- or organ- threatening disease which is defined by courses of 1 gram per day for 3 days monthly for 6 months, with 0.5-1.5 mg of oral prednisone per kilogram between pulses, to control both renal and extra-renal manifestations. It is usually used as initial management of active nephritis, sole therapy to avoid cumulative adverse effects of long-term daily corticosteroid therapy, or regimen for exacerbations of severe cases not responsive to daily oral steroids [17,18].

Severe COPD exacerbations

Intravenous corticosteroids are helpful in the treatment of severe exacerbations of COPD. Corticosteroid therapy can improve lung function (FEV1) and hypoxemia (PaO2), reduces recovery time, ICU stay, cost of admission and may reduce the risk of early relapse [19]. The optimal dose and duration of steroids in COPD exacerbations are unknown. According to a recent meta-analysis the low-dose regimen (initial dose 30-80 mg/day of prednisolone) is proper for treating COPD exacerbations. However, the high-dose group did not show obviously higher risk of side effects [20].

We included the recommendation of the Systemic Corticosteroids in Chronic Obstructive Pulmonary Disease Exacerbations (SCCOPE) trial [21].

Methylprednisiolone succinate IV 125 mg every 6 hours for 3 days than 60 mg daily for 4 days than 40 mg daily for 4 days than 20 mg daily for 4 days.

Severe asthma exacerbation

In severe asthma there is airway obstruction and airway inflammation. In order to reduce the inflammation systemic corticosteroids must be included as part of the regimen in all patients with acute severe asthma.

Receptor-binding affinities of lung corticosteroid receptors are reduced in the face of airway inflammation, that's why multiple daily dosing of systemic corticosteroids for the initial therapy of acute asthma exacerbations appears necessary. As in severe COPD exacerbations, the optimal dose and duration of steroids in severe asthma exacerbations are unknown. The oral and IV routes are equally effective, so that the oral route may be used if patients can swallow. However, in ICU settings patients are intubated and mechanically ventilated so we prefer to use the intravenous form [16].

Regarding the duration a 7 day-day course in adults has been found to be as effective as 14-day course [22].

The National Institutes of Health (NIH) guidelines recommend 120 to 180 mg/day of prednisone, prednisolone, or methylprednisolone in 3 or 4 divided doses for 48 hours and then 60 to 80 mg/day until peak expiratory flow rate (PEFR) reaches 70% of predicted. The anti- inflammatory effect of corticosteroids as measured by improvement in pulmonary function is not immediate and can take up to 24 hours to occur [23].

Brain edema

Four types of cerebral edema are present: the vasogenic cerebral edema that results from an increased permeability of the endothelium of cerebral capillaries to albumin and other plasma proteins due to the breakdown of the tight endothelial junctions; the cytotoxic cerebral edema in which the blood brain barrier is not affected but there is imbalance in cellular metabolism that weaken the functioning of the sodium and potassium pump in the glial cell membrane; the osmotic cerebral edema that results when the blood becomes diluted; and the interstitial cerebral edema that result in obstructive hydrocephalus.

Glucocorticoids are very effective in reducing the vasogenic edema that occurs in many clinical conditions like inflammatory conditions, tumors, and other disorders. However, steroids are not helpful to treat cytotoxic edema and are harmful in patients with brain ischemia [24]. In patients with severe head injury the use of glucocorticoids are not recommended for improving outcome or reducing Intracranial pressure (ICP) [25].

Dexamethasone is the preferred agent due to its very low mineralocorticoid activity. The usual initial dose is 10 mg intravenously or orally, followed by 4 mg every 6 hours [25].

Corticosteroids should be tapered within 2 to 3 weeks. This can be done by decreasing the dose by 50% every 4 days [25].

Anaphylaxis

There are many theoretical benefits of using steroids in patients with anaphylaxis. However, there are no placebo-controlled trials to confirm these assumed benefits of steroids in anaphylaxis. The use of prednisone 1 mg/kg up to 50 mg orally or hydrocortisone 1.5-3 mg/kg IV is suggested [26].

Pulmonary fibrosis

The latest international evidence-based guideline on the diagnosis and management of idiopathic pulmonary fibrosis (IPF) that was published in 2011 recommended against the use of corticosteroid monotherapy in patients with IPF. Also the recommendation for corticosteroids in patients with acute exacerbation of IPF is weak; that is, corticosteroids should be used in the majority of patients with acute exacerbation of IPF, but not using corticosteroids may be a reasonable choice in a minority [27]. Corticosteroids (e.g. prednisone, methylprednisolone) are used in the majority of patients who suffer an acute exacerbation of IPF, usually in pulse doses. We recommend using methyl prednisolone pulse therapy (1000 mg/day for 3 days, 500 mg/day for 2 days, 250 mg/day for 2 days, 125 mg/day for 2 days, and 80 mg/day for 2 days), followed by oral prednisolone (1 mg per kilogram per day, reduced by about 20% each week) [28].

Thyroid storm

The benefits of steroids in thyroid storm are mainly blocking T4-to- T3 conversion and prophylaxis against relative adrenal insufficiency.

Hydrocortisone 300 mg intravenous loading followed by 100 mg every 8 hours [29].

Myxedema

In myxedema there is a possibility of secondary hypothyroidism and associated hypopituitarism, so hydrocortisone should be administered until adrenal insufficiency is excluded. Intravenous hydrocortisone should be given at a dosage of 100 mg every eight hours. Not treating adrenal insufficiency with hydrocortisone may precipitate adrenal crisis. Before therapy a random cortisol level should be drawn, and if not depressed, the hydrocortisone can be stopped without tapering [30].

Brain dead patients who are candidates for organ donation

Methylprednisolone 15 mg/kg IV every 24 hours as part of the triple hormonal therapy that includes the use of levothyroxine and vasopressin infusion [31].

Conclusions

Corticosteroids are one of the most common medications that are used for a variety of indications in the intensive care units. Due to the diverse adverse effects of corticosteroids that affect the morbidity and mortality of critically ill patients and because of the high number of medication errors that are associated with these medications, we wrote this review that can be used as a guide for health care professionals who are taking care of critically ill patients that are receiving corticosteroids. This review covers mainly the most common indications of corticosteroids in ICU and also how to taper corticosteroids according to the best evidence that recommends their use. Many other indications of corticosteroids are not covered like autoimmune hemolytic anemia, prevention and treatment of rejection of transplanted organs, hypercalcemia and many others because their incidence in the ICUs is rare.

Competing Interests

The authors declare no financial, professional, political, personal, religious, ideological, academic, intellectual, commercial or other relationship that would be a conflict of interest in the interpretation of any information related to this review.

References

1. Katzung BG (2007) Basic and Clinical Pharmacology. (10th edn). New York, NY: McGraw-Hill Companies Inc.

2. Dellinger RP, Levy MM, Rhodes A, Annane D, Gerlach H, et al. (2013) Surviving Sepsis Campaign: International Guidelines for Management of Severe Sepsis and Septic Shock. Critical Care Medicine 41: 580-637.

3. Lee CH, Peng MJ, Wu CL (2007) Dexamethasone to prevent postextubation airway obstruction in adults: a prospective, randomized, double-blind, placebo-controlled study. Critical Care 11: R72.

4. Lacy CF, Armstrong LL, Goldman MP, Leonard L (2010) Lance:Drug Information Handbook, 18th ed. Hudson, Ohio, Lexi-Comp, Inc.

5. Roberts RJ, Welch SM, Devlin JW (2008) Corticosteroids for Prevention of Postextubation Laryngeal Edema in Adults. Ann Pharmacother 42: 686-691.

6. Fan T, Wang G, Mao B, Xiong Z, Zhang Y, Liu X, Wang L, Yang S (2008) Prophylactic administration of parenteral steroids for preventing airway complications after extubation in adults: meta-analysis of randomised placebo controlled trials. BMJ 337:a1841.

7. Bracken MB, Shepard MJ, Collins WF, Holford TR, Young W, et al. (1990) A randomized, controlled trial of methylprednisolone or naloxone in the treatment of acute spinal-cord injury. Results of the Second National Acute Spinal Cord Injury Study. NEngl J Med 322: 1405-1411.

8. Khilnani GC, Hadda V (2011) Corticosteroids and ARDS: A review of treatment and prevention evidence. Lung India 28: 114–119.

9. Meduri GU, Golden E, Freire AX, Taylor E, Zaman M, et al. (2007) Methylprednisolone Infusion in Early Severe ARDS. CHEST 131: 954-963.

10. Tunkel AR, Hartman BJ, Kaplan SL, et al. (2004) Practice Guidelines for the Management of Bacterial Meningitis. Clinical Infectious Diseases 39. 1267–1284.

11. Hoffman O and Weber RJ (2009) Review: Pathophysiology and treatment of bacterial meningitis. TherAdvNeurolDisord 2: 401-412.

12. Thwaites G, Fisher M, Hemingway C, Scott G, Solomon T, et al. (2009) British Infection Society guidelines for the diagnosis and treatment of tuberculosis of the central nervous system in adults and children. Journal of Infection 59: 167-187.

13. Prasad K, Singh MB (2008) Corticosteroids for managing tuberculous meningitis. Cochrane Database of Systematic Reviews, Issue 1.

14. Mayosi BM (2002) Interventions for treating tuberculous pericarditis. Cochrane Database of Systematic Reviews, Issue 4.

15. Jose G Castro, Maya Morrison-Bryant (2010) Management of Pneumocystis Jiroveciipneumonia in HIV infected patients: current options, challenges and future directions. HIV/AIDS - Research and Palliative Care 2: 123–134.

16 Dipiro J, Talbert B, Yee GC, Matzke GR, Wells BG, Posey LM (2008) Pharmacotherapy: A Pathophysiologic Approach, 7th edition, New York, McGraw-Hill

17. Paget SA, Gibofsky A, Beary JF (2000) Manual of Rheumatology & Outpatient Orthopedic Disorders. Lippincott Williams & Wilkins

18. Sinha A, Bagga A (2008) Pulse steroid therapy. Indian Journal of Pediatrics 75: 1057-1066.

19. (2014) Management of exacerbations: GOLD (Global Initiative for Chronic Obstructive Lung Disease)

20. Cheng T, Gong Y, Guo Y, Cheng Q, Zhou M, Shi G, Wan H (2013) Systemic corticosteroid for COPD exacerbations, whether the higher dose is better? A meta-analysis of randomized controlled trials. ClinRespir J 7: 305-318.

21. Erbland ML, Deupree RH, Niewoehner DE (1998) Systemic Corticosteroids in Chronic Obstructive Pulmonary Disease Exacerbations (SCCOPE): rationale and design of an equivalence trial. Veterans Administration Cooperative Trials SCCOPE Study Group. Control Clin Trials 19: 404-417.

22. Hasegawa T, Ishihara K, Takakura S, Fujii H, Nishimura T, Okazaki M, Katakami N, et al. (2000) Duration of systemic corticosteroids in the treatment of asthma exacerbation; a randomized study. Intern Med 39: 794-797.

23. National Asthma Education and Prevention Program. Clinical practice guidelines: expert panel report. Guidelines for the diagnosis and management of asthma. Bethesda (MD): National Institutes of Health, National Heart, Lung, and Blood Institute. 1997. Publication No. 97– 4051.

24. Rabinstein AA (2006) Treatment of Cerebral Edema. The Neurologist 12: 59-73.

25. Kaal EC, Vecht CJ (2004) The management of brain edema in brain tumors. Current Opinion in Oncology 16: 593-600.

26. Brown AFT (2009) Current management of anaphylaxis. Emergencias 21: 213-223.

27. Raghu G, Collard HR, Egan JJ, Martinez FJ, Behr J, et al. (2011) An Official ATS/ERS/JRS/ALAT Statement: Idiopathic Pulmonary Fibrosis: Evidence-based Guidelines for Diagnosis and Management. American Journal Of Respiratory And Critical Care Medicine 183: 788-824.

28. Horita N, Akahane M, Okada Y, Kobayashi Y, Arai T, et al. (2011) Tacrolimus and Steroid Treatment for Acute Exacerbation of Idiopathic Pulmonary Fibrosis. Intern Med 50: 189-195.

29. Bahn RS , Burch HB, Cooper DS, Garber JR, M. Greenlee MC, et al. (2011) Hyperthyroidism Management Guidelines. EndocrPract 17: 3.

30. Wall CR (2000) Myxedema Coma: Diagnosis and Treatment. AmFam Physician 62: 2485-2490.

31. Shemie SD, Ross H, Pagliarello J, Baker AJ, Greig PD, et al. (2006) Organ donor management in Canada: recommendations of the forum on Medical Management to Optimize Donor Organ Potential. CMAJ 174:S13-32.

5

Autocrine/Paracrine Insulin-like Growth Factor Binding Protein-3 Acts as Pro-apoptotic Factor for Leydig cells in the Rat Testis

Eugenia Colón[1,2,*], Christine Carlsson-Skwirut[1], Konstantin V Svechnikov[1] and Olle Söder[1]

[1]Department of Woman and Child Health, Paediatric Endocrinology Unit, Astrid Lindgren Children's Hospital, Karolinska Institute and University Hospital, SE 17176 Stockholm, Sweden
[2]Department of Pathology and Cytology, Sodersjukhuset, Karolinska Institute and University Hospital, SE 11883 Stockholm, Sweden

Abstract

The secretory insulin-like growth factor-binding protein-3 (IGFBP-3) induces apoptosis via both insulin-like growth factor-I (IGF-I)-dependent and -independent mechanisms. Here, we have examined the effects of IGFBP-3 on Leydig cell apoptosis, proliferation and steroidogenesis. Immunohistochemical analysis of testes of rats at different ages revealed that IGFBP-3 is expressed first after 20 days of postnatal life and is present at a high level in the adult testis. In addition, Western blotting showed that the expression of IGFBP-3 in Leydig cells isolated from 60-day-old rats is higher than in 40-day-old animals. The rate of DNA synthesis (as assessed by incorporation of ^{3}H-thymidine *in vitro*) in Leydig cells from 40-day-old rats is reduced by IGFBP-3, which also blocks the promotion of cell survival by IGF-I. Moreover, IGFBP-3 induces apoptosis in Leydig cells and, at the same time, attenuates the anti-apoptotic action of IGF-I. Furthermore, IGF-I stimulates secretion of IGFBP-3, -4, and -2 by Leydig cells. The pro-inflammatory cytokine tumor necrosis factor- α induces apoptosis in these same cells and increases their secretion of IGFBP-3 and IGFBP-4.

These findings provide the first evidence that IGFBP-3 acts as a pro-apoptotic effector of Leydig cells and can also block the positive effect of IGF-I on cell survival. In addition, IGFBPs appear to modulate interactions between IGF-I and pro-inflammatory cytokines in the testis, suggesting possible participation of these proteins in processes such as testicular inflammation and cancer.

Keywords: IGFBP-3; IGFBP-2; PPP; Leydig cells; Steroidogenesis; IGF-I; IGF-IR

Introduction

Insulin-like growth factors (IGFs) are involved in cell metabolism, growth, differentiation, and survival (1) in most organs, including those of the reproductive axis [1-3]. The activities of these factors are regulated by a family of six high affinity-binding proteins (IGFBP-1–6), which determine IGF bioavailability in circulating fluids and the cellular environment [1,4,5].

IGFBP-3 is the most abundant circulating IGF-binding protein and mediates IGF independent actions on cell survival and apoptosis [6,7]. In the testis, IGFs and IGFBPs are localized in the same cells that express LH and FSH receptors [8-10]. IGFBP-2 and -3 are the most abundant IGFBPs in this organ [9] and large amounts of IGFBP-3 are produced by Sertoli and Leydig cells [9,11]. Both FSH and (Bu)2cAMP markedly lower IGFBP-3 levels in Sertoli cells [11] and this binding protein can either inhibit or enhance the effects on Leydig cells steroidogenesis depending on the surrounding conditions [9,12].

The involvement of IGFBP-3 in steroidogenesis, development, and tumor growth in the testis is poorly understood. Previous investigations have revealed that IGFBP-3, -4, and -2 are predominantly expressed by Leydig cells [9]. It has been proposed that IGFBP-3 also potentiates the inhibitory effects of cytokines on steroidogenesis [9,12]. Both IGFBP-3 and -4 have been reported to be down-regulated in testicular seminomas [13], allowing more rapid tumor growth.

How the apoptotic effects of IGFBP-3 are mediated in the testis is largely unclear. It was described previously that IGFBP-3 can induce apoptosis via an intrinsic apoptotic pathway [14]. Apoptotic stimuli lead to an increase in the permeability of the outer mitochondrial membrane and promote the release of cytochrome c into the cytosol. Cytochrome c binds to apoptotic protease-activating factor-1 and caspase-9, promoting the activation of caspase-3 [15]. Members of the Bcl-2 family have been shown to influence this process [16].

Apoptosis can also be induced via an extrinsic pathway that involves ligand-mediated activation of death receptors, such as the TNF receptor 1 (TNFR1). Upon binding of TNFα to the TNFR1, an intracellular death effectors complex is formed, consisting of adaptor molecules, such as Fas-associated death domain protein and an inactive precursor form of caspase-8 [17]. Formation of this complex leads to cleavage of caspase-8 into active subunits and the subsequent proteolysis of downstream substrates. Activation of the transcription factor nuclear factor-kB (NFkB) by nuclear translocation elicits a potent survival signal and blocks this death receptor-mediated apoptotic pathway [18].

Following secretion, IGFBP-3 is well known to inhibit growth via both IGF-I-dependent and -independent pathways [6,7]. Such effects have been observed with different types of cells, including prostate and breast cancer cells [7,19,20]. The possible independent effects of IGFBP-3 on Leydig cell function have not been studied.

IGFBP-3 levels are regulated by multiple factors, including cytokines. We and others have demonstrated the relation between cytokines and binding proteins in Leydig cells [8,9,21]. The inhibitory effects of IL-1β and IL-1α on Leydig cell steroidogenesis is partially

*Corresponding author: Colón E, Department of Pathology and Cytology, Sodersjukhuset, Karolinska Institute and University Hospital, SE 11883 Stockholm, Sweden, E-mail: eugenia.colon@ki.se

mediated by the stimulation of IGFBP-2 and -3, suggesting that these cytokines utilize common pathways. Cytokines are generated under both normal and pathological circumstances and have been implicated in the pathogenesis of diseases such as inflammation and cancer in the testis [21-23]. Previous experiments from our group have demonstrated the constitutive production of both IL-1α and IL-18 by the testis [23,24]. IL-18 is a defense factor in the male gonad and IL-1α can stimulate or inhibit steroidogenesis depending on the surrounding conditions [12,21].

The testis is a site of IGF-I biosynthesis and action; high levels of IGFBP-3 are expressed in normal testis [8,25]. IGF-I mRNA and protein, as well as specific IGF-I receptors, are present in the testis and have been localized in Leydig, peritubular and germ cells [26]. Testicular levels of IGF-I peak during the fourth week postpartum at the beginning of the pubertal rise in testosterone secretion [26]. Since IGFBP-3 regulates IGF-I bioavailability and IGF-I is involved in the processes of differentiation, steroidogenesis, and apoptosis in Leydig cells, we studied the modulation of IGFBPs on the effects of IGF-I at the time of IGF-I peak expression in the testis.

Recently, the independent actions of IGFBP-3 on apoptosis have been described in other model systems. At present, little is known about the independent actions of IGFBP-3 and its interactions with pro-inflammatory cytokines in the testis. In this study, we investigated the influence of IGFBP-3 on Leydig cell function and apoptosis, as well as the regulation of the secretion of this binding protein by IGF-I and certain pro-inflammatory cytokines.

Materials and Methods

Reagents

Dulbecco's Modified Eagle's Medium (DMEM)-Ham's nutrient mixture F-12, Modified Eagle's Medium (MEM), Hank's Balanced Salts Solution (HBSS) without Ca^{2+} or Mg^{2+}, and penicillin and streptomycin were purchased from Invitrogen (Life Technologies, Inc. Paisley, UK). Bovine serum albumin (BSA) (fraction V), Percoll, HEPES and collagenase type I (Sigma-Aldrich St. Louis, MO) were used to isolate Leydig cells, which were subsequently treated with recombinant rat IGF-I, IGF-II, IGFBP-3, (GroPep Limited, Adelaide, Australia) IL-1β, IL18 and/or TNFα (R&D Systems, Abingdon, UK). The Cell Proliferation Reagent WST-1 (Roche Diagnostics, Penzberg, Germany), was employed to assess cell viability and the Analysis of DNA Fragmentation by Cell Death Detection ELISA^{plus} (Roche Diagnostics, Meylan, France), kit to monitor apoptosis.

Western blotting was performed with anti-α-tubulin (Santa Cruz Biotechnology Inc., CA, USA), anti IGFBP-3 (GroPep Limited, Adelaide, Australia), and anti-caspase 3 (Santa Cruz Biotechnology Inc., CA, USA) antibodies. The cyclolignan PPP (picropodophyllin); (a kind gift from Dr Olle Larsson and Dr Magnus Axelson) was synthesized and recrystallized to obtain a final purity of 99.7% and dissolved physiological in saline (5 μM) or DMSO (0.5 mM) prior to addition to the medium of cell cultures [27].

Experimental animals

Testes and Leydig cells were obtained from 10-, 20-, 40- and 60-day-old male Sprague-Dawley rats (B&K Laboratories, Sollentuna, Sweden), employing five animals in each age group, as described below. These animals were provided with a standard pellet diet and water ad libitum. All animal experiments were conducted in accordance with institutional guidelines and approved in advance by the local ethics committee for animal experimentation (N 218/05).

Immunocytochemistry

For each age group five testes, one from each animal, were stained with primary antibodies directed towards IGFBP-3 (see above) together with the HRP-Streptavidin complex (Rabbit Immunocruz staining system, Santa Cruz Biotechnology, Inc., USA), in accordance with the manufacturer's instructions. In brief, tissue sections were deparaffinized and then placed in Tris-buffered saline containing 0.05% Tween-20 (pH 7.6) (TBS/T) for 5 min. Thereafter, the antigen was retrieved by placing the tissues in 10 mM citrate buffer, pH 6.0, after which endogenous peroxidase activity was blocked by incubation with 3% H_2O_2 for 30 min. Subsequently, the sections were incubated overnight at 4°C with anti-IGFBP-3 (at a dilution of 1:50), followed by sequential exposure for 1 hour each to a biotinylated secondary antibody and a peroxidase-conjugated streptavidin complex. Thereafter, staining with 3,3-diaminobenzidine tetrahydrochloride (Peroxidase Substrate Kit, SK-4100, Vector Laboratories, Inc.) resulted in a brown color localized in the cytoplasm and clearly distinguishable from the unstained background. The specificity of the antibody towards IGFBP-3 was confirmed by incubation of parallel sections with non-immune rabbit IgG at the same dilution (negative control). All sections were then counterstained with Mayer's hematoxylin, dehydrated and mounted under a coverslip with resin (Permount, SP15–100, Fisher Scientific Co. USA).

Finally, 10 separated fields in each of three non-adjacent sections from each testis were examined for staining employing a Nikon Eclipse E800 microscope (40-fold magnification; Nikon, Inc., Melville, NY) equipped with a SPOT RT digital camera (Diagnostic Instruments, Inc., Nikon, Inc., Melville, NY) and interfaced with a computer.

Isolation and culture of Leydig cells

Leydig cells from rats 40 days (immature Leydig cells) and older (60 days, adult Leydig cells) were prepared according to the procedure developed by Klinefelter et al. [28], as described earlier [2,29]. The corresponding cells from 10-day-old rats (progenitor Leydig cells) were obtained as described by Khan [30]. The purity of these Leydig cell preparations was 90%, as demonstrated by specific histochemical staining for 3-hydroxysteroid dehydrogenase [31], 11βhydroxysteroid dehydrogenase [32], anti-cytokeratin pan antibody for Sertoli cells [33], together with ED2 staining for macrophages [34]. Examination of Trypan blue exclusion revealed that cell viability was routinely greater than 96%.

Subsequently, 1.5×10^4 cells in a total volume of 200 μl were usually plated in each individual well of 96-well plates (Falcon, USA) and then incubated for 24 hours at 34°C. At this point, the culture medium was replaced by fresh medium containing IGFBP-3 (1-100 ng/ml) and/or IGF-I (10-100 ng/ml) [21] and thereafter incubated for an additional 24 hours. In the case of Western ligand blotting $2x10^6$ cells were incubated in each well of 6-well plates (Falcon, USA) for 24 hours, following which the culture medium was replaced by fresh medium with or without IGF-I (10 ng/ml), IGF-II (10 ng/ml) [21], IL-1β [29], IL-18 (100 ng/ml) [23], TNFα (10 ng/ml) and/or PPP (100 nmol/L) [35] and incubated for an additional 24 h.

Quantification of DNA synthesis by Leydig cells *in vitro*

After culturing of 96-well plates as described above, Leydig cells isolated from 10-40-days-old rats were labeled for the final 4 hours of culture with ^{3}H-thymidine (1 μCi per well; Amersham Pharmacia

Biotech, Little Chalfont, UK) and the radioactivity incorporated (cpm) was subsequently determined using a Beckman scintillation spectrometer. In each individual experiment triplicate or quadruplicate cell cultures were subjected to each treatment and three independent experiments were performed.

Determination of the number of viable Leydig cells in cultures

The numbers of viable Leydig cells in each culture were determined employing the WST-1 procedure (Roche Diagnostics GmbH, Mannheim, Germany), as described previously [2]. Accordingly, following treatment of Leydig cells in culture with IGFBP-3 (1-100 ng/ml) and /or IGF-I (100 ng/ml), 100 μl serum-free DMEM and 10 μl WST-1 were added to each well and the increase in absorption at 450 nm monitored for 60 min.

Determination of Leydig cell apoptosis *in vitro*

The extent of apoptosis occurring in cultured Leydig cells was assessed with an ELISA kit designed for both qualitative and quantitative photometric determination of cytoplasmic levels of histone-associated DNA fragments. In this case Leydig cells (1.5×10^4 per well) were cultured on 96-well plates for 24 hours, and then treated with IGFBP-3 (1-100 ng/ml), IGF-I (10-100 ng/ml) and/or TNFα (10 ng/ml) for an additional 24 hours. For treatments involving both IGF-I and TNFα, IGF-I was added 30 min prior to the cytokine. Following incubation, attached cells were harvested and centrifuged at 1500 rpm for 6 min, after which the resulting pellets were subjected to the ELISA procedure in accordance with the manufacturer's instructions. The level of cytoplasmic nucleosomes in treated cells was calculated as a percentage of the corresponding value for untreated cells.

Western blotting

The levels of the IGFBP-3 and caspase-3 were analyzed by PAGE/Western blotting. For this purpose cells were washed twice with PBS and then disrupted by sonication in a lysis buffer. Protein transfer and blocking was performed as described previously [21]. The PVDF membrane was stained with 5% Ponceau S for 5 minutes in order to confirm equal transfer of different proteins. In all cases α-tubulin was used as an internal control for loading.

Incubation with antibodies was performed in accordance with the manufacturer's specifications and, after additional washing; bound antibody was labeled with donkey anti-rabbit or sheep anti-mouse IgG secondary antibodies conjugated with horseradish peroxidase (Amersham Pharmacia Biotech). Finally, for detection by enhanced chemiluminescence these blots were incubated with ECL Plus Western blotting agent and then exposed to ECL Hyperfilm (Amersham Pharmacia Biotech). In accordance with the manufacturer's instructions stripping and reanalysis of the membranes were also accomplished.

Western ligand blotting

IGFBPs were examined by Western ligand blotting in the manner as originally described by Hossenlopp et al. (36) with minor modifications. Conditioned media from primary cultures of Leydig cells incubated in the absence or presence of IGF-I (10 ng/ml), IGF-II (10 ng/ml), IL-1β (10 ng/ml), IL-18 (100 ng/ml) and/or TNF α (10 ng/ml) and/or 100 nmol/L PPP for 24 hours were collected for this purpose. When present, PPP was added to the culture medium 1 hour prior to the addition of IGF-I.

Briefly, normal rat serum (5 μl), recombinant human IGFBP-2 (40 ng), or an aliquot of the medium from Leydig cell cultures (100 μl) was diluted with non-reducing sample buffer containing sodium dodecyl sulfate for separation by SDS-PAGE (12% gels). The resulting bands were electroblotted onto nitrocellulose filters (with a pore size of 0.45 μm) in a Hoefer Semi-Dry Transphor unit at 200 mA (Amersham Biosciences) during 1 hour. Thereafter, the filters were treated sequentially with 0.1% Tween 20 in Tris-buffered saline (pH 7.6) (TBS-T) and 1% BSA in TBS-T, and subsequently probed with 125I-labeled IGF-I dissolved in TBS-T containing 1% BSA (2×10^6 cpm/50 ml). Next, the filters were washed with TBS-T, dried, and subjected to autoradiography. Finally, each band was analyzed by densitometry and its level expressed as the fold-increase in relationship to the corresponding control band.

Determination of androgen production

Conditioned media collected from the various cell cultures described above were stored at -20°C prior to being assayed for testosterone and 5α-androstane-3α, 17β-diol, the predominant androgens synthesized by immature Leydig cells. Testosterone was determined employing a Coat-a-Count RIA kit, with a cross-reactivity for 5α-androstane-3α, 17β-diol of 0.4% (Diagnostic Products Corp., Los Angeles, CA), in accordance with the manufacturer's instructions. 5α-androstane-3α, 17β-diol was quantitated by RIA using specific antiserum (Cosmo Bio Co. LTD., Tokyo, Japan) and radiolabeled 5α-[9, 11,-3H (N)] androstane-3α, 17β-diol (specificity radio activity=40 Ci/mmol; NEN Life Science Products, Boston, MA) with a cross-reactivity for testosterone of 0.2%.

Statistical analyses

All data are presented as mean values ± SD. Comparison of androgen levels (i.e., the sum of the levels of 5α-androstane-3α, 17β-diol and testosterone) was performed using a one-way repeated measures analysis of variance ANOVA, together with Tukey's post-hoc test for pair-wise comparisons. Rates of cell proliferation, the degrees of cell survival and death, and the values obtained by western and western ligand blotting were compared utilizing one-way repeated measures analysis of variance ANOVA, employing the Holm-Sidak procedure for all pair-wise multiple comparisons. In all cases a p value of <0.05 was considered to be statistically significant.

Results

Western blotting analysis and cellular distribution of IGFBP-3 expression during postnatal testicular development

Immunohistochemical analysis of the testis of rats at different ages revealed that staining for IGFBP-3 increased from 10-60 days of postnatal age (Figures 1A-1K). On postnatal day 10 no expression of IGFBP-3 was found (Figure 1A), at 20 days of age, Leydig cells (LC) stained positively for IGFBP-3 (Figure 1C); at 60 days of age Leydig cells (LC) also stained positively (Figures 1H-1J). These findings are in good agreement with the results of Western blotting (Figure 2), which revealed that expression of IGFBP-3 by cultures of Leydig cells isolated from 60-day-old rat testis was 3.2 -fold higher than in the case of 20-day-old testis and 2.3-fold higher than that of testis of 40-day-old rats (Figure 2).

The influence of IGFBP-3 on the survival and DNA synthesis of rat Leydig cells in culture

We studied the possible direct and indirect action of IGFBP-3 on proliferation and viability in progenitor Leydig cells and immature Leydig cells. We wanted to study the relation between the rising of IGF-I and the levels of IGFBP-3 at this time of development. The effect

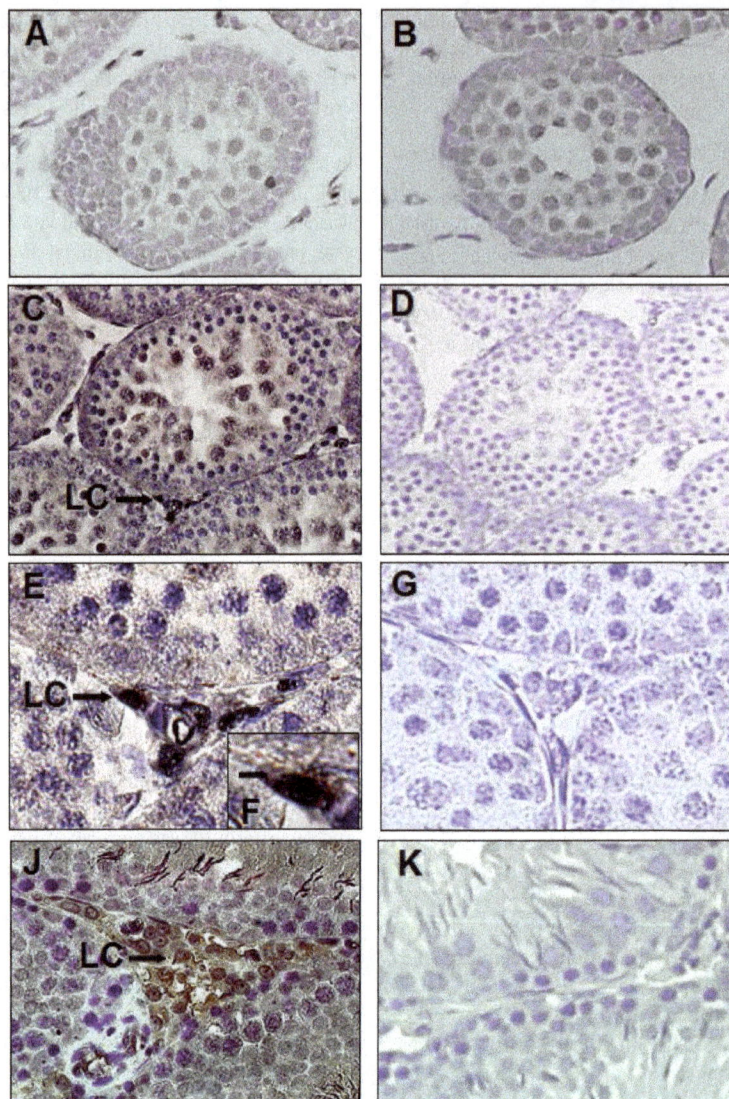

Figure 1: Immunohistochemical detection of IGFBP-3 in the testis of rats of different ages. (A) The testis of the 10-day-old rat demonstrated no staining for IGFBP-3. (B) Negative control for (A), involving incubation with non-immune rabbit IgG at the same dilution as the antibody (see the Materials and Methods). (C) In the testis of the 20-day-old rat, Leydig cells (LC) (indicated by arrows) in the interstitial compartment expressed IGFBP-3. (D) Negative control for (C), performed as in (B). (E, F) The interstitial compartment of testes from 20-day-old rats, arrows indicate Leydig cells (LC). (G) Negative control for E. (J) Two-fold higher magnification of interstitial compartment of the testis of adult (60-day-old) rats with arrows indicating Leydig cells staining positively for IGFBP-3. (K) Negative control for (J), performed as in (B). Levels of magnification: A, B, E, G, J, K: 60X; C, D: 40X; F: 100X.

of IGFBP-3 on the proliferation and viability of cultured Leydig cells isolated from 10 and 40-day-old rats were measured. DNA synthesis by untreated Leydig cells isolated from 10-day-old rats, declined spontaneously during the 48-hour culture period (Figure 3A). In the presence of IGF-I, the initial rate of this synthesis was maintained, while IGFBP-3 (1-100 ng/ml), either alone or in combination with IGF-I had no effect on this parameter (Figure 3A). IGFBP-3 had also no effect on cell viability at this age (Figure 3B).

In the case of cultured Leydig cells from 40-day-old rats, IGF-I (100 ng/ml) also prevented the spontaneous decline in the rate of DNA synthesis (as assessed by incorporation of [³H]TdR into DNA between hours 44 and 48 of incubation), but in these cultures IGFBP-3 reduced the rate of DNA synthesis (at a concentration of 100 ng/ml) and blocked the action of IGF-I (at 10-100 ng/ml) (Figure 3C).

The viability of cultures of Leydig cells isolated from 40-day-old rats (as assessed by the WST-1 procedure) mirrored the incorporation of [³H]TdR (Figure 3D). Thus, with no treatment, the number of viable cells remaining following 48 hours of incubation was 35% lower than the initial number and IGF-I prevented this loss of viable cells (Figure 3D). IGFBP-3 (100 ng/ml) inhibited this promotion of survival by IGF-I.

To understand the kinetics of the action of IGFBP-3 on Leydig cell viability we tested the action of IGFBP-3 at different time points (0. 12, 24 h). IGFBP-3 was able to decrease the survival effect of IGF-I on Leydig cells (Figure 4A).

To clarify the action of IGFBP-3 in Leydig cells at this stage of development (immature Leydig cells) we studied the possible apoptotic effect. IGFBP-3 enhanced apoptosis, as well as attenuating the reduction

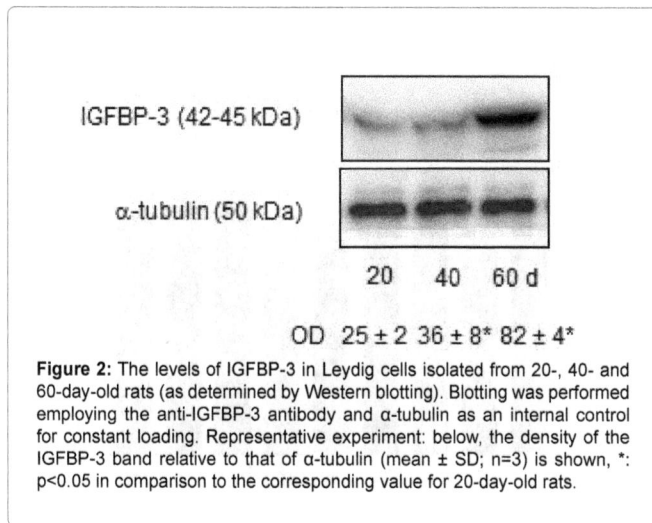

Figure 2: The levels of IGFBP-3 in Leydig cells isolated from 20-, 40- and 60-day-old rats (as determined by Western blotting). Blotting was performed employing the anti-IGFBP-3 antibody and α-tubulin as an internal control for constant loading. Representative experiment: below, the density of the IGFBP-3 band relative to that of α-tubulin (mean ± SD; n=3) is shown, *: $p<0.05$ in comparison to the corresponding value for 20-day-old rats.

in apoptosis caused by IGF-I (Figure 4B). To elucidate the mechanism of action of IGFBP-3 we tested the activation of caspase-3 at different time points. The result showed that exposure to IGFBP-3 (100 ng/ml) during 24h is associated with cleavage of caspase-3 into active fragments (20 and 17 kDa) (Figure 4C).

Relation between steroidogenesis and secretion of IGFBPs

Since the main function of Leydig cells is the production of androgens we tested the action of IGFBP-3 on steroidogenesis and the influence of IGFBP-3 on IGF-I stimulated Leydig cells. In culture of Leydig cells isolated from 40-day-old rats, IGFBP-3 itself decreased the total level of androgens present and furthermore attenuated the stimulation of steroidogenesis by IGF-I (Figure 5A).

Subsequently, we stimulated Leydig cells with IGF-I to investigate the effect of this peptide on IGFBPs secretion. The pattern of secretion of the IGFBPs by untreated and treated Leydig cells was examined employing Western ligand blotting with radioactive IGF-I as a probe. This procedure revealed a double band with an apparent molecular weight of 42-45 kilo Dalton (kDa), another band at 30 kDa and an additional band at 24 kDa, corresponding to IGFBP-3, IGFBP-2 and IGFBP-4 respectively, as demonstrated by previous investigations [21]. The finding demonstrated that the enhanced production of androgens by IGF-I (Figure 5A) was associated with more extensive secretion of IGFBP-2 and IGFBP-3 (Figure 5B).

To investigate the possible role played by IGF-IR in IGFBPs secretion, we treated cells with IGF-I or IGF-II in the absence or presence of a selective inhibitor of IGF-IR, the cyclolignan PPP. IGF-II was used in this context since it acts as an IGF-IR agonist at high concentration, thus serving as a positive control to IGF-I action. Pre-treatment with PPP [27], prevented the enhanced secretion of all investigated IGFBPs induced by IGF-I or IGF-II (Figure 5C).

Effects of IL-1β, IL-18 and TNFα on secretion of IGFBPs by Leydig cells

Previously it has been demonstrated that IL-1β and TNFα can modulate the expression of IGFBPs in the testis. To further characterize the regulation of binding protein secretion by cytokines and growth factors in Leydig cells, the effects of IL-1β, IL-18 and TNFα alone were examined.

As shown in Figure 6A, IL-1β by itself stimulated the secretion of IGFBP-3 and diminished the level of IGFBP-2 in the medium of these same cultures. IL-18 alone stimulated the secretion of IGFBP-3 and IGFBP-2 (Figure 6A).

TNFα stimulated the secretion of IGFBP-3 and IGFBP-4 by Leydig cells from 40-day-old-rats (Figure 6B). Furthermore, the induction of apoptosis in these Leydig cells by TNFα could be substantially prevented by pre-treatment with IGF-I (Figure 6C).

Discussion

The involvement of IGFBP-3 in steroidogenesis, development and tumor growth in the testis is poorly understood. In the present investigation we demonstrated that IGFBP-3 is expressed in a developmental fashion in the rat testis and for the first time, that IGFBP-3 itself induces apoptosis in Leydig cells by activating caspase-3 in a manner dependent on the stage of development. Furthermore, this binding protein blocks the promotion by IGF-I of the survival of rat Leydig cells from 40-days-old rats in cultures. Apparently, expression of IGFBP-3 plays an important role in the development of the testis and may influence the numbers of cells present in the mature testis.

IGFBP-3 induces apoptosis via both IGF-dependent and–independent mechanisms [6]. Interestingly, we found that IGFBP-3 does not induce apoptosis in Leydig cells isolated from 10-days-old rats (progenitor Leydig cells) but clearly induce apoptosis in Leydig cells isolated from 40-days-old rats (immature Leydig cells). These results suggest a developmental action of IGFBP-3 that may be explained by the pattern of expression of IGFBP-3, the possible developmental expression of the IGFBP-3 receptor or a relationship with the expression of IGF-IR in Leydig cells [36].

IGFBP-3 may inhibit cell growth by induction of apoptosis either indirectly, by sequestering insulin-like growth factors away from the insulin-like growth factor receptor, or directly via a putative IGFBP-3 receptor and/or translocation to the nucleus. At present, the identity of IGFBP-3 receptor is not well established [19,37,38].

Previous data demonstrate that IGFBP-3 can exert its actions on target cells in several ways: (a) inducing apoptosis; (b) regulating the cell cycle; and (c) possible cross-talk with major signal transduction pathways. Possible mechanisms for intrinsic apoptotic pathway of IGFBP-3 involve, in part, increasing of the ratio of pro-apoptotic (Bax and Bad) to anti-apoptotic (Bcl-2 and Bcl-XL) proteins and rising of caspase-3 activity [39]. Our results suggest that IGFBP-3 may induce the activation of caspase-3 at 12 h or earlier after start of incubation and that the increased activity at this time point was related with lower viability.

The testis is a site of IGF-I production and action [25]. Testicular levels of IGF-I peak during the fourth week postpartum, at the start of the pubertal rise in testosterone secretion [25]. The expression of IGFBP-3 in Leydig cells is high at this point of development and it is known that IGFBP-3 serves as an important regulator of IGF-I activity. We suggest that the action of IGF-I in differentiation, proliferation and apoptosis in the testis is modulated by IGFBP-3 and maybe also by other IGFBPs, and that this modulation is necessary for the proper function of IGF-I. Furthermore, we observed here that pre-treatment with PPP, a selective inhibitor of IGF-IR, attenuated the stimulation by IGF-I and IGF-II on IGFBPs secretion by Leydig cells, suggesting that IGF-IR plays a key role in this process.

Postnatally, the proliferative capacity of the Leydig cell lineage

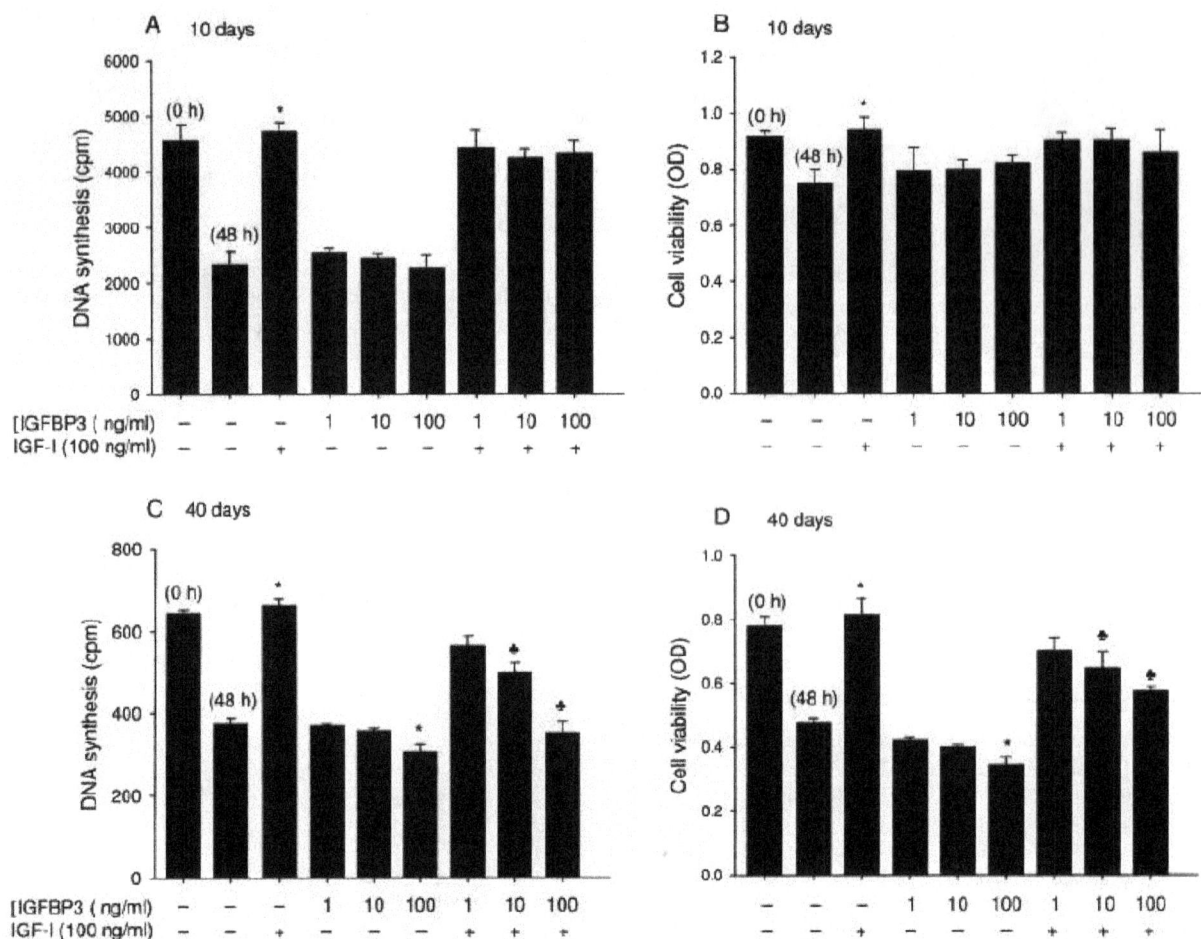

Figure 3: Effects of IGFBP-3 and/or IGF-I on DNA synthesis (A, C), and cell viability (B, D) in cultures of Leydig cells isolated from 10- and 40-day-old rats. Leydig cells were isolated, cultured and treated as described in the Materials and Methods. All values shown represent means ± SD for three independent experiments. (A, 10d) (C, 40d) Incorporation of ^{3}H-thymidine by untreated cells at the beginning of the culture period i.e., between 0 and 4 hours of culture, and by both untreated and treated cells between hours 44 and 48 of incubation (48 h). *: p<0.05 compared to the 48-hour value for untreated control cells. ♣: p<0.05 compared to the 48-hour value for cells exposed to IGF-I.
(B, 10d) (D, 40d) The numbers of viable cells as assessed employing the WST-1 procedure. Following treatment (see above), 10 μl of the WST-1 reagent was added to each well (containing 1.5 × 10^4 cells); the incubation continued for an additional 60 minutes at 37° C; and finally, the absorption of the culture medium at 450 nm was determined. OD=optical density units. *: p<0.05 compared to the 48-hour value for untreated control cells, ♣: p<0.05 compared to the 48-hour value for cells exposed to IGF-I.

is suppressed during the transition from progenitor Leydig cells to immature Leydig cells, a process that seems to be under genetic control [40]. The developmental expression of IGFBP-3 also suggests that this protein is involved in the process of development and perhaps in the reduced capacity of proliferation. IGFBP-3 may also be involved in the regulation of androgen production. Previously, it has been demonstrated that IGFBP-3 inhibits stimulation of Leydig cell steroidogenesis by IGF-I and mediates the inhibitory action of IL-1β and TNFα on steroidogenesis [8,12]. These findings are strongly supported by the present data. In order to investigate the function of IGFBP-3 under inflammatory conditions and the possible action on the extrinsic pathway of apoptosis in the testis, we studied the effect of TNFα on IGFBPs expression and apoptosis. Our data suggest that a rise in IGFBP-3 is involved in the apoptotic action of TNFα in Leydig cells. Additionally, the apoptotic effect of TNFα could be prevented by pre-treatment with IGF-I, suggesting a cross-talk between the pathways involved in the actions of both of these substances. The protective effect

of IGF-I on TNFα induced apoptosis has also been observed in other model systems, including the neuronal SH-SY5Y cell line [41,42]. This suggests that IGFBP-3 may also play a role in mediating extrinsic apoptotic pathways in cells that are sensitive to the actions of TNF-α.

Pro-inflammatory cytokines are apparently involved in certain pathological process in the testis. For instance, local levels of TNFα and IL-1β are elevated, following ischemia/reperfusion of this organ, suggesting that these cytokines are early mediators of ischemia/reperfusion-induced testicular injury [22]. There are clear differences in the individual effects of these cytokines on secretion of IGFBPs by Leydig cells, indicating that they have different roles to play. Previously, TNFα was found to attenuate the stimulatory action of IGF-I on the level of FSH receptors on Sertoli cells [43] demonstrating that IGF-I plays a role in the functioning of these cells as well. Our findings suggest the existence of antagonistic interactions between TNFα and IGF-I with respect to their effects. The present findings clearly indicate that IGFBPs

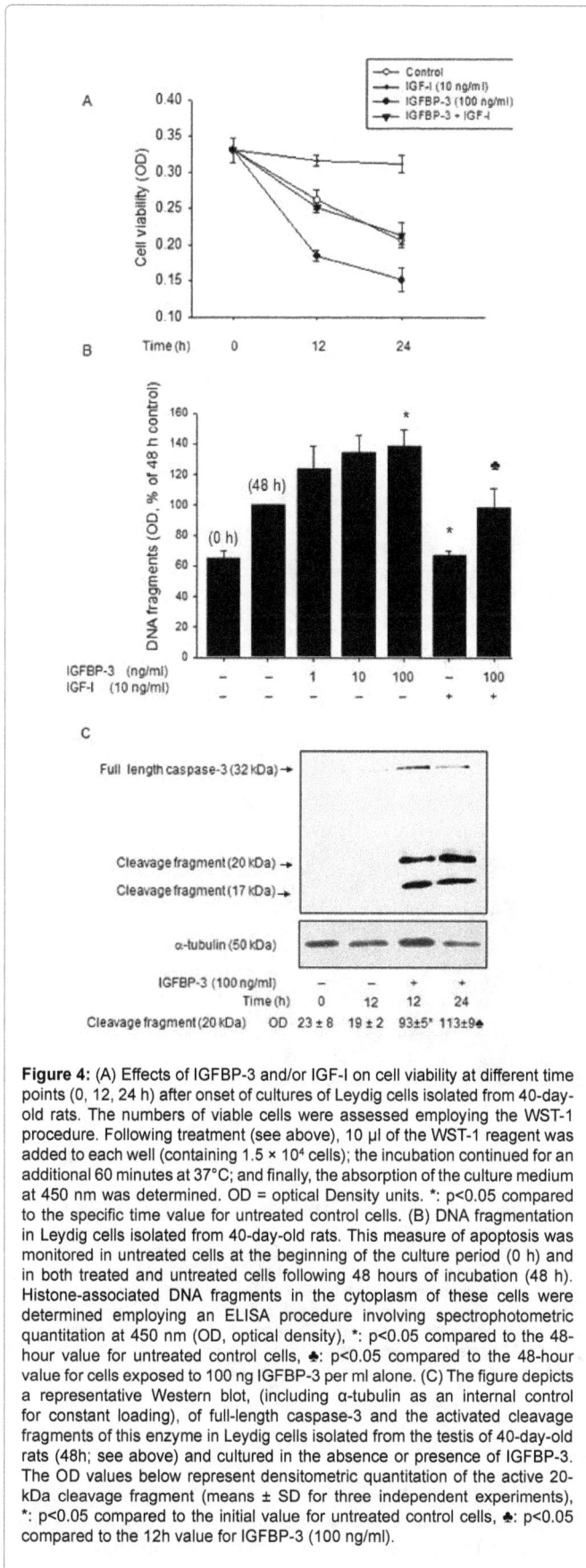

Figure 4: (A) Effects of IGFBP-3 and/or IGF-I on cell viability at different time points (0, 12, 24 h) after onset of cultures of Leydig cells isolated from 40-day-old rats. The numbers of viable cells were assessed employing the WST-1 procedure. Following treatment (see above), 10 μl of the WST-1 reagent was added to each well (containing 1.5×10^4 cells); the incubation continued for an additional 60 minutes at 37°C; and finally, the absorption of the culture medium at 450 nm was determined. OD = optical Density units. *: p<0.05 compared to the specific time value for untreated control cells. (B) DNA fragmentation in Leydig cells isolated from 40-day-old rats. This measure of apoptosis was monitored in untreated cells at the beginning of the culture period (0 h) and in both treated and untreated cells following 48 hours of incubation (48 h). Histone-associated DNA fragments in the cytoplasm of these cells were determined employing an ELISA procedure involving spectrophotometric quantitation at 450 nm (OD, optical density), *: p<0.05 compared to the 48-hour value for untreated control cells, ♣: p<0.05 compared to the 48-hour value for cells exposed to 100 ng IGFBP-3 per ml alone. (C) The figure depicts a representative Western blot, (including α-tubulin as an internal control for constant loading), of full-length caspase-3 and the activated cleavage fragments of this enzyme in Leydig cells isolated from the testis of 40-day-old rats (48h; see above) and cultured in the absence or presence of IGFBP-3. The OD values below represent densitometric quantitation of the active 20-kDa cleavage fragment (means ± SD for three independent experiments), *: p<0.05 compared to the initial value for untreated control cells, ♣: p<0.05 compared to the 12h value for IGFBP-3 (100 ng/ml).

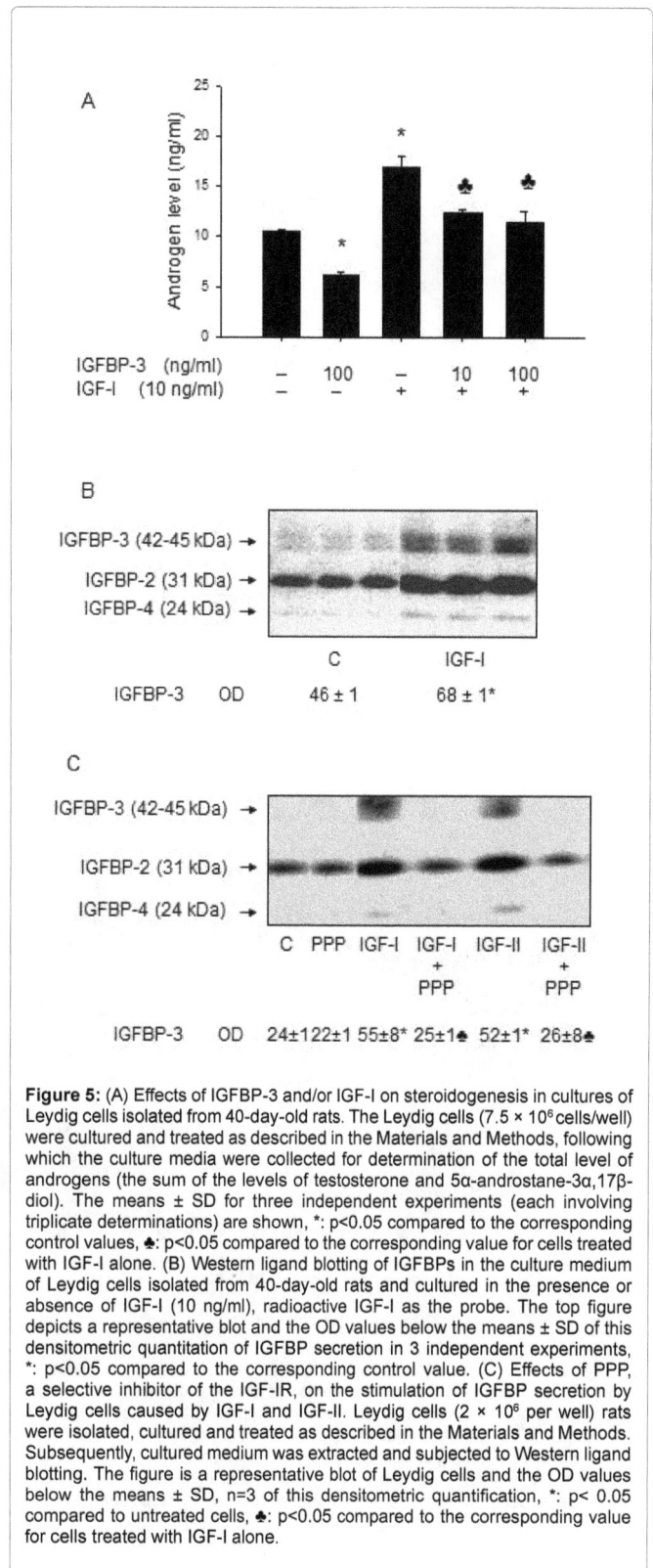

Figure 5: (A) Effects of IGFBP-3 and/or IGF-I on steroidogenesis in cultures of Leydig cells isolated from 40-day-old rats. The Leydig cells (7.5×10^6 cells/well) were cultured and treated as described in the Materials and Methods, following which the culture media were collected for determination of the total level of androgens (the sum of the levels of testosterone and 5α-androstane-3α,17β-diol). The means ± SD for three independent experiments (each involving triplicate determinations) are shown, *: p<0.05 compared to the corresponding control values, ♣: p<0.05 compared to the corresponding value for cells treated with IGF-I alone. (B) Western ligand blotting of IGFBPs in the culture medium of Leydig cells isolated from 40-day-old rats and cultured in the presence or absence of IGF-I (10 ng/ml), radioactive IGF-I as the probe. The top figure depicts a representative blot and the OD values below the means ± SD of this densitometric quantitation of IGFBP secretion in 3 independent experiments, *: p<0.05 compared to the corresponding control value. (C) Effects of PPP, a selective inhibitor of the IGF-IR, on the stimulation of IGFBP secretion by Leydig cells caused by IGF-I and IGF-II. Leydig cells (2×10^6 per well) rats were isolated, cultured and treated as described in the Materials and Methods. Subsequently, cultured medium was extracted and subjected to Western ligand blotting. The figure is a representative blot of Leydig cells and the OD values below the means ± SD, n=3 of this densitometric quantification, *: p< 0.05 compared to untreated cells, ♣: p<0.05 compared to the corresponding value for cells treated with IGF-I alone.

are under paracrine regulation by pro-inflammatory cytokines in the testis, linking inflammation to metabolic events, including regulation of steroidogenesis. Previous results from our group indicate that IL-18, which is produced constitutively by germ cells, may serve as a host

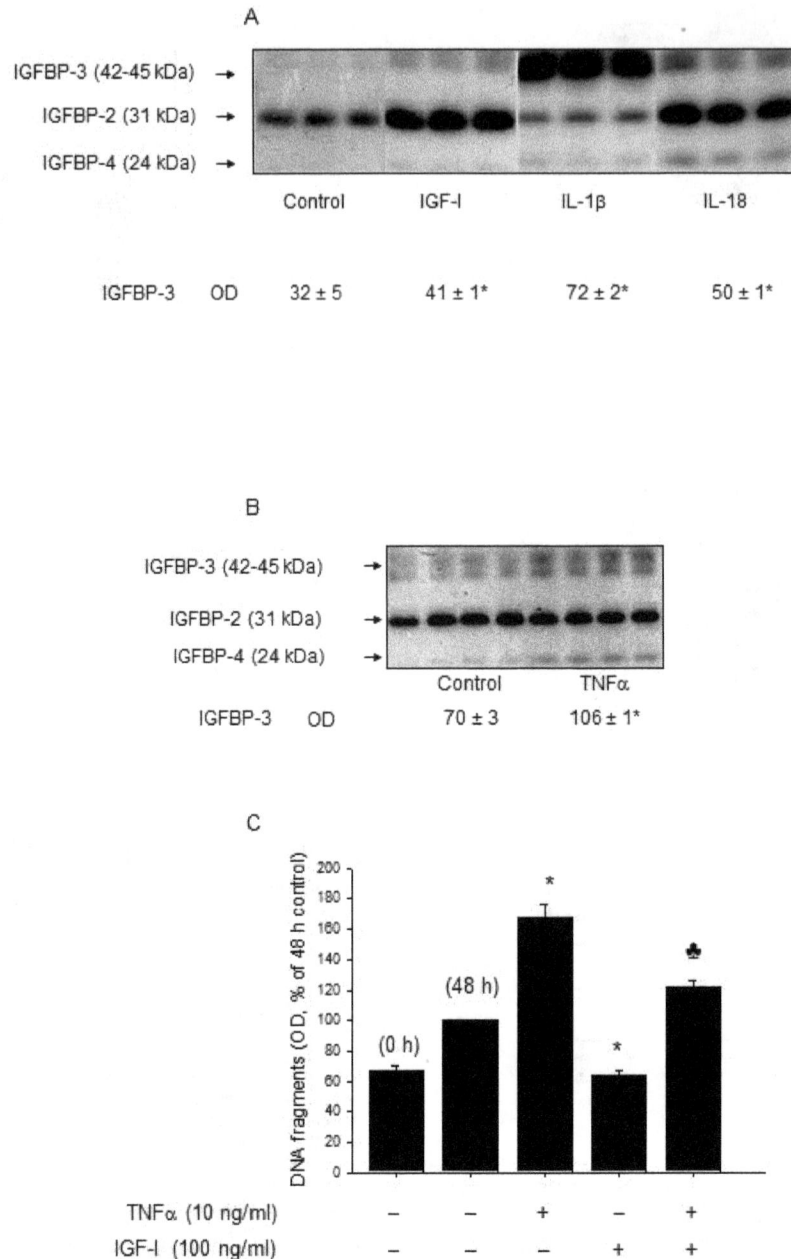

Figure 6: (A) Influence of IL-1b, IL-18 and IGF-I alone on the secretion of IGFBPs by Leydig cells isolated from 40-day-old rats. The cells were isolated, cultured (2 × 10⁶ per well) and treated as described in the Materials and Methods. The figures depicts representative Western ligand blots of extracts of the culture media, while the OD values below document the means ± SD of the densitometric values obtained in three independent experiments, *: p<0.05 compared to untreated cells. (B) Effects of TNFa on the secretion of binding proteins in Leydig cells from 40-day-old rats. The cells isolated were cultured (2 × 10⁶ per well) and treated as described in the Materials and Methods. Representative Western ligand blotting of extracts of culture media, while the OD values underneath document the means ± SD of the densitometric values, n=4 of densitometric quantitation of these blots, *: p<0.05 compared to the untreated cells (48 h). (C) Effects of TNFa on apoptosis in Leydig cells from 40-day-old rats. Apoptosis in untreated Leydig cells at the beginning of the culture period (0h) and in both treated and untreated cells following 48 hours of incubation (48 h). The cytoplasmic levels of histone-associated DNA fragments in these cells were determined by an ELISA procedure involving spectrophotometric quantitation at 450 nm. *: p<0.05 compared to the 48h value for untreated control cells; ♣: p<0.05 compared to TNFa treated cells.

defense factor in the male gonad [23]. Our present results indicate that IGFBPs modulate the function of this cytokine in the testis. IL-18, also produced constitutively by the rat testis [44], and IL-1β increase the secretion of IGFBP-3 [21] indicating that they occupy common signaling pathways and suggesting a possible role of IGFBP-3 in certain

inflammatory conditions.

In summary, we demonstrate here that IGFBP-3 is expressed in a developmentally regulated fashion in the testis, where it induces apoptosis in Leydig cells in a manner that is also dependent on the stage of their development. IGFBP-3 blocks the promotion of survival by IGF-I and the secretion of this binding protein is regulated by cytokines. We propose that IGFBPs may play an important role in the regulation of Leydig cell numbers and development in the testis and thus may affect the total capacity of androgen biosynthesis.

References

1. LeRoith D, Roberts CT Jr (2003) The insulin-like growth factor system and cancer. Cancer Lett 195:127-137.

2. Colon E, Strand ML, Carlsson-Skwirut C, Wahlgren A, Svechnikov KV, et al. (2006) Anti-apoptotic factor humanin is expressed in the testis and prevents cell-death in leydig cells during the first wave of spermatogenesis. J Cell Physiol 208: 373-385.

3. Lin T, Wang D, Nagpal ML, Chang W (1994) Human chorionic gonadotropin decreases insulin-like growth factor-I gene transcription in rat Leydig cells. Endocrinology 134: 2142-2149.

4. LeRoith D, Werner H, Beitner-Johnson D, Roberts CT Jr (1995) Molecular and cellular aspects of the insulin-like growth factor I receptor. Endocr Rev 16: 143-163.

5. LeRoith D, Werner H, Neuenschwander S, Kalebic T, Helman LJ (1995) The role of the insulin-like growth factor-I receptor in cancer. Ann N Y Acad Sci 766: 402-408.

6. Cohen P (2006) Insulin-like growth factor binding protein-3: insulin-like growth factor independence comes of age. Endocrinology 147: 2109-2111.

7. Rajah R, Valentinis B, Cohen P (1997) Insulin-like growth factor (IGF)-binding protein-3 induces apoptosis and mediates the effects of transforming growth factor-beta1 on programmed cell death through a p53- and IGF-independent mechanism. J Biol Chem 272: 12181-12188.

8. Lin T, Haskell J, Vinson N, Terracio L (1986) Characterization of insulin and insulin-like growth factor I receptors of purified Leydig cells and their role in steroidogenesis in primary culture: a comparative study. Endocrinology 119: 1641-1647.

9. Lin T, Wang D, Nagpal ML, Shimasaki S, Ling N (1993) Expression and regulation of insulin-like growth factor-binding protein-1, -2, -3, and -4 messenger ribonucleic acids in purified rat Leydig cells and their biological effects. Endocrinology 132: 1898-1904.

10. Zhou J, Bondy C (1993) Anatomy of the insulin-like growth factor system in the human testis. Fertil Steril 60: 897-904.

11. Smith EP, Dickson BA, Chernausek SD (1990) Insulin-like growth factor binding protein-3 secretion from cultured rat sertoli cells: dual regulation by follicle stimulating hormone and insulin-like growth factor-I. Endocrinology 127: 2744-2751.

12. Wang D, Nagpal ML, Shimasaki S, Ling N, Lin T (1995) Interleukin-1 induces insulin-like growth factor binding protein-3 gene expression and protein production by Leydig cells. Endocrinology 136: 4049-4055.

13. Neuvians TP, Gashaw I, Hasenfus A, Hacherhacker A, Winterhager E, et al. (2005) Differential expression of IGF components and insulin receptor isoforms in human seminoma versus normal testicular tissue. Neoplasia 7: 446-456.

14. Bernardi P, Petronilli V, Di Lisa F, Forte M (2001) A mitochondrial perspective on cell death. Trends Biochem Sci 26: 112-117.

15. Li P, Nijhawan D, Budihardjo I, Srinivasula SM, Ahmad M, et al. (1997) Cytochrome c and dATP-dependent formation of Apaf-1/caspase-9 complex initiates an apoptotic protease cascade. Cell 91: 479-489.

16. Gross A, McDonnell JM, Korsmeyer SJ (1999) BCL-2 family members and the mitochondria in apoptosis. Genes Dev 13: 1899-18911.

17. Ashkenazi A, Dixit VM (1998) Death receptors: signaling and modulation. Science 281: 1305-1308.

18. Beg AA, Baltimore D (1996) An essential role for NF-kappaB in preventing TNF-alpha-induced cell death. Science 274: 782-784

19. Liu B, Lee KW, Anzo M, Zhang B, Zi X, et al. (2006) Insulin-like growth factor-binding protein-3 inhibition of prostate cancer growth involves suppression of angiogenesis. Oncogene.

20. Oh Y, Muller HL, Pham H, Rosenfeld RG (1993) Demonstration of receptors for insulin-like growth factor binding protein-3 on Hs578T human breast cancer cells. J Biol Chem 268: 26045-26048.

21. Colon E, Svechnikov KV, Carlsson-Skwirut C, Bang P, Soder O (2005) Stimulation of steroidogenesis in immature rat Leydig cells evoked by interleukin-1alpha is potentiated by growth hormone and insulin-like growth factors. Endocrinology 146: 221-230.

22. Lysiak JJ, Nguyen QA, Kirby JL, Turner TT (2003) Ischemia-reperfusion of the murine testis stimulates the expression of proinflammatory cytokines and activation of c-jun N-terminal kinase in a pathway to E-selectin expression. Biol Reprod 69: 202-210.

23. Strand ML, Wahlgren A, Svechnikov K, Zetterstrom C, Setchell BP, et al. (2005) Interleukin-18 is expressed in rat testis and may promote germ cell growth. Mol Cell Endocrinol 240: 64-73.

24. Jonsson CK, Zetterstrom RH, Holst M, Parvinen M, Soder O (1999) Constitutive expression of interleukin-1alpha messenger ribonucleic acid in rat Sertoli cells is dependent upon interaction with germ cells. Endocrinology 140: 3755-3761.

25. Wang G, Hardy MP (2004) Development of leydig cells in the insulin-like growth factor-I (igf-I) knockout mouse: effects of igf-I replacement and gonadotropic stimulation. Biol Reprod 70: 632-639.

26. Moore A, Chen CL, Davis JR, Morris ID (1993) Insulin-like growth factor-I mRNA expression in the interstitial cells of the rat testis. J Mol Endocrinol 11: 319-324.

27. Vasilcanu D, Girnita A, Girnita L, Vasilcanu R, Axelson M, et al. (2004) The cyclolignan PPP induces activation loop-specific inhibition of tyrosine phosphorylation of the insulin-like growth factor-1 receptor. Link to the phosphatidyl inositol-3 kinase/Akt apoptotic pathway. Oncogene 23: 7854-7862.

28. Klinefelter GR, Hall PF, Ewing LL (1987) Effect of luteinizing hormone deprivation in situ on steroidogenesis of rat Leydig cells purified by a multistep procedure. Biol Reprod 36: 769-783.

29. Svechnikov KV, Sultana T, Soder O (2001) Age-dependent stimulation of Leydig cell steroidogenesis by interleukin-1 isoforms. Mol Cell Endocrinol 182: 193-201.

30. Khan SA, Khan SJ, Dorrington JH (1992) Interleukin-1 stimulates deoxyribonucleic acid synthesis in immature rat Leydig cells in vitro. Endocrinology 131: 1853-1857.

31. Payne AH, Downing JR, Wong KL (1980) Luteinizing hormone receptors and testosterone synthesis in two distinct populations of Leydig cells. Endocrinology 106: 1424-1429.

32. Wang GM, Ge RS, Latif SA, Morris DJ, Hardy MP (2002) Expression of 11beta-hydroxylase in rat Leydig cells. Endocrinology 143: 621-626.

33. Petersen C, Boitani C, Froysa B, Soder O (2001) Transforming growth factor-alpha stimulates proliferation of rat Sertoli cells. Mol Cell Endocrinol 181: 221-227.

34. Schlatt S, de Kretser DM, Hedger MP (1999) Mitosis of resident macrophages in the adult rat testis. J Reprod Fertil 116: 223-228.

35. Colon E, Zaman F, Axelson M, Larsson O, Carlsson-Skwirut C, et al. (2007) Insulin-like growth factor-I is an important antiapoptotic factor for rat leydig cells during postnatal development. Endocrinology 148: 128-139.

36. Hossenlopp P, Seurin D, Segovia-Quinson B, Hardouin S, Binoux M (1986) Analysis of serum insulin-like growth factor binding proteins using western blotting: use of the method for titration of the binding proteins and competitive binding studies. Anal Biochem 154: 138-143.

37. Buckbinder L, Talbott R, Velasco-Miguel S, Takenaka I, Faha B, et al. (1995) Induction of the growth inhibitor IGF-binding protein 3 by p53. Nature 377: 646-649.

38. Butt AJ, Fraley KA, Firth SM, Baxter RC (2002) IGF-binding protein-3-induced growth inhibition and apoptosis do not require cell surface binding and nuclear translocation in human breast cancer cells. Endocrinology 143: 2693-2699.

39. Butt AJ, Firth SM, King MA, Baxter RC (2000) Insulin-like growth factor-binding protein-3 modulates expression of Bax and Bcl-2 and potentiates p53-independent radiation-induced apoptosis in human breast cancer cells. J Biol Chem 275: 39174-39181.

40. Ge RS, Dong Q, Sottas CM, Chen H, Zirkin BR, et al. (2005) Gene expression in rat leydig cells during development from the progenitor to adult stage: a cluster analysis. Biol Reprod 72: 1405-1415.

41. Kenchappa P, Yadav A, Singh G, Nandana S, Banerjee K (2004) Rescue of TNFalpha-inhibited neuronal cells by IGF-1 involves Akt and c-Jun N-terminal kinases. J Neurosci Res 76: 466-474.

42. Wang JY, Grabacka M, Marcinkiewicz C, Staniszewska I, Peruzzi F, et al. (2006) Involvement of alpha1beta1 integrin in insulin-like growth factor-1-mediated protection of PC12 neuronal processes from tumor necrosis factor-alpha-induced injury. J Neurosci Res 83: 7-18.

43. Besset V, Le Magueresse-Battistoni B, Collette J, Benahmed M (1996) Tumor necrosis factor alpha stimulates insulin-like growth factor binding protein 3 expression in cultured porcine Sertoli cells. Endocrinology 137: 296-303.

44. Wahab-Wahlgren A, Holst M, Ayele D, Sultana T, Parvinen M, et al. (2000) Constitutive production of interleukin-1alpha mRNA and protein in the developing rat testis. Int J Androl 23: 360-365.

6

Dehydroepiandrosterone, Over-studied but Under-used in the Treatment of Vascular Remodeling Diseases

Roxane Paulin and Sébastien Bonnet*

Department of Medicine, Laval University, Centre de Recherche du CHUQ, Hôtel-Dieu de Québec, Québec City, QC, Canada

Abstract

Vascular remodeling is characterized by a narrowing of the lumen of the vessels, resulting in decreased blood flow, increased pressure and heart failure. This process is found in diseases like atherosclerosis, restenosis after angioplasty, transplants coronary disease, systemic and pulmonary hypertensive vascular disease, and is stimulated by elevated levels of cholesterol, inflammation, oxidative stress, excess of vasodilating molecules and growth factors. Efficient treatments able to fix or prevent the progression of this process are still missing. The hormone dehydroepiandrosterone (DHEA), which levels decrease with aging while cardiovascular risks increase, was hypothesized to have a role in the pathophysiology of vascular diseases. Despite the fact that numerous properties such as fat-reducing, anti-oxidant, vasodilating, anti-inflammatory and anti-proliferative have emerged from two decade of studies, DHEA remain clinically underused in the treatment of vascular remodeling diseases. The lack of understanding of the exact mechanism of action and some controversial epidemiological studies are not foreign to the fact that DHEA is shunned. Nonetheless, we believe that DHEA cannot be ignored since promising results were obtained pre-clinically and clinically in the treatment of vascular remodeling diseases. We are probably close to understand the function of this molecule, especially by its action as a peroxisome proliferator, and it will be a shame to deprive patient of a way to improve their quality of life, or worst a way to extend their survival.

Introduction

Inward inappropriate vascular remodeling is a common feature of several diseases like atherosclerosis, restenosis after angioplasty, transplants coronary disease, systemic and pulmonary hypertensive vascular disease [1] causing a narrowing of the lumen and decreasing maximal flow rates. The arterial wall is composed of three independent layers: a monolayer of endothelial cells (ECs) called intima, a main layer composed by vascular smooth muscle cells (VSMCs), the media, and a network of connective tissue, the adventitia. Under physiological conditions, VSMCs are quiescent, contractile and non-migratory. Remodeling occurs in response to various stimuli that disrupt the usually ordered multilayered structure of the wall by activating VSMCs. Elevated cholesterol levels, inflammation, oxidative stress, excess of vasodilating molecules and growth factor are potent stimuli that are found in these diseases. Most of these molecules bind receptors and enhance cascades of signal transduction resulting in a pro-proliferative, survival, constricted, migratory and invasive phenotype of the VSMCs. This abnormal VSMC's phenotype plays a critical role in the thickening of vessel wall, the rearrangements of cellular and non-cellular elements and/or the formation of neointima or atherosclerotic plaque.

Dehydroepiandrosterone (DHEA) is an adrenal steroid circulating abundantly as a sulfate conjugated form DHEA-S [2]. DHEA-S reaches a maximal plasma level between 15 and 25 years old and the following decline in DHEA-S [3-5] has been related to aging-associated diseases development [6-10]. DHEA is a potent uncompetitive inhibitor of the first enzyme in the pentose phosphate pathway (PPP), the mammalian glucose-6-phosphate deshydrogenase (G6PDH). Studies performed on Sardinian males bearing a Mediterranean variant of G6PDH deficiency, support the hypothesis that reduced G6PDH activity has a beneficial affect on age-related disease development. Indeed, these individuals arbor reduced mortality rates from cerebrovascular and cardiovascular diseases and seems to be more likely to achieve centenarian [11]. Since almost a century, numerous hypothesis have emerged on the possible role of DHEA(-S) in the pathophysiology of vascular diseases, especially coronary heart diseases, atherosclerosis, carotid stenosis and Pulmonary Hypertension. Number of studies using DHEA as therapy exploded at the end of the eighties. These studies, while showing an efficient impact of DHEA in the reduction of remodeling processes [12-14], failed to demonstrate the exact mechanism by which the molecule act. Hormone replacement therapy using DHEA and DHEA-S in elderly has even been discussed [10,15-17] without concretization. The original enthusiasm has been replaced by sober skepticism, as many questions remain unanswered. Moreover epidemiologic studies were controversial concerning the hypothesis of an inverse correlation between the diseases manifestation and the serum level of DHEA(S), and showed dramatic differences according to sex and diseases end-point for example [18-21]. Close to two decades after, without clarification of the exact mechanism of action of the molecule, several properties of DHEA such as fat-reducing, anti-oxidant, vasodilating, anti-inflammatory and anti-proliferative properties have emerged, increasing again the interest for the treatment of cardiovascular diseases. We propose in this review to make an overview of the findings supporting the fact that DHEA could be an important therapeutic strategy in the treatment of vascular diseases, explaining how DHEA can works and to discuss why DHEA remain clinically underused as therapy.

***Corresponding author:** Dr. Sébastien Bonnet, Centre de Recherche de L'Hôtel-Dieu de Québec, 10 rue McMahon, Québec, QC, G1R2J6, Canada, E-mail: sebastien.bonnet@crhdq.ulaval.ca

DHEA Cholesterol/Fat Reducing Properties

Low-density lipoproteins (LDL), also called bad cholesterol, are known to promote cardiovascular diseases and particularly atherosclerosis. This syndrome begins by damage to the endothelium leading to a chronic inflammatory response in the walls of arteries by expression of various adhesion molecules and cytokines, which promote the migration of circulating leukocytes, such as monocytes, T lymphocytes and dendrites into the sub-endothelial space of the artery [22]. Oxidized-LDL are implicated in the initiation of inflammatory processes [23] as migrating mononuclear leukocytes incorporate oxidized-LDL to become foam cells, which accumulate in the sub-endothelial space due to an impaired emigration. Foam cells secrete oxygen-free radicals as well as various cytokines that further accelerate inflammation [24-26]. VSMCs migrate into the neointima and secrete matrix proteins to stabilize the plaque [27-29]. Instability in the cap may lead to rupture and subsequent thrombus formation.

In humans and rodents, DHEA administration have been described to result in a substantial decrease in body fat mass, fat accumulation and decreased body weight [30-34]. As a G6PDH inhibitor, DHEA inhibits the production of NADP [35]. NADPH is involved in numerous metabolic pathways such as fatty acid, phospholipid, cholesterol and steroid synthesis and its reduced production lead to decreased fatty acid production and subsequent reduction of LDL production. In these conditions, less LDL can be oxidized and fewer atheromas would be formed [36]. Indeed, DHEA has been found to have an inhibitory effect on cholesterol ester accumulation induced by AcLDL in cultured macrophage cells (5774-l cells) [37], but the mechanism was poorly understood.

DHEA is known as a peroxisome proliferator able to induce many genes through peroxisome proliferator-activated receptors (PPAR) [38]. Once activated, the isoform PPARα represses activation of enzymes involved in fat synthesis [39,40]. DHEA can be implicated in lowers triglycerides production and in less fat deposition through its effect on PPARα. In adipose tissue the predominant isoform of PPAR is PPARγ, a nuclear hormone receptor and a ligand-activated transcription factor that binds specifically to PPAR response elements in the promoter regions of target genes and regulates the transcription of many adipocyte-specific genes [41,42]. DHEA has been shown to induce PPARγ gene expression by over 2.5-fold in adipose tissue of DHEA-treated rats. DHEA-induced PPARγ activation may lead to an increase in lipolysis rate, increased flux of fatty acids through the β-oxidation pathway and a decrease in de novo lipogenesis rate in adipose tissue, accompanied by an increase in energy expenditure [43].

DHEA Anti-oxidant and Anti-inflammatory Properties

Another recent study hypothesized that DHEA may affect the oxidized LDL-induced inflammatory response. Indeed, DHEA administration was shown to modulate the expression of inflammatory molecules in human umbilical vein endothelial cells (HUVECs) injured by oxidized LDL, like up-regulating nitric oxide production and down-regulating malondialdehyde, adhesion molecules VCAM-1, ICAM and E-selectin. This was attributed in part to a DHEA-dependant inhibition of NF-κB and a subsequent attenuation of inflammation [44]. Indeed, multiple genes involved in monocyte/endothelial interaction such as vascular cell adhesion molecule-1 (VCAM-1) and monocyte chemotactic protein-1 (MCP-1) contain in their promoters NF-κB binding sites [45]. DHEA-dependant inhibition of NF-κB is not surprising considering the fact that PPARα

has been shown to antagonize NF-κB signaling pathway involved in the vascular inflammation of atherosclerosis [46,47]. This hypothesis was formulated by Altman et al. whom showed that DHEA(-S)-dependant VCAM-1 decreased expression could be partially restored by using the PPARα inhibitor MK866 [48]. These findings furnish important clues on DHEA mechanism of actions and demonstrate a significant role for DHEA(-S) in the prevention of inflammatory processes in the endothelium.

DHEA Vasodilating Properties

A constricted state of VSMCs in wall arteries is also a factor increasing the inward narrowing of the vessels. In pulmonary arterial hypertension (PAH), distal arteries are particularly constricted and this phenomenon plays a critical role in the global rise of pressure observed in the pulmonary vasculature. Several mechanisms are implicated in this abnormal constricted state. First, an imbalance between vasoconstricting and vasodilating factors levels have been measured in the serum of PAH patients [49-51], with an abnormal downregulation of vasodilating molecules like nitric oxide and an overexpression of vasoconstricting molecules like endothelin-1 [52-54]. There are also evidences showing a decrease in gene expression and function of K_v channels [55] as well as a decrease in BK_{Ca} protein expression [56] resulting in membrane depolarization and enhanced contraction.

Ratios of cellular reducing factor, such as $NADP^+/NADPH$ and GSH/GSSG are known to open Kv and BK_{Ca} channels and hyperpolarize plasma membrane [57-59]. Following this principle, again as an inhibitor of the PPP and able to modify these ratio (Figure 1), DHEA was hypothesized to have vasodilating properties. DHEA was found to efficiently inhibit hypoxic pulmonary vasoconstriction, at least in part by opening BK_{Ca} channels in pulmonary VSMCs [60-62]. Western Blot analysis of arterial pulmonary extract showed that the BK_{Ca}-subunit expression is upregulated after DHEA treatment compared to chronic hypoxia rats [63]. By using specific K^+ channel inhibitors, it was identified that only K_v channels are positively implicated in DHEA-dependent relaxation of VSMCs. DHEA also prevents and reverses chronic hypoxia induced pulmonary hypertension in rats by BK_{Ca} opening.

Vascular tone is also controled by cyclic guanosine 3', 5'-monophosphate (cGMP), a factor generated in the vasculature via two main guanylate cyclase: cytosolic soluble guanylate cyclase (sGS) and membrane-bound particulate guanylate cyclase (pGC) [64]. sGC serves as a receptor for biologically active gas nitric oxide (NO) [65,66] and cGMP is generated by sGC following this interaction. DHEA has been reported to increase sGC protein expression and activity and by improving pulmonary artery vasodilator responsiveness to NO [67]. DHEA effects on sGC may not be direct but again, secondary to PPP inhibition and increased levels H_2O_2 production that have been reported to stimulate sGC and increase cGMP in vasculature [68,69]. Finally, activation of the RhoA/ROCK signaling pathway contributes to vasoconstriction in VSMCs, a pathway that plays an important role in the pathogenesis of PAH. Chronic DHEA treatments in PAH rat model were described to decrease RhoA/ROCK signaling pathway activity by multiple mechanisms, including preservation of sGC expression and inhibition of ROCK cleavage [70].

DHEA Anti-proliferative Properties

In diseases like restenosis and PAH, the proliferative phenotype of VSMCs is critical in the inward narrowing of the vessel. Some enzymes, essential for cell cycle progression like multifunctional Ca^{2+}/CaM-

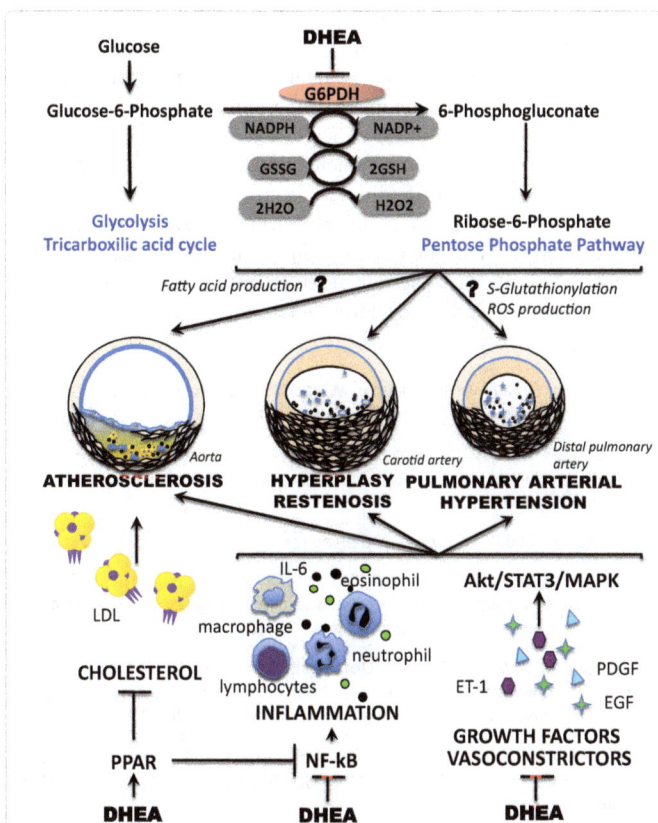

Figure 1: Vascular remodeling diseases are characterized by an inappropriate inward narrowing of the vessels that obstruct the lumen and decrease the flow. In artherosclerosis, there is an important role of "bad cholesterol" low-density lipoprotein (LDL) that once oxidized, is incorporated by leucocytes (monocytes, lymphocytes...) to form foam cells that and accumulate in the sub-endothelial space due to an impaired migration. Vascular smooth muscle cells (VSMCs) migrate into the neointima and secrete matrix proteins to stabilize the plaque. Instability in the cap may lead to rupture and subsequent thrombus formation. In hyperplasia and pulmonary arterial hypertension, the narrowing is due to increased VSMCs constriction, proliferation and survival, fulfilling the internal space. Pro-inflammatory molecules, vasoconstrictors and growth factors play a critical role in the enhancement of this inappropriate VSMCs phenotype. Dehydroepiandrosterone (DHEA), that has been described to have anti-cholesterol, anti-proliferative, anti-inflammatory and vasodilating properties appear to be beneficial in the treatment of vascular remodeling diseases. Nonetheless, the exact mechanism by which DHEA acts is still unclear. Several evidences suggest that DHEA is a peroxisome proliferator. Through PPAR factors activation, several genes implicated in lipid metabolism are expressed, dereasing LDL accumulation. PPARα is also implicated in inhibition of inflammation by antagonize NF-κB. Moreover PPAR factors are able to enhance the expression of genes like glutaredoxin (GRX1), playing an important role in the downregulation of tyrosine phosphorylation, like for the PDGF receptor, and glutathionylation, a post transcriptional modification that could be implicated in DHEA-dependant inhibition of signaling factors such as Akt, STAT3 and NF-κB. Originally, DHEA was described as an inhibitor of the glucose 6-phosphate deshydrogenase (G6PDH), whose role in vascular remodeling processes is unknown. However, G6PDH inhibition is known to change NADPH ratio, whose reduced levels lead to decreased fatty acid production and subsequent reduction of LDL production; GSH ratio, which is also implicated in protein glutathionylation; and reactive oxygen species (ROS) production implicated in enhanced vasdilatation. Thus, DHEA-dependant G6PDH inhibition could also be beneficial in the treatment of vascular remodeling diseases.

dependent protein kinase, calcineurin and spindle pole body protein are Ca²⁺/CaM-dependent, inactive in absence of Ca²⁺/CaM [71]. Ca²⁺ is also able to act directly on transcription factors (such as DREAM) or indirectly through protein phosphatase (calcineurin/NFAT) or kinases (CaM kinases/CREB, PKC/NFκB) to induce the activation of numerous

target genes. Thus, the ability of DHEA to induce dilatation and to release cytosolic Ca²⁺ may also play important roles in cell proliferation. Nonetheless, DHEA is also recognized for anti-proliferative properties through its actions on pro-proliferative factors. DHEA treatment of human aortic SMC inhibits PDGF-induced MAPK activation [72]. In human internal mammary artery, DHEA significantly decreases PDGF-induced ERK1 kinase activity in a dose-dependant manner [73]. We also showed recently, in human carotid VSMC, that DHEA could inhibit PDGF induced-Akt activation [74]. These results were confirmed *in vivo* by a decrease of vascular remodeling in the rat model of balloon-injured carotid treated with DHEA, showing the potential of DHEA as therapeutic for restenosis. It was demonstrated that PDGF-induced proliferation is inhibited by DHEA through a GSH/GRX1 mechanism [75], GRX1 playing an important role in PDGF signal regulation by a downregulation of tyrosine phosphorylation of the PDGF receptor [76]. This is in agreement with previous findings showing that GRX1 and γ-Glutamylcysteine synthetase (γ-GCS) display a PPAR response element in their promoter and are up-regulated at the transcriptional level by PPARα.

We have recently demonstrated the critical role of the Src/STAT3 (Signal transducer and activator of transcription 3) axis in PAH, that enhance NFAT (Nuclear Factor of Activated T-cells) expression and activation through a Pim1 (Provirus integration site for Moloney murine leukemia virus) dependant mechanism [77]. STAT3 has also been showed as a regulator of the Bone morphogenic protein receptor 2 (BMPR2) [78], which is recognized as a hallmark of PAH [79,80]. An association between DHEA treatment and decreased STAT3 activation in regenerative rat liver [81] has been previously described and make us hypothesized that DHEA could also reverse PAH by STAT3 inhibition. Indeed, we demonstrated *in vitro* and *in vivo* that DHEA treatments decrease Src/STAT3 activation in PAH and restore several STAT3-downstream targets aberrantly expressed in PAH, such as BMPR2, Survivin, Pim1 and NFATc2[82]. Nonetheless, the mechanism by which DHEA decreases STAT3 activation remains unknown. Once again, the PPAR family of proteins could be implicated in this mechanism as it has been demonstrated that activation of PPARγ, which is downregulated in PAH[83], have an inhibitory effect on STAT3[84-86]. A direct physical protein-protein interaction occurs between PPARγ and the active form of STAT3, resulting in a decreased transcriptional activity of STAT3. Moreover, the PPARγ agonist ciglitazone has been showed to decrease the level of STAT3 phosphorylation in glioblastoma cell lines, correlated with an increased expression of STAT3 inhibitors like the Suppressor of cytokine signaling (SOCS) 3 and the Protein inhibitor of activated STAT3 (PIAS3) [87]. PPARγ agonists rosiglitazone and pioglitazone that have been used in the treatment of PAH patients were associated with adverse cardiovascular events [88], thus DHEA may offers an alternative therapeutic approach.

Discussion

Whereas several studies have strong evidences in vitro and in vivo showing that DHEA have several beneficial effects for the treatment of vascular remodeling, DHEA is still clinically poorly used. The first reason that can explain this skepticism is in part due to controversial epidemiologic studies. Nonetheless, these studies are often performed by measurement of endogenous DHEAS, and never on DHEA directly, which is understandable considering the fact that DHEAS is the circulatory form of DHEA, more stable and no representative/correlative to DHEA levels and variations. DHEA present diurnal variations [89,90] and the metabolic clearance of DHEAS is lower than the DHEA one [91]. These parameters should be considered in the future in order to avoid mis-conclusion about the inverse correlation between DHEA levels and vascular remodeling diseases frequency.

Another reason is the lack of knowledge regarding the exact mechanism of action of the molecule. I think that DHEA has lost credibility by the fact that it has been considered as a "miracle drug". Moreover, the scientific community is more and more dedicated to avoid side effect of treatments, and successfully accomplish this step is easier when the implicated molecular and signaling mechanisms are well known. The skepticism was thus replaced by fear of a long-term tragic side effect. Close to 30 years after the first studies, no specific toxicity has been described for DHEA, and we are close to define the exact action of DHEA. Known as a G6PDH inhibitor, it is believe that DHEA major effects are independent of this property. DHEA synthetic analogues 8354 and 8356, are 37-fold and 144-fold stronger inhibitors of G6PDH respectively than natural DHEA. However, they have less effect for example on CE accumulation, compare to natural DHEA [37]. Moreover, the role of G6PDH in vascular remodeling diseases is unclear. Some report described that G6PDH is implicated in VSMCs contractility [92-94] but it is not clearly established that this pathway is aberrantly expressed in vascular remodeling diseases. Thus, DHEA effects may not actually be related to the inhibition/rescue of G6PDH and associated pathways.

As described above, a lot of the DHEA effects can be associated to PPAR activation. PPARα has been shown to decrease fat accumulation, by enhancing enzyme involved in fat synthesis [39,40], regulates the transcription of lipolytic genes [41,42]. PPARα is also implicated in inhibition of inflammation by antagonize NF-κB [44-48]. And finally, by enhancing the transcription of multiple genes like GRX1, PPARα seems to play an important role the downregulation of tyrosine phosphorylation, like for the PDGF receptor [76]. We are now in rights to ask the tantalize question: Does this mechanism of reduced tyrosine phosphorylation can be implicated as well in the inhibition of Akt, STAT3, NF-κB and other transcription factor?

STAT3 is in part regulated by glutathionylation, a reversible and redox-sensitive post-translational modification occurring under oxidative stress. Glutathionylation of STAT3 decreases its affinity as a substrate for enzymatic phosphorylation and abrogates STAT3-specific DNA binding [95]. Glutathionylation depends on Glutaredoxin (GRX) and thioredoxin levels (deglutathionylation enzymes) and on the increase in the cellular GSH/GSSG ratio, which also exert a reversible action on protein S-glutathionylation. Interestingly Akt[96], NFκB [97], and other protein like eNOS or MEKK1[98,99] are also subject to glutathionylation. This mechanism of regulation may be a masterpiece in the understanding of DHEA effect as a peroxysome proliferator.

Concerning DHEA vasodilatator properties, since Src and STAT3 is known as K+ channels inhibitors/Ca²⁺ channel opener [100-104] their inhibition by DHEA in PAH could explain how DHEA upregulates K_v and BK_{Ca} channels [63]. The large panel of DHEA action is probably secondary to the effect on a masterpiece like PPAR factors and repercussion of this signal downstream. Nonetheless, the implication of PPAR in all these processes is only speculative and has to be confirmed. It will be interesting that future studies dedicated to increase the knowledge on DHEA effect on vascular diseases take a look on PPAR implication.

DHEA is orally available, relatively cheap and without known side effects. Because DHEA is a naturally occurring substance, it belongs to the public domain and cannot be patented. Therefore, pharmaceutical companies are not rushing to invest millions of dollars on clinical trials to determine the effectiveness of DHEA. However, a wide range of small-scale studies has been conducted on DHEA for many years and for many diseases, and the findings show great promise for the value of DHEA. Interestingly, pharmaceutical firms have tested some synthetic forms of DHEA. With the development of the knowledge on DHEA properties, we will maybe see the development of interesting synthetic molecules that will reconcile DHEA and industry.

References

1. Heeneman S, Sluimer JC, Daemen MJ (2007) Angiotensin-converting enzyme and vascular remodeling. Circ Res 10: 441-454.

2. Parker CR (1999) Dehydroepiandrosterone and dehydroepiandrosterone sulfate production in the human adrenal during development and aging. Steroids 64: 640-647.

3. Baulieu EE (2002) Androgens and aging men. Mol Cell Endocrinol 198: 41-49.

4. Bélanger A, Candas B, Dupont A, Cusan L, Diamond P, et al. (1994) Changes in serum concentrations of conjugated and unconjugated steroids in 40- to 80-year-old men. J Clin Endocrinol Metab 79: 1086-1090.

5. Labrie F, Bélanger A, Cusan L, Gomez JL, Candas B (1997) Marked decline in serum concentrations of adrenal C19 sex steroid precursors and conjugated androgen metabolites during aging. J Clin Endocrinol Metab 82: 2396-2402.

6. Barrett-Connor E, Khaw KT, Yen SS (1986) A prospective study of dehydroepiandrosterone sulfate, mortality, and cardiovascular disease. N Engl J Med 315: 1519-1524.

7. Schriock ED, Buffington CK, Hubert GD, Kurtz BR, Kitabchi AE, et al. (1988) Divergent correlations of circulating dehydroepiandrosterone sulfate and testosterone with insulin levels and insulin receptor binding. J Clin Endocrinol Metab 66: 1329-1331.

8. Schwartz AG, Pashko L, Whitcomb JM (1986) Inhibition of tumor development by dehydroepiandrosterone and related steroids. Toxicol Pathol 14: 357-362.

9. Casson PR, Andersen RN, Herrod HG, Stentz FB, Straughn AB, et al. (1993) Oral dehydroepiandrosterone in physiologic doses modulates immune function in postmenopausal women. Am J Obstet Gynecol 169: 1536-1539.

10. Morales AJ, Nolan JJ, Nelson JC, Yen SS (1994) Effects of replacement dose of dehydroepiandrosterone in men and women of advancing age. J Clin Endocrinol Metab 78: 1360-1367.

11. Cocco P, Todde P, Fornera S, Manca MB, Manca P, et al. (1998) Mortality in a cohort of men expressing the glucose-6-phosphate dehydrogenase deficiency. Blood 91: 706-709.

12. Gordon GB, Bush DE, Weisman HF (1988) Reduction of atherosclerosis by administration of dehydroepiandrosterone. A study in the hypercholesterolemic New Zealand white rabbit with aortic intimal injury. J Clin Invest 82: 712-720.

13. Arad Y, Badimon JJ, Badimon L, Hembree WC, Ginsberg HN (1989) Dehydroepiandrosterone feeding prevents aortic fatty streak formation and cholesterol accumulation in cholesterol-fed rabbit. Arteriosclerosis 9: 159-166.

14. Eich DM, Nestler JE, Johnson DE, Dworkin GH, Ko D, et al. (1993) Inhibition of accelerated coronary atherosclerosis with dehydroepiandrosterone in the heterotopic rabbit model of cardiac transplantation. Circulation 87: 261-269.

15. Yen SS, Morales AJ, Khorram O (1995) Replacement of DHEA in aging men and women. Potential remedial effects. Ann N Y Acad Sci 774: 128-142.

16. Weksler ME (1996) Hormone replacement for men. BMJ 312: 859-860.

17. Shomali ME (1997) The use of anti-aging hormones. Melatonin, growth hormone, testosterone, and dehydroepiandrosterone: consumer enthusiasm for unproven therapies. Md Med J 46: 181-186.

18. Barrett-Connor E, Goodman-Gruen D (1995) The epidemiology of DHEAS and cardiovascular disease. Ann N Y Acad Sci 774: 259-270.

19. Barrett-Connor E Goodman-Gruen D (1995) Dehydroepiandrosterone sulfate does not predict cardiovascular death in postmenopausal women. The Rancho Bernardo Study. Circulation 91: 1757-1760.

20. LaCroix AZ, Yano K, Reed DM (1992) Dehydroepiandrosterone sulfate, incidence of myocardial infarction, and extent of atherosclerosis in men. Circulation 86: 1529-1535.

21. Contoreggi CS, Blackman MR, Andres R, Muller DC, Lakatta EG, et al. (1990) Plasma levels of estradiol, testosterone, and DHEAS do not predict risk of coronary artery disease in men. J Androl 11: 460-470.

22. Rocha VZ, Libby P (2009) Obesity, inflammation, and atherosclerosis. Nat Rev Cardiol 6: 399-409.

23. Steinberg D (2002) Atherogenesis in perspective: hypercholesterolemia and inflammation as partners in crime. Nat Med 8: 1211-1217.

24. Aviram M, Rosenblat M, Etzioni A, Levy R (1996) Activation of NADPH oxidase required for macrophage-mediated oxidation of low-density lipoprotein. Metabolism 45: 1069-1079.

25. Marumo T, Schini-Kerth VB, Fisslthaler B, Busse R (1997) Platelet-derived growth factor-stimulated superoxide anion production modulates activation of transcription factor NF-kappaB and expression of monocyte chemoattractant protein 1 in human aortic smooth muscle cells. Circulation 96: 2361-2367.

26. Griendling KK, Sorescu D, Ushio-Fukai M (2000) NAD(P)H oxidase: role in cardiovascular biology and disease. Circ Res 86: 494-501.

27. Lusis AJ (2000) Atherosclerosis. Nature 407: 233-241.

28. Newby AC, Zaltsman AB (1999) Fibrous cap formation or destruction--the critical importance of vascular smooth muscle cell proliferation, migration and matrix formation. Cardiovasc Res 41: 345-360.

29. Geng YJ, Libby P (2002) Progression of atheroma: a struggle between death and procreation. Arterioscler Thromb Vasc Biol 22: 1370-1380.

30. Nestler JE, Barlascini CO, Clore JN, Blackard WG (1988) Dehydroepiandrosterone reduces serum low density lipoprotein levels and body fat but does not alter insulin sensitivity in normal men. J Clin Endocrinol Metab 66: 57-61.

31. Cleary MP, Zabel T, Sartin JL (1988) Effects of short-term dehydroepiandrosterone treatment on serum and pancreatic insulin in Zucker rats. J Nutr 118: 382-387.

32. Cleary MP, Zisk JF (1986) Anti-obesity effect of two different levels of dehydroepiandrosterone in lean and obese middle-aged female Zucker rats. Int J Obes 10: 193-204.

33. Tagliaferro AR, Davis JR, Truchon S, Van Hamont N (1986) Effects of dehydroepiandrosterone acetate on metabolism, body weight and composition of male and female rats. J Nutr 116: 1977-1983.

34. Mohan PF, Ihnen JS, Levin BE, Cleary MP (1990) Effects of dehydroepiandrosterone treatment in rats with diet-induced obesity. J Nutr 120: 1103-1114.

35. Lopez, A, Krehl WA (1967) A possible interrelation between glucose-6-phosphate dehydrogenase and dehydroepiandrosterone in obesity. Lancet 2: 485-487.

36. Watson RR, Huls A, Araghinikuam M, Chung S (1996) Dehydroepiandrosterone and diseases of aging. Drugs Aging 9: 274-291.

37. Taniguchi S, Yanase T, Kobayashi K, Takayanagi R, Nawata H (1996) Dehydroepiandrosterone markedly inhibits the accumulation of cholesteryl ester in mouse macrophage J774-1 cells. Atherosclerosis 126: 143-154.

38. Yamada J, Sakuma M, Ikeda T, Fukuda K, Suga T (1991) Characteristics of dehydroepiandrosterone as a peroxisome proliferator. Biochim Biophys Acta 1092: 233-243.

39. Tang X, Ma H, Zou S, Chen W (2007) Effects of dehydroepiandrosterone (DHEA) on hepatic lipid metabolism parameters and lipogenic gene mRNA expression in broiler chickens. Lipids 42: 1025-1033.

40. Schoonjans K, Staels B, Auwerx J (1996) Role of the peroxisome proliferator-activated receptor (PPAR) in mediating the effects of fibrates and fatty acids on gene expression. J Lipid Res 37: 907-925.

41. Schoonjans K, Staels B, Auwerx J (1996) The peroxisome proliferator activated receptors (PPARS) and their effects on lipid metabolism and adipocyte differentiation. Biochim Biophys Acta 1302: 93-109.

42. Auwerx J, Schoonjans K, Fruchart JC, Staels B (1996) Regulation of triglyceride metabolism by PPARs: fibrates and thiazolidinediones have distinct effects. J Atheroscler Thromb 3: 81-89.

43. Karbowska J, Kochan Z (2005) Effect of DHEA on endocrine functions of adipose tissue, the involvement of PPAR gamma. Biochem Pharmacol 70: 249-257.

44. Wang L, Hao Q, Wang YD, Wang WJ, Li DJ (2011) Protective effects of dehydroepiandrosterone on atherosclerosis in ovariectomized rabbits via alleviating inflammatory injury in endothelial cells. Atherosclerosis 214: 47-57.

45. 45   Collins T, Read MA, Neish AS, Whitley MZ, Thanos D, et al. (1995) Transcriptional regulation of endothelial cell adhesion molecules: NF-kappa B and cytokine-inducible enhancers. FASEB J 9: 899-909.

46. Delerive P, De Bosscher K, Besnard S, Vanden Berghe W, Peters JM, et al. (1999) Peroxisome proliferator-activated receptor alpha negatively regulates the vascular inflammatory gene response by negative cross-talk with transcription factors NF-kappaB and AP-1. J Biol Chem 274: 32048-32054.

47. Rival Y, Bénéteau N, Taillandier T, Pezet M, Dupont-Passelaigue E, et al. (2002) PPARalpha and PPARdelta activators inhibit cytokine-induced nuclear translocation of NF-kappaB and expression of VCAM-1 in EAhy926 endothelial cells. Eur J Pharmacol 435: 143-151.

48. Altman R, Motton DD, Kota RS, Rutledge JC (2008) Inhibition of vascular inflammation by dehydroepiandrosterone sulfate in human aortic endothelial cells: roles of PPARalpha and NF-kappaB. Vascul Pharmacol 48: 76-84.

49. Csiszar A, Labinskyy N, Olson S, Pinto JT, Gupte S, et al. (2009) Resveratrol prevents monocrotaline-induced pulmonary hypertension in rats. Hypertension 54: 668-675.

50. Schermuly RT, Dony E, Ghofrani HA, Pullamsetti S, Savai R, et al. (2005) Reversal of experimental pulmonary hypertension by PDGF inhibition. J Clin Invest 115: 2811-2821.

51. Frasch HF, Marshall C, Marshall BE (1999) Endothelin-1 is elevated in monocrotaline pulmonary hypertension. Am J Physiol 276: 304-310.

52. Rubens C, Ewert R, Halank M, Wensel R, Orzechowski HD, et al. (2001) Big endothelin-1 and endothelin-1 plasma levels are correlated with the severity of primary pulmonary hypertension. Chest 120: 1562-1569.

53. Giaid A, Yanagisawa M, Langleben D, Michel RP, Levy R, et al. (1993) Expression of endothelin-1 in the lungs of patients with pulmonary hypertension. N Engl J Med 328: 1732-1739.

54. Stewart DJ, Kubac G, Costello KB, Cernacek P (1991) Increased plasma endothelin-1 in the early hours of acute myocardial infarction. J Am Coll Cardiol 18: 38-43.

55. Michelakis ED, McMurtry MS, Wu XC, Dyck JR, Moudgil R, et al. (2002) Dichloroacetate, a metabolic modulator, prevents and reverses chronic hypoxic pulmonary hypertension in rats: role of increased expression and activity of voltage-gated potassium channels. Circulation 105: 244-250.

56. Bonnet S, Savineau JP, Barillot W, Dubuis E, Vandier C, et al. (2003) Role of Ca(2+)-sensitive K(+) channels in the remission phase of pulmonary hypertension in chronic obstructive pulmonary diseases. Cardiovasc Res 60: 326-336.

57. Lee KT, Tan IK (1975) A general colorimetric procedure using oxidized chlorpromazine hydrochloride for the estimation of enzymes dependent on NADH/NAD+ and NADPH/NADP+ systems. Mikrochim Acta 64: 139-150.

58. Weir EK, Archer SL (1995) The mechanism of acute hypoxic pulmonary vasoconstriction: the tale of two channels. FASEB J 9: 183-189.

59. Michelakis ED, Reeve HL, Huang JM, Tolarova S, Nelson DP, et al. (1997) Potassium channel diversity in vascular smooth muscle cells. Can J Physiol Pharmacol 75: 889-897.

60. Farrukh IS, Peng W, Orlinska U, Hoidal JR (1998) Effect of dehydroepiandrosterone on hypoxic pulmonary vasoconstriction: a Ca(2+)-activated K(+)-channel opener. Am J Physiol 274: 186-195.

61. Peng W, Hoidal JR, Farrukh IS (1999) Role of a novel KCa opener in regulating K+ channels of hypoxic human pulmonary vascular cells. Am J Respir Cell Mol Biol 20: 737-745.

62. Sachin AG, Kai-Xun L, Takao O, Koichi S, Masahiko O, et al. (2002) Inhibitors of pentose phosphate pathway cause vasodilation: involvement of voltage-gated potassium channels. J Pharmacol Exp Ther 301: 299-305.

63. Bonnet S, Dumas-de-La-Roque E, Bégueret H, Marthan R, Fayon M, et al. (2003) Dehydroepiandrosterone (DHEA) prevents and reverses chronic hypoxic pulmonary hypertension. Proc Natl Acad Sci U S A 100: 9488-9493.

64. Münzel T, Feil R, Mülsch A, Lohmann SM, Hofmann F, et al. (2003) Physiology and pathophysiology of vascular signaling controlled by guanosine 3',5'-cyclic monophosphate-dependent protein kinase [corrected]. Circulation 108: 2172-2183.

65. Friebe A, Koesling D (2003) Regulation of nitric oxide-sensitive guanylyl cyclase. Circ Res 93: 96-105.

66. Moncada S, Higgs EA (2006) The discovery of nitric oxide and its role in vascular biology. Br J Pharmacol 147: 193-201.

67. Oka M, Karoor V, Homma N, Nagaoka T, Sakao E, et al. (2007) Dehydroepiandrosterone upregulates soluble guanylate cyclase and inhibits hypoxic pulmonary hypertension. Cardiovasc Res 74: 377-387.

68. Sato A, Sakuma I, Gutterman DD (2003) Mechanism of dilation to reactive oxygen species in human coronary arterioles. Am J Physiol Heart Circ Physiol 285: 2345-2354.

69. Fujimoto S, Asano T, Sakai M, Sakurai K, Takagi D, et al. (2001) Mechanisms of hydrogen peroxide-induced relaxation in rabbit mesenteric small artery. Eur J Pharmacol 412: 291-300.

70. Homma N, Nagaoka T, Karoor V, Imamura M, Taraseviciene-Stewart L, et al. (2008) Involvement of RhoA/Rho kinase signaling in protection against monocrotaline-induced pulmonary hypertension in pneumonectomized rats by dehydroepiandrosterone. Am J Physiol Lung Cell Mol Physiol 295: 71-78.

71. Means AR (1994) Calcium, calmodulin and cell cycle regulation. FEBS Lett 347: 1-4.

72. Yoshimata T, Yoneyama A, Jin-no Y, Tamai N, Kamiya Y (1999) Effects of dehydroepiandrosterone on mitogen-activated protein kinase in human aortic smooth muscle cells. Life Sci 65: 431-440.

73. Williams MR, Ling S, Dawood T, Hashimura K, Dai A, et al. (2002) Dehydroepiandrosterone inhibits human vascular smooth muscle cell proliferation independent of ARs and ERs. J Clin Endocrinol Metab 87: 176-181.

74. Bonnet S, Paulin R, Sutendra G, Dromparis P, Roy M, et al. (2009) Dehydroepiandrosterone reverses systemic vascular remodeling through the inhibition of the Akt/GSK3-{beta}/NFAT axis. Circulation 120: 1231-1240.

75. Urata Y, Goto S, Kawakatsu M, Yodoi J, Eto M, et al. DHEA attenuates PDGF-induced phenotypic proliferation of vascular smooth muscle A7r5 cells through redox regulation. Biochem Biophys Res Commun 396: 489-494.

76. Kanda M, Ihara Y, Murata H, Urata Y, Kono T, et al. (2006) Glutaredoxin modulates platelet-derived growth factor-dependent cell signaling by regulating the redox status of low molecular weight protein-tyrosine phosphatase. J Biol Chem 281: 28518-28528.

77. Paulin R, Courboulin A, Meloche J, Mainguy V, Dumas de la Roque E, et al. (2011) Signal transducers and activators of transcription-3/pim1 axis plays a critical role in the pathogenesis of human pulmonary arterial hypertension. Circulation 123: 1205-1215.

78. Brock M, Trenkmann M, Gay RE, Michel BA, Gay S, et al. (2009) Interleukin-6 modulates the expression of the bone morphogenic protein receptor type II through a novel STAT3-microRNA cluster 17/92 pathway. Circ Res 104: 1184-1191.

79. Zakrzewicz A, Hecker M, Marsh LM, Kwapiszewska G, Nejman B, et al. (2007) Receptor for activated C-kinase 1, a novel interaction partner of type II bone morphogenetic protein receptor, regulates smooth muscle cell proliferation in pulmonary arterial hypertension. Circulation 115: 2957-2968.

80. Tada Y, Majka S, Carr M, Harral J, Crona D, et al. (2007) Molecular effects of loss of BMPR2 signaling in smooth muscle in a transgenic mouse model of PAH. Am J Physiol Lung Cell Mol Physiol 292: 1556-1563.

81. Kopplow K, Wayss K, Enzmann H, Mayer D (2005) Dehydroepiandrosterone causes hyperplasia and impairs regeneration in rat liver. Int J Oncol 27: 1551-1558.

82. Paulin R, Meloche J, Jacob MH, Bisserier M, Courboulin A, et al. (2011) Dehydroepiandrosterone inhibits the Src/STAT3 constitutive activation in Pulmonary Arterial Hypertension. Am J Physiol Heart Circ Physiol 301: 798-809.

83. Hansmann G, Wagner RA, Schellong S, Perez VA, Urashima T, et al. (2007) Pulmonary arterial hypertension is linked to insulin resistance and reversed by peroxisome proliferator-activated receptor-gamma activation. Circulation 115: 1275-1284.

84. Wang LH, Yang XY, Zhang X, Huang J, Hou J, et al. (2004) Transcriptional inactivation of STAT3 by PPARgamma suppresses IL-6-responsive multiple myeloma cells. Immunity 20: 205-218.

85. Kim HJ, Rho YH, Choi SJ, Lee YH, Cheon H, et al. (2005) 15-Deoxy-delta12,14-PGJ2 inhibits IL-6-induced Stat3 phosphorylation in lymphocytes. Exp Mol Med 37: 179-185.

86. Ji JD, Kim HJ, Rho YH, Choi SJ, Lee YH, et al. (2005) Inhibition of IL-10-induced STAT3 activation by 15-deoxy-Delta12,14-prostaglandin J2. Rheumatology (Oxford) 44: 983-988.

87. Ehrmann J, Strakova N, Vrzalikova K, Hezova R, Kolar Z (2008) Expression of STATs and their inhibitors SOCS and PIAS in brain tumors. In vitro and in vivo study. Neoplasma 55: 482-487.

88. Juurlink DN, Gomes T, Lipscombe LL, Austin PC, Hux JE, et al. (2009) Adverse cardiovascular events during treatment with pioglitazone and rosiglitazone: population based cohort study. BMJ 339: 2942.

89. Rosenfeld RS, Hellman L, Roffwarg H, Weitzman ED, Fukushima DK, et al. (1971) Dehydroisoandrosterone is secreted episodically and synchronously with cortisol by normal man. J Clin Endocrinol Metab 33: 87-92.

90. Nieschlag E, Loriaux DL, Ruder HJ, Zucker IR, Kirschner MA, et al. (1973) The secretion of dehydroepiandrosterone and dehydroepiandrosterone sulphate in man. J Endocrinol 57: 123-134.

91. Baulieu EE (1996) Dehydroepiandrosterone (DHEA): a fountain of youth? J Clin Endocrinol Metab 81: 3147-3151.

92. Ata H, Rawat DK, Lincoln T, Gupte SA (2011) Mechanism of glucose-6-phosphate dehydrogenase-mediated regulation of coronary artery contractility. Am J Physiol Heart Circ Physiol 300: 2054-2063.

93. Gupte RS, Ata H, Rawat D, Abe M, Taylor MS, et al. (2011) Glucose-6-phosphate dehydrogenase is a regulator of vascular smooth muscle contraction. Antioxid Redox Signal 14: 543-558.

94. Matsui R, Xu S, Maitland KA, Hayes A, Leopold JA, et al. (2005) Glucose-6 phosphate dehydrogenase deficiency decreases the vascular response to angiotensin II. Circulation 112: 257-263.

95. Xie Y, Kole S, Precht P, Pazin MJ, Bernier M (2009) S-glutathionylation impairs signal transducer and activator of transcription 3 activation and signaling. Endocrinology 150: 1122-1131.

96. Wang J, Pan S, Berk BC (2007) Glutaredoxin mediates Akt and eNOS activation by flow in a glutathione reductase-dependent manner. Arterioscler Thromb Vasc Biol 27: 1283-1288.

97. Liao BC, Hsieh CW, Lin YC, Wung BS (2010) The glutaredoxin/glutathione system modulates NF-kappaB activity by glutathionylation of p65 in cinnamaldehyde-treated endothelial cells. Toxicol Sci 116: 151-163.

98. Chen CA, Wang TY, Varadharaj S, Reyes LA, Hemann C, et al. (2010) S-glutathionylation uncouples eNOS and regulates its cellular and vascular function. Nature 468: 1115-1118.

99. Cross JV, Templeton DJ (2004) Oxidative stress inhibits MEKK1 by site-specific glutathionylation in the ATP-binding domain. Biochem J 381: 675-683.

100. Nitabach MN, Llamas DA, Thompson IJ, Collins KA, Holmes TC (2002) Phosphorylation-dependent and phosphorylation-independent modes of modulation of shaker family voltage-gated potassium channels by SRC family protein tyrosine kinases. J Neurosci 22: 7913-7922.

101. Alioua A, Mahajan A, Nishimaru K, Zarei MM, Stefani E, et al. (2002) Coupling of c-Src to large conductance voltage- and Ca2+-activated K+ channels as a new mechanism of agonist-induced vasoconstriction. Proc Natl Acad Sci U S A 99: 14560-14565.

102. Dey D, Shepherd A, Pachuau J, Martin-Caraballo M (2011) Leukemia inhibitory factor regulates trafficking of T-type Ca2+ channels. Am J Physiol Cell Physiol 300: 576-587.

103. Trimarchi T, Pachuau J, Shepherd A, Dey D, Martin-Caraballo M (2009) CNTF-evoked activation of JAK and ERK mediates the functional expression of T-type Ca2+ channels in chicken nodose neurons. J Neurochem 108: 246-259.

104. Hu XQ, Singh N, Mukhopadhyay D, Akbarali HI (1998) Modulation of voltage-dependent Ca2+ channels in rabbit colonic smooth muscle cells by c-Src and focal adhesion kinase. J Biol Chem 273: 5337-5342.

7

Exercise, Science and Designer Doping: Traditional and Emerging Trends

Graham MR[1], Davies B[2], Grace FM[3], Evans PJ[4] and Baker JS[3]

[1]Sport and Exercise Science, Institute of Health, Medical Science and Society Science, Glyndwr University, Wrexham, Wales, UK, LL11 2AW
[2]Health and Exercise Science, University of Glamorgan, Pontypridd, Wales, UK, CF83 1DL
[3]Exercise Science, University of the West of Scotland, Hamilton, Scotland, ML3 OJB
[4]Department of Endocrinology, Royal Gwent Hospital, Newport, Wales, UK, NP20 2UB

Abstract

The list of doping agents is enormous, and for the majority, any beneficial sporting effect is contentious. The World Anti-Doping Agency (WADA) and United Kingdom (UK) Anti-Doping have difficulty detecting the peptide hormones, growth hormone (GH), insulin-like growth factor-1 (IGF-I), insulin and erythropoietin (Epo), because they require blood analysis. Only in the last two years has an athlete been convicted of taking GH, which is still being used as a doping agent because the window for detection is so brief. This positive test was not contested, which suggests that science may be winning the war on drugs. Athletes appear to have ceased taking insulin, because of its life-threatening acute effects, and in recent years no adverse analytical findings have been reported for this drug.

"Older" doping agents, which are known to enhance performance in sport, include testosterone and their derivatives, anabolic steroids.

The pharmaceutical industry continues to manufacture new medicines, pushing back the boundaries in combating wasting disease states and the ageing process, but is inadvertently producing the latest generation of doping agents. This will challenge anti-doping scientists.

WADA's banned list also includes fibroblast growth factors, hepatocyte growth factor, mechano growth factors, platelet-derived growth factor, vascular-endothelial growth factor which may promote muscle, tendon or ligament development, vascularisation, energy utilisation, regenerative capacity and fibre type. Athletes will use whatever they believe works, but can only use what is available. Internet companies offer these anabolic products, but their veracity cannot be proven.

There are questions that need to be answered? Are these products available to athletes, do they enhance performance, are athletes really taking them and are they so difficult to detect. The internet has made them available to anyone with a credit card and it appears that if they are cycled correctly, unless an athlete is caught in possession of them, the opportunity of proving a case of doping is almost impossible.

Keywords: Anabolic steroids; Epo; GH; IGF-I; Insulin; Mechano growth factor; Myostatin

Introduction

The involvement of sport's scientists in elite sport has led them to develop improved nutrition, physiological and psychological techniques but also to be significantly implicated in the development and use of performance enhancing drugs [1]. East German scientists were involved in the state-sponsored systematic doping of athletes in the former East Germany [2]. American scientists have also been concerned in the dissemination of performance and image enhancing drugs used in international sport. Dr John Ziegler, originally developed the androgenic anabolic steroid (AAS) Methandrostenolone (Dianabol) which was released in the USA in 1958 by the pharmaceutical giant, Ciba. Ziegler pioneered its athletic use as an aid to muscle growth by bodybuilders, administering it to USA weightlifting champion Bill March in 1959 when he was the physician to the USA Weightlifting team [3]. This appears to be the first documented use of AAS in sport [4]. The emphasis and rewards placed on winning and breaking world records has made this liaison between sporting performance and science almost inextricable.

In 1960, Danish cyclist, Knut Jensen, was the first athlete to die in Olympic competition due to doping, during the 100 km team time trial race. His autopsy revealed traces of amphetamine [5]. British cyclist

Tom Simpson, whose motto was "if it takes ten to kill you, take nine and win....." was the first death caused by doping in the Tour de France, in 1967. Two tubes of amphetamines and a further empty tube were found in the rear pocket of his racing jersey. His autopsy revealed traces of amphetamine, alcohol and the diuretic frusemide.

In 1967 to combat doping, the International Olympic Commitee (IOC) established a Medical Commission which provided three fundamental principles: protection of the health of athletes, respect for medical and sport ethics, and equality for all competing athletes [6].

At that time the list of banned substances included narcotic analgesics, stimulants and alcohol. Although it was suspected that AAS were being used at this time, testing methods were insufficiently developed to warrant their inclusion. The first compulsory doping controls were at the Winter Olympic Games in Grenoble, France in 1968 [7]. In the 1984 Olympics, some team doctors were involved in exploiting the doping regulations. Team doctors had to fill in

*Corresponding author:** Graham MR, Sport and Exercise Science, Institute of Health, Medical Science and Society Science, Glyndwr University, Wrexham, Wales, UK, LL11 2AW, E-mail: drgraham.ac.uk@live.co.uk

declarations for all athletes using specific drugs perceived to be performance enhancing. If competitors produced a doctor's certificate stating that they needed a drug for health reasons, they would not be disqualified, if drug checks proved positive. Following a large number of positive urinalyses some teams provided medical certificates covering the whole team [8]. This identified the deception that physicians were prepared to be concerned in to win at any cost. One of the drugs in this instance was a beta-blocker, which could in fact impede performance, in endurance events.

Convictions of celebrity athletes for doping offences and their subsequent confessions has identified the extent of their subterfuge [9-14].

The authorities are partly to blame. Zero tolerance and a lifetime ban for any offence, would be a far greater deterrent than a two year ban, for the first adverse analytical finding (AAF), a two year to lifetime ban for second or subsequent violations and a four year to lifetime ban for trafficking. The World Anti-Doping Agency (WADA) have written extensive documents, euphemising the fact that they are prepared to offer "deals" with offending dopers in an attempt to identify the provenance of these doping agents and suppliers [15].

When rewards for athletic success are so great, human nature is such that certain individuals will always succumb to fruit of the forbidden tree. Athletes are more concerned with failure than they are about adverse health effects as a consequence of cheating [16].

Doping could be halted overnight if the sanctions were severe enough.

Specific questions need to be answered. Do these agents really enhance performance? Are they harmful? Are they detectable? This short review will assess current doping agents being used, whether they have the desired effect, and whether athletes can beat "the test".

Anabolic Steroids

Androgenic anabolic steroids (AAS) are a group of synthetic compounds similar in chemical structure to the natural anabolic steroid testosterone (see Figure 1) [17]. In 1969, the first application of radioimmunoassay (RIA) for the measurement of steroids in biological fluids was published [18].

The IOC Medical Commission acted by the introduction of AAS as a banned class in 1974 following the development of a screen for the 17α-alkylated orally active drugs, in the biological medium of urine. Any presumptive positive samples could then be analysed by gas chromatography-mass spectrometry (GC-MS) for confirmatory identification [19]. The advantages that GC/MS screen provided, resulted in the replacement of RIA, which is today's accepted method.

AAS detection has always been problematic. They are abused by athletes during training and are not taken during the actual competitive period, in an attempt to avoid detection. Since oral preparations are cleared from the body between 2-14 days following withdrawal, and water soluble "injectables" after 4 weeks, it is possible to use these agents during periods of intensive training and test negative. In 1982, the IOC test for detection of testosterone administration was based on the GC/MS determination of the urinary ratio of testosterone (T) to its 17 α-epimer, epitestosterone (E), following glucuronide hydrolysis, commonly referred to as T/E ratio [20]. In healthy men and women, the T/E ratio is approximately 1. Supraphysiological doses of testosterone cause an increase in the ratio as a result of increased excretion of testosterone. The T/E ratio may be augmented as a consequence of dose-dependent inhibition of testicular steroidogenesis. When supraphysiological doses of testosterone are taken, suppression of luteinising hormone secretion decreases urinary epitestosterone glucuronide. The WADA Medical Code stipulates that if a ratio of T/E is greater than 4, it is mandatory that the relevant medical authority conducts an investigation before the sample is declared positive. Investigations include a review of T/E results from previous tests, subsequent tests and also results of any serum endocrine investigations. The athlete will then be monitored at least monthly for three months. However, an athlete may have a physiological increased ratio being a natural biological outlier [21]. In the case of a T/E ratio ≥4, isotope ratio mass spectrometry (IRMS) can determine the exogenous administration [22].

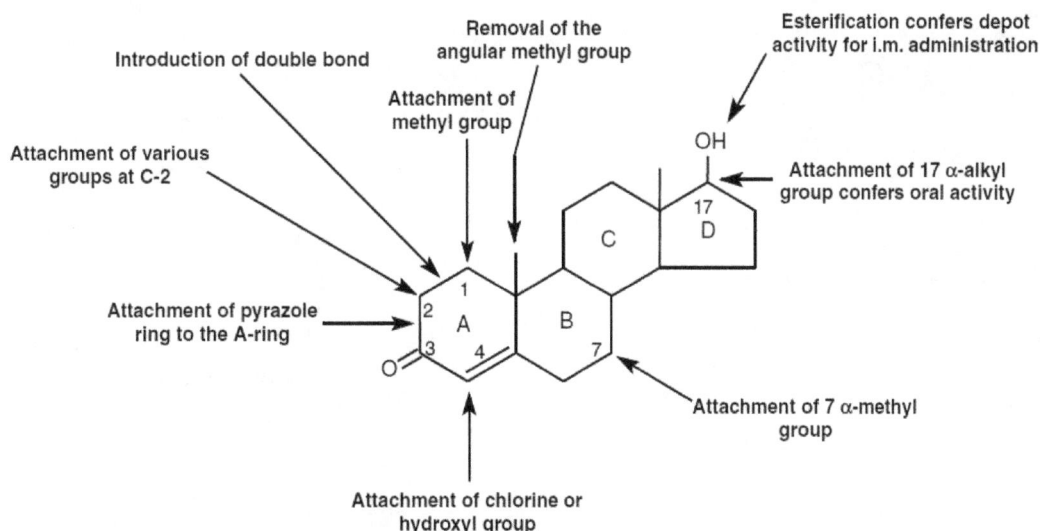

IM = intramuscular

Figure 1: The structure of testosterone and structural modifications to the A- and B-rings of this steroid molecule that increase anabolic activity. Substitution at C-17 confers oral or depot activity (Reproduced with permission from Kicman and Gower, 2003).

Do AAS Enhance Performance?

AAS were proven only as recently as 1996 to increase muscle mass and strength in adult males [23]. Extrapolation of these effects to the sporting arena is not in doubt and is the reason why they are still the most common AAS in anti-dope testing today [24].

The prevalence of AAS use, the risks to an athlete's health and the methods used to detect them by urinalysis are well documented in the literature [25].

Accessibility

The price of genuine AAS and their restriction due to their classification under the misuse of drugs act, 1971, has initiated an enormous counterfeit market. The most popular AAS are presented in 10 ml multi-dose vials, claiming to have very high concentrations of active ingredients. Multiple websites offer AAS, at varying prices [26]. A large majority of these counterfeit products are made in unlicensed laboratories in countries where the law is more permissive than the UK or USA, such as Mexico, China and Thailand. The dangers associated with such products are patently obvious. Table 1 identifies genuine prescription medicines, which are AAS and have been used as doping agents and the cost to the National Health Service in the UK. Table 2 identifies potential counterfeit AAS that are currently used by bodybuilders, weightlifters, powerlifters and rugby players, available from other sources, including internet companies.

Growth Hormone (GH)

The somatotroph cells in the anterior pituitary synthesise and secrete the polypeptide human growth hormone (hGH) which appears to have been isolated in 1944 [27] and then manufactured by recombinant DNA technology in the mid 1980's producing recombinant human growth hormone (rhGH) [28]. It is secreted as a 191-amino-acid, 4-helix bundle protein, weighing 22,000 daltons (70-80%) and a less abundant 176-amino-acid form, weighing 20,000 daltons (20-30%) [29]. See Figure 2 for GH three-dimensional configuration.

Athletes have been trying to extrapolate postulated benefits to achieve physical improvement since 1982 [30]. Its powerful effects in GH deficiency (GHD) were proven in 1989 [31] and these effects were also experienced in elderly men aged 60 years of age in 1990 [32].

Its seizure of rhGH in the possession of Chinese swimmers at the 1998 World Swimming Championships and again discovery of possession by cyclists at the Tour de France cycling event in 1998 have proven its abuse at an elite level [33].

Does rhGH Enhance Performance?

Extensive research with rhGH on non-competitive athletes has produced controversial results. Contemporary evidence appears to contradict the proven anabolic effect of rhGH in deficiency, in drug naïve healthy human muscle, in males (mean age of 28 years) [33]. Nor

Product	Pharmaceutical Manufacturer	Manufacturers Price	Mode of delivery
Sustanon 250® (testosterone propionate 30 mg, testosterone phenylpropionate 60 mg, testosterone isocaproate 60 mg, and testosterone decanoate 100 mg) 250 mg/1 ml	Organon	net price 1-mL amp =£2.45	Intramuscular
Testosterone enantate 250 mg/1 ml	Non-Proprietary (Generic)	net price 1-mL amp = £13.33	Intramuscular
Deca-Durabolin® (nandrolone decanoate) 50 mg/1 ml	Organon	net price 1-mL amp = £3.17	Intramuscular
Testosterone propionate (Virormone®) 50 mg/1 ml	Nordic	net price 2-mL amp = £4.50	Intramuscular
Testosterone undecanoate (Nebido) 250mg/1 ml	Bayer Schering	net price 4-mL amp = £76.70	Intramuscular
Restandol® Testocaps (testosterone undecanoate) 40 mg/capsule	Organon	net price 30-cap pack = £8.55; 60-cap pack = £17.10	Oral
Pro-Viron® (mesterolone) 25 mg/tablet	Bayer Schering	Net price 30-tab pack = £4.19	Oral
Striant® SR (testosterone tablet) 30 mg/tablet	(The Urology Co.)	net price 60-tab pack = £45.84	Mucoadhesive buccal tablets / Sublingual
Intrinsa® (Testosterone patch) (self-adhesive, releasing testosterone 300 mcg/24 hours)	Warner Chilcott	net price 8-patch pack = £26.91	Transdermal
Testim® (Testosterone gel 50 mg/5 gm)	Ferring	net price (testosterone 50 mg/5 g tube) 30-tube pack = £32.00	Transdermal
Testogel® (Testosterone gel) 50 mg/5 gm sachet	Bayer Schering	net price 30-sachet pack = £31.11	Transdermal
Tostran® (testosterone gel 2%) (10 mg/metered application)	ProStrakan	net price 60-gm multidose dispenser = £26.67	Transdermal
Testosterone 100 mg	Organon	net price 100 mg = £7.40; 200 mg = £13.79	Implant

Table 1: Prescription only Medicines, Testosterone and Esters used in hormone replacement

Product	Black-market Pharmaceutical Manufacturer	Black-market Wholesale Price	Black-market Retail Price
Anabolic Steroid Hormones (IM)			
Sustanon 250 mg (1 ml)	Generic (non-proprietary)/ Organon (Pakistan)	£1.75	£2.5
Testosterone enanthate 250 mg (1 ml)	Generic (non-proprietary)/ Apex/Prochem/Dragon/British Dragon, Pharmaceuticals	£2	£3.5
Testosterone 400 (testosterone propionate, cypionate and enanthate) (10 mls)	Generic (non-proprietary)/ Apex/Prochem/Dragon/British Dragon, Pharmaceuticals	£18	£30
Nandrolone 300 mg/ml (10 mls)	Generic (non-proprietary)/ Apex/Prochem/Dragon/British Dragon, Pharmaceuticals	£19	£30
Masteron (Drostanolone Propionate) 100mg/ml (10 mls)	Generic (non-proprietary)/ Apex/Prochem/Dragon/British Dragon, Pharmaceuticals	£20	£30
Virormone (Testosterone propionate) (100-125mg/ml) (10 mls)	Generic (non-proprietary)/ Apex/Prochem/Dragon/British Dragon, Pharmaceuticals	£14	£20
Testosterone cypionate 100mg/ml (10 mls)	Generic (non-proprietary)/ Apex/Prochem/Dragon/British Dragon, Pharmaceuticals	£17	£25
Trenbolone acetate; Trenbolone enanthate (150 mg/ml) (10 mls)	Generic (non-proprietary)/ Apex/Prochem/Dragon/British Dragon, Pharmaceuticals	£20	£30
Parabolon (trenbolone hexahydrobenzylcarbonate) (75-150 mg/ml) (10 mls)	Negma		
Equitest 400 (testosterone undecanoate 240 mg, boldenone undecanoate 160 mg/ml) (10 mls)	Prochem	£20	£30
Super-tren 2000 (methyltrienolone 2000 mcg/ml) (10 mls)	Prochem	£27	£50
Anabolic Steroid Hormones (Oral)			
Primobol 50 (Methenolone tablets) 50 mg/tablet 30 tabs	British Dragon Pharmaceuticals	£38	£50
Anavar/Oxanobol (oxandrolone) 10-50 mg/tablet 60 tabs	Generic (non-proprietary)/ Apex/Prochem/Dragon/British Dragon, Pharmaceuticals	£38	£50
Winstrol (stanozolol) 10-50mg/tablet 50 tabs	Generic (non-proprietary)/ Apex/Prochem/Dragon/British Dragon, Pharmaceuticals	£28	£35
Androlic/Anadrol/Oxydrol (Oxymetholone tablets) 50mg/tablet 60 tablets	Generic (non-proprietary)/ Apex/Prochem/Dragon/British Dragon, Pharmaceuticals	£28	£60
Dianabol/Methanobol/DBol (Methandienone/ Methandrostenolone) 10mg/tablet (500 tablets)	Generic (non-proprietary)/ Apex/Prochem/Dragon/British Dragon, Pharmaceuticals	£40	£55
Peptide Hormones			
Hygetropin (rhGH) 100 IU	Hygene Biopharm Co.,Ltd.	£100	£140
GenLei® Jintropin™ (rhGH) 100 IU	Gene Science Pharmaceutical Co., Ltd.	£100	£140
Turbovital (rhIgf-1) 1000 mcg	Hygene Biopharm Co.,Ltd.	£200	£285
Growth Hormone Secretagogues			
Hexarelin/Sermorelin/Ipamorelin (growth hormone releasing hormone) 2mg/amp	ProPeptides Co., Ltd	£24	£50
Myostatin inhibitor			
Follistatin 344 (5 mcg)	Southern Research Co., Ltd	£62	£100

Table 2:

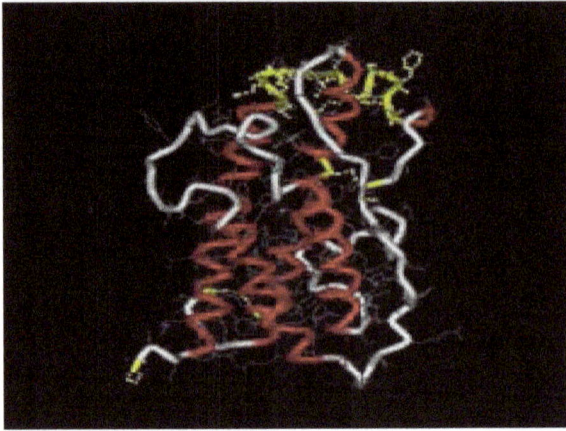

Figure 2: The growth hormone somatropin, in its correct 22-kD-hGH form. Three-dimensional structure, generated from the protein data base SWISS PROT. Structural data supplied with the help of the program RasMol. The n-terminal amino acid (at the bottom left hand corner) is marked yellow, as are the disulphide bridges (and the sequence range missing on the 20 kDa hGH variant). The ranges with an α-Helix-structure are marked in red.

did it appear to improve athletic performance in females (mean age of 25 years) and males (mean age of 27 years) [34].

Administration of rhGH caused no further increase in muscle mass or strength, than that provided by resistance training in experienced male weight lifters (mean age of 22 years) attempting to further increase muscle mass [35].

Difficulties appear to have arisen in targeting an appropriate dose range that would promote muscle protein anabolism and not cause adverse effects, counteracting performance enhancement.

In contrast, a study was conducted on experienced male weight lifters, who were former AAS users (mean age of 31 years) that improved endurance performance, power and strength [36]. The beneficial effects were believed to have occurred because of AAS withdrawal inducing a state of catabolism, which was rectified by rhGH administration. Catabolism was identified by low results for insulin-like growth factor-1 (IGF-I) the surrogate marker of endogenous GH production [37]. Such research suggests that senescence or pharmaceutically induced catabolism are two conditions that may benefit from rhGH administration, in a sporting context.

Detection of rhGH

The current official method employed by WADA cannot detect pituitary hGH by blood or urine. Replacement GH is no longer derived from cadaver pituitaries, by pharmaceutical companies, because of the risk of Creutzfeldt-Jakob disease transmission. This is an incurable degenerative neurological disorder transmitted by contaminated harvested human brain products, which is invariably fatal. However unless an athlete can obtain purified cadaver pituitary, rhGH is the only form of the agent available.

RhGH is currently undetectable by urinalysis. Detection is by blood analysis and relies on the difference between the isoforms of hGH. Endogenous hGH comprises 70%, 22 Kilodaltons (KDa) and 30%, 20 KDa, whereas rhGH is 100% 22 KDa [38]. RhGH induces the production of IGF-I and markers of collagen metabolism, type 3 pro-collagen (P-III-P), using mathematical equations which are different for males and females, but this has not yet been accepted by WADA

[39]. These GH-2000 formulae show reasonable sensitivity, with false-positive rates of ≤1 in 10,000, but WADA will not adopt immunoassays they do not own, to prevent commercial companies changing their immunoassays. This is a political decision, not based on scientific discovery and is delaying a robust test which can withstand legal challenge.

A method of cycling the drug, one week on, one week off, using half strength doses can have significant effects on performance whilst thwarting the current detection techniques of the authorities [36].

Table 3 identifies genuine rhGH and Table 4 identifies potential counterfeit rhGH from internet companies.

GHRelin (Growth Hormone Secretagogues)

Growth hormone releasing hormone (GHRH) induces the synthesis and secretion of growth hormone, and somatostatin suppresses the secretion of growth hormone. Growth hormone is also regulated by ghrelin, a growth hormone secretagogue-receptor ligand that is synthesized mainly in the gastrointestinal tract [40]. Twice daily administration of ghrelin improved exercise capacity and left ventricular function in patients with chronic heart failure [41].

This knowledge has initiated the development of companies purporting to sell growth hormone secretagogues, such as sermorelin and its analogues (See Table 4).

Insulin-like Growth Factor-1 (IGF-I)

The insulin-like growth factors (IGFs) are proteins with high sequence similarity to insulin. They are part of a complex system that cells use to communicate with their environment. IGF-I is mainly secreted by the liver and is induced by GH secretion [37]. IGF-I induces cell proliferation and is thought to inhibit apoptosis [42] .

It consists of 70 amino acids in a single chain with three intra-molecular disulfide bridges. IGF-I has a molecular weight of 7,649 daltons. It displays homology to proinsulin, the precursor of insulin [43].

IGF-I mediates some of the metabolic actions of GH and has both GH-like and insulin-like actions. Both GH and IGF-I have a net anabolic effect enhancing whole body protein synthesis, improving anthropometry in GHD. Both hormones have been used in catabolism and have been effective in counteracting the protein wasting effects of glucocorticoids. IGF-I administration improves insulin sensitivity, whereas GH therapy can cause compensatory hyperinsulinaemia.

Insulin-like growth factor-2 (IGF-2) is thought to be a primary growth factor required for early development while IGF-I expression is required for achieving maximal growth.

Factors that are known to cause variation in the levels of IGF-I in the circulation, include genetic make-up, diurnal variation, age, sex, exercise status, stress levels, nutrition and disease state.

IGF-I has an involvement in regulating neurogenesis, myelination, synaptogenesis, and dendritic branching and neuroprotection after neuronal damage. The IGF-I level reflects the secretory activity of GH and is a marker for identification of normal GH production [44]. Levels of IGF-I are at their peak during late adolescence and decline throughout adulthood, mirror imaging GH [45].

The stability of the IGF-I molecule, following administration by injection, has been enhanced by combining it with one of its binding proteins (BP). It is commercially available as rhIGFBP-3 which also limits adverse effects.

No athlete has yet tested positive for rhIGF-I and published knowledge of its use in sport is limited. Tests for detecting it are currently being processed and consequently athletes have switched to doping with rhIGF-I as opposed to rhGH.

Its effect on physical exercise and anthropometry is being investigated, based on similar measurement of markers as rhGH action, with the hope of being available in time for the 2012 Olympics [46].

The concomitant administration of rhGH and rhIGF-I in GH resistant states has been shown to be synergistic and have effects that are far greater than either alone [44]. Athletes believe that the combination is more powerful than double of either alone and lower doses of either will limit detection (personal communications). Such beliefs appear to be supported by contemporary research [39,44].

Table 3 identifies genuine rhIGF-I and Table 4 identifies potential counterfeit rhIGF-I from internet companies.

Erythropoietin (Epo)

Erythropoietin (Epo) is a glycoprotein hormone (40% carbohydrate) with a molecular weight of 32-39 KDa that controls erythropoiesis, in the bone marrow. It is produced mainly by the peri-tubular capillary endothelial cells in the kidney but also in the liver.

Synthetic or pharmaceutical erythropoietins, Epoetins (Epos) or recombinant human erythropoietins (rhEpos), consist of epoetin alfa, beta, theta, and zeta. These erythropoiesis-stimulating agents (ESAs) are commercially available and are used to treat symptomatic anaemia associated with erythropoietin deficiency in chronic renal failure, to increase the yield of autologous blood in normal individuals and to shorten the period of symptomatic anaemia in patients receiving cytotoxic chemotherapy.

Darbepoetin is a hyperglycosylated derivative of epoetin; it has a longer half-life and can be administered less frequently than epoetin.

Methoxy polyethylene glycol-epoetin beta is a continuous erythropoietin receptor activator that is used for the treatment of symptomatic anaemia associated with chronic kidney disease. It has a longer duration of action than epoetin. The increase in red blood cell production is considered to be performance enhancing in endurance sports, such as middle or long distance running, cycling, skiing and swimming.

Detection of rhEpo

RhEpo was directly identified by urinalysis in 2000, when a test developed based on immunoelectrophoresis and double blotting (IEF/DB), was endorsed by the IOC and subsequently WADA [47]. It uses changes in the Epo isoform profile as detected by isoelectric focusing in polyacrylamide slab gels (IEF-PAGE).

The problem in detection has always been that the duration of the effect on performance is greater than the duration of any haematological changes associated with rhEpo use. Following discontinuation, red cell mass gradually returns to its original state but can take weeks, leaving an open window where there is no evidence of use but where performance is enhanced [48].

Testing for rhEpo in urine appears to be wrought with difficulties because the amount of endogenous Epo in urine, (urinary human epo, uhEpo) is extremely low [49]. The permeability of the renal tubules to Epo is complex. Exercise-induced renal ischaemia in conjunction with post-exercise proteinuria appears to affect the clearance of this peptide hormone. Also, by injecting microdoses of rhEpo, the window of detection can be reduced to as little as 12-18 hours post-injection [50].

Research on subjects who adminstered rhEpo for four weeks, with two weeks of "boosting", followed by two weeks of "maintenance" and a cessation period of three weeks, provided divisive results. A WADA "Laboratory A" determined rhEpo use in all subjects during the boosting period, whereas WADA "Laboratory B" found no use, with

Product	Pharmaceutical Manufacturer	Manufacturers Price	Mode of delivery
Genotropin® (somatropin/rhGH) two-compartment cartridge containing powder for reconstitution	Pharmacia	net price 5.3-mg (16-unit) cartridge = £122.87; 12-mg (36-unit) cartridge = £278.20	Subcutaneous/Intramuscular
Humatrope® (somatropin/rhGH) two-compartment cartridge containing powder for reconstitution	Lilly	net price 6-mg (18-unit) cartridge =£108.00; 24-mg (72-unit) cartridge = £432.00	Subcutaneous/Intramuscular
Norditropin® SimpleXx prefilled solution (somatropin 3.3 mg; 10 units/mL	Novo Nordisk	net price 1.5-mL (5-mg, 15-unit) cartridge = £106.35; 1.5-mL (15-mg, 45-unit) cartridge = £319.05	Subcutaneous/Intramuscular
Increlex® (Mecasermin 10 mg/mL; Recombinant human insulin-like growth factor-1; rhIGF-1)	Ipsen	net price 4-mL vial = £605.00	Subcutaneous/Intramuscular
Eprex® (prefilled syringe, epoetin alfa) (Recombinant human erythropoietin; rhEpo)	Janssen-Cilag	net price 1000 units = £5.53; 40 000 units = £265.48	Subcutaneous/Intravenous
NeoRecormon® (prefilled syringe, epoetin beta) (Recombinant human erythropoietin; rhEpo)	Roche	net price 500 units = £3.75; 30 000 units = £224.69	Subcutaneous/Intravenous
Aranesp® Erythropoetin; darbepoetin alfa, 25 micrograms/mL	Amgen	net price 0.4 mL (10 micrograms) = £14.68; 1 mL (500 micrograms) = £734.05	Subcutaneous/Intravenous

Table 3: Prescription only Medicines, Peptide hormones used in hormone replacement.

one sample to be negative, and the remaining seven to be suspicious. The detection rates decreased throughout the maintenance and post period when total haemoglobin mass and exercise performance were elevated. During this period, "*Laboratory A*" found only two of 24 samples to be positive and three to be suspicious, and "*Laboratory B*" found no positive or suspicious samples. This study demonstrated a poor correlation in test results comparing two WADA-accredited laboratories. Consequently, after the initial rhEpo "boosting" period the power to detect rhEpo use during the maintenance and post periods appeared minimal [51].

The development of new ESAs, has required advanced methods for detecting the abuse of these substances. Blood markers became crucial, because synthetic Epos, harvested in animal cells, were best confirmed in serum after immunoaffinity purification. With the development of "Dynepo" (manufactured in cultured human, not animal cells), the additional application of sodium dodecylsulfate-polyacrylamide gel electrophoresis (SDS-PAGE) became necessary. The development of the haematological "athlete's biological passport" is the most recent advancement in indirect testing for ESA doping. Longitudinal monitoring of blood profiles by comparing athletes' individual hematological values against their own historical baselines rather than a population-derived threshold enhances the efficacy of indirect testing.

Recent developments in "dope testing" for Epo include molecular mass-based methods. The molecular mass of most rhEpos is higher than for uhEpo, which can be shown by SDS-PAGE [52].

Consequently from 2006, Epo tests at the Olympics have been conducted on both blood and urine, in an attempt to identify dopers, but the method officially adopted by WADA for the confirmation of rhEpo, is still urinalysis and still based on a combination of IEF/DB and distinguishes between endogenous erythropoietin and rhEpo isoforms.

Any false-positive Epo test concerns that researchers had up to this period [53] were contested and refuted relying on scientific analytical rigour [54].

Does rhEpo Enhance Performance?

RhEpo can be administered subcutaneously or intravenously and has performance-enhancing effects due to the powerful stimulation of red blood cell production, improving maximal oxygen uptake ($\dot{V}O_2$max) thereby increasing delivery of oxygen to the exercising skeletal muscle.

It has been shown to increase maximal aerobic power [55] and $\dot{V}O_2$max [48]. Cyclists have confessed to using it throughout their career demonstrating the difficulty in detecting it and their belief in its performance enhancement [56].

However, there are dangers to the exercising athlete using rhEpo. Arterial systolic blood pressure (SBP) at rest remains unaltered before and after rhEpo admin. During submaximal exercise at 200 watts, corresponding to an average of approx 50% of $\dot{V}O_2$max SBP increases markedly from 177 to 191 mmHg, increasing stress on the heart during heavy strenuous and prolonged exercise [57]. During competition cycling and running, the average energy turn-over is often in the range of 75-85% of $\dot{V}O_2$max for long periods.

Athletes who abuse recombinant human erythropoietin (rhEPO) only want to pass the finishing line in first place and have no consideration for any potential health consequences [58]. Exercise in healthy non-doped individuals, elevates packed cell volume and the

dehydration associated with intense exercise can exacerbate blood viscosity which may expose previously undiagnosed cardiovascular abnormalities.

The use of rhEpo in chronic aerobic exercise, mimicking a sports doping model in rats, resulted in a sudden death episode during the eighth week, of a ten week trial [59]. The aetiology of death was suggested to be an elevation of packed cell volume, resulting in hyperviscosity, hypertension, cardiac hypertrophy, sympathetic and serotinergic overactivity. Post-mortem examination identified cerebral vascular congestion, left ventricular hypertrophy, and congestive hepatopathy caused by right-sided heart failure, which reinforced the hypothesis that there were several patho-physiological effects from rhEpo abuse.

Table 3 identifies genuine rhEpo and Table 4 identifies potential counterfeit rhEpo from an internet company.

MGF (IGF-I Ec peptide)

Muscle development must be under the control of local growth factors because if a specific muscle is mechanically overloaded, as in resistant exercise, it is that muscle and not all the muscles that undergo hypertrophy. Mechano growth factor (MGF) has been identified and appears to be derived from the IGF-I gene and has a unique C-terminal peptide (IGF-I Ec peptide). It has a molecular weight of 2868 daltons. After resistance exercise, which may cause disruption and damage to the myofibril cell membranes, the IGF-I gene predominantly produces the IGF-I splice variant IGF-I Ec peptide (MGF) which activates muscle stem (satellite) cells or muscle progenitor cells that provide the extra nuclei required for muscle hypertrophy, repair and maintenance. The appearance of MGF also up-regulates new protein synthesis. After this initial splicing of IGF-I into MGF, production then switches towards producing a systemic release of IGF-I Ea from the liver, which also up-regulates protein synthesis. The expression of IGF-I splice variants, over the course of the regeneration of muscle, following stress, is thought to be the primary anabolic mechanism by which the body repairs injuries or produces new muscle. Sarcopaenia and dystrophic muscle appear to have an impaired ability to express MGF or refresh the satellite cell pool [60].

Unlike mature IGF-I, the distinct E domain of MGF inhibits terminal differentiation whilst increasing myoblast proliferation. Blocking the IGF-I receptor with a specific antibody indicates that the function of MGF E domain is mediated via a different receptor, providing localised tissue adaptation and suggesting why loss of muscle mass occurs in the elderly and in dystrophic muscle in which MGF production is markedly affected [61]. Such potential has attracted the attention of commercial companies claiming to be able to manufacture such peptide hormones for athletic abuse. MGF is available commercially as an injectable peptide, and can be purchased from internet sites. It corresponds to the 24 most C-terminal residues of IGF-IEb, a different splice variant isoform of IGF-I and has anecdotally been shown to increase local muscle growth and cellular proliferation. However, no analogous peptide product of the IGF-I gene has been identified or isolated from cultured cells [62].

Research in humans, with MGF is currently under consideration.

Table 4 identifies a potential counterfeit MGF from an internet company.

A Myostatin Inhibitor (Follistatin)

Myostatin is a transforming growth factor-β (TGF-β) family member that plays an essential role in regulating skeletal muscle growth.

Product	Black-market Pharmaceutical Manufacturer	Black-market Wholesale Price	Black-market Retail Price
Peptide Hormones (Administration by Subcutaneous Injection)			
Hygetropin (rhGH) 100 IU	Hygene Biopharm Co.,Ltd.	£100	£140
GenLei® Jintropin™ (rhGH) 100 IU	Gene Science Pharmaceutical Co., Ltd.	£100	£140
Turbovital (rhIgf-1) 1000 mcg	Hygene Biopharm Co.,Ltd.	£200	£285
Growth Hormone Secretagogues			
Hexarelin/Sermorelin/Ipamorelin (growth hormone releasing hormones) 2mg/amp	ProPeptides Co., Ltd	£24	£50
Recombinant Human Erythropoietin-Alpha	Prospec Protein Specialist	5µg £32; 50µg £82; 1mg £940	5µg £50; 50µg £100; 1mg £1200
Myostatin inhibitor			
Follistatin 344 (5 mcg/amp)	Southern Research Co., Ltd	£62	£100
Mechano Growth Factor			
MGF (C-terminal) 2 mg amp	Peptide Labs Research Peptides	£18	£50

Key: amp = ampoule; rhGH = recombinant human growth hormone; rhIgf-1 = recombinant human insulin-like growth factor-1

Table 4: Counterfeit Peptide Hormone Doping Agents.

It acts as a negative regulator of skeletal muscle mass. Pharmacological agents capable of blocking myostatin activity may have applications for promoting muscle growth in human disease. Follistatin, also known as activin-binding protein is a peptide hormone, in humans, encoded by the FST gene. Follistatin is an autocrine glycoprotein that is expressed in nearly all tissues. It is part of the inhibin-activin-follistatin axis and is produced by folliculostellate (FS) cells of the anterior pituitary. In the tissues activin has a strong role in cellular proliferation, thereby making follistatin the safeguard against uncontrolled cellular proliferation and also allowing it to function as an instrument of cellular differentiation. Both of these roles are vital in tissue rebuilding and repair.

Follistatin has been assessed for its role in regulation of muscle growth in mice, as an antagonist to myostatin [63]. demonstrated that inhibition of myostatin, either by genetic elimination (knockout mice) or by increasing the amount of follistatin, resulted in greatly increased muscle mass. Mice that lack the gene that makes myostatin have roughly twice the amount of body muscle as normal. But mice without myostatin that also overproduce follistatin have about four times as much muscle as normal mice [64]. In 2009, research with Macaque monkeys demonstrated that regulating follistatin via gene therapy also resulted in muscle growth and increases in strength [65].

Such research paves the way for future control of disease states, but the application for the use of a myostatin inhibitor in sport is all too evident. There is currently no scientific proof that such a drug can benefit sport's performance in humans, however, multiple internet companies wax lyrical about the benefits of their products.

Table 4 identifies a potential counterfeit myostatin inhibitor (Follistatin 344) from an internet company.

Conclusion

The existence of high rewards from competitive sport will always predispose the more vulnerable athlete to experiment with the latest ergogenic aid or designer doping agent.

The presence of the internet would appear to be an effective market-place for the acquisition of such products and to negate the requirement of a personal physician. However, there are few safeguards to confirm the veracity of these agents and to protect such individuals willing to risk life and limb, in pursuit of gold.

Despite the increased intensity in anti-doping, a level playing field even exists for the cheating dope! Following the "accidental" ingestion of a banned substance by the less discerning athlete, a sport scientist is often required as an expert, to contest any charge of wrong-doing by a prosecuting authority [66].

References

1. Waddington I (1996) The development of sports medicine. Sociology of Sport 13: 176-196.

2. Franke WW, Berendonk B (1997) Hormonal doping and androgeniization of athletes: a secret program of the German Democratic Republic Goverment. Clin Chem 43: 1262-1279.

3. Todd T (1987) Anabolic steroids: the gremlins of sport. J Sport Hist 14: 87-107.

4. Fair JD (1993) Isometrics or Steroids? Exploring New Frontiers of Strength in the Early 1960s. Journal of Sport History 20: 1-24.

5. http://sportsanddrugs.procon.org/view.resource.php?resourceID=002366.

6. http://www.olympic.org/medical-commission.

7. Mottram DR (1999) Banned drugs in sport. Does the International Olympic Committee (IOC) list need updating? Sports Med 27: 1-10.

8. Donohoe T, Johnson N (1986) Foul play: Drug Abuse in Sports. Oxford: Blackwell Scientific Publications.

9. http://www.nytimes.com/keyword/ben-johnson.html

10. http://www.timesonline.co.uk/tol/sport/more_sport/athletics/article3942201.ece

11. http://news.bbc.co.uk/sport1/hi/olympics/athletics/7403158.stm

12. http://www.telegraph.co.uk/sport/othersports/drugsinsport/7293877.html

13. http://www.cyclingweekly.co.uk/news/latest/519647.html

14. http://www.perthnow.com.au/sport/marion-jones-letter-of-confession/story-e6frg1wu-1111114586262; http://www.sportsscientists.com/2007/10/marion-jones-self-confessed-drug-user.html

15. http://www.wada-ama.org/Documents/World_Anti-Doping_Program/WADP-The-Code/WADA_Anti-Doping_CODE_2009_EN.pdf.

16. Bamberger M, Yaeger D (1997) Over the edge. Sports Illustrated 14: 62-70.

17. Kicman AT, Gower DB (2003) Anabolic steroids in sport: biochemical, clinical and analytical perspectives. Ann Clin Biochem 40: 321-356.

18. Brooks RV, Firth RG, Sumner NA (1975) Detection of anabolic steroids by radioimmunoassay. Br J Sports Med 9: 89-92.

19. Ward RJ, Shackleton CH, Lawson AM (1975) Gas chromatographic mass spectrometric methods for the detection and identification of anabolic steroid drugs. Br J Sports Med 9: 93-97.

20. Oftebro H (1992) Evaluating an abnormal urinary steroid profile. Lancet 339: 941-942.

21. Garle M, Ocka R, Palonek E, Björkhem I (1996) Increased urinary testosterone epitestosterone ratios found in Swedish athletes in connection with a national control program: evaluation of 28 cases. J Chromatogr B Biomed Appl 687: 55-59.

22. Becchi M, Aguilera R, Farizon Y, Flament MM, Casabianca H, et al. (1994) Gas chromatography/combustion/isotope-ratio mass spectrometry analysis of urinary steroids to detect misuse of testosterone in sport. Rapid Commun Mass Spectrom 8: 304-308.

23. Bhasin S, Storer TW, Berman N, Callegari C, Clevenger B, et al. (1996) The effects of supraphysiologic doses of testosterone on muscle size and strength in normal men. N Engl J Med 335: 1-7.

24. http://www.wada-ama.org/en/Resources/Q-and-A/Lab-Statistics-Report/html.

25. Graham MR, Davies B, Grace FM, Kicman A, Baker JS (2008) Anabolic steroid use: patterns of use and detection of doping. Sports Med 38: 505-525.

26. http://www.premium-steroids.com/index.php?main_page=product_info&products_id=59.

27. Li CH, Evans HM (1944) The Isolation of Pituitary Growth Hormone. Science 99: 183-184.

28. Fryklund L (1986) Current research on recombinant human growth hormone and the related growth factors, IGF-I and GRF. Acta Paediatr Scand Suppl 325: 85-89.

29. Baumann G (1991) Growth hormone heterogeneity: genes, isohormones, variants, and binding proteins. Endocr Rev 12: 424-449.

30. Duchaine D (1982) Underground Steroid Handbook, 1st ed. California: HLR Technical Books 84: 30.

31. Salomon F, Cuneo RC, Hesp R, Sönksen PH (1989) The effects of treatment with recombinant human growth hormone on body composition and metabolism in adults with growth hormone deficiency. N Engl J Med 321: 1797-1803.

32. Rudman D, Feller AG, Nagraj HS, Gergans GA, Lalitha PY, et al. (1990) Effects of human growth hormone in men over 60 years old. N Engl J Med 323: 1-6.

33. Wallace JD, Cuneo RC, Baxter R, Orskov H, Keay N, et al. (1999) Responses of the growth hormone (GH) and insulin-like growth factor axis to exercise, GH administration, and GH withdrawal in trained adult males: a potential test for GH abuse in sport. J Clin Endocrinol Metab 84: 3591-3601.

34. Berggren A, Ehrnborg C, Rosén T, Ellegård L, Bengtsson BA, et al. (2005) Short-term administration of supraphysiological recombinant human growth hormone (GH) does not increase maximum endurance exercise capacity in healthy, active young men and women with normal GH-insulin-like growth factor I axes. J Clin Endocrinol Metab 90: 3268-3273.

35. Yarasheski KE, Zachweija JJ, Angelopoulos TJ, Bier DM (1993) Short-term growth hormone treatment does not increase muscle protein synthesis in experienced weight lifters. J Appl Physiol 74: 3073-3076.

36. Graham MR, Baker JS, Evans P, Kicman A, Cowan D, Hullin D, et al. (2008) Physical effects of short term rhGH administration in abstinent steroid dependency. Hormone Research 69: 343-354.

37. Le Roith D, Scavo L, Butler A (2001) What is the role of circulating IGF-I? Trends Endocrinol Metab 12: 48-52.

38. Wu Z, Bidlingmaier M, Dall R, Strasburger CJ (1999) Detection of doping with human growth hormone. Lancet 353: 895.

39. Powrie JK, Bassett EE, Rosen T, Jørgensen JO, Napoli R, et al. (2007) Detection of growth hormone abuse in sport. Growth Horm IGF Res 17: 220-226.

40. Kojima M, Hosoda H, Date Y, Nakazato M, Matsuo H, Kangawa K (1999) Ghrelin is a growth-hormone-releasing acylated peptide from stomach. Nature 9: 656-660.

41. Nagaya N, Moriya J, Yasumura Y, Uematsu M, Ono F, et al. (2004) Effects of ghrelin on left ventricular function, exercise capacity, muscle wasting in patients with chronic heart failure. Circulation 110: 3674-3679.

42. O'Reilly KE, Rojo F, She QB, Solit D, Mills GB, et al. (2006) mTOR inhibition induces upstream receptor tyrosine kinase signaling and activates Akt Cancer Res 66: 1500-1508.

43. Rinderknecht E, Humbel RE (1978) The amino acid sequence of human insulin-like growth factor I and its structural homology with proinsulin. J Biol Chem 253: 2769-2776.

44. Mauras N, Haymond MW (2005) Are the metabolic effects of GH and IGF-I separable. Growth Horm IGF Res 15: 19-27.

45. Milani D, Carmichael JD, Welkowitz J, Ferris S, Reitz RE, et al. (2004) Variability and reliability of single serum IGF-I measurements: impact on determining predictability of risk ratios in disease development. J Clin Endocrinol Metab 89: 2271-2274.

46. Guha N, Sönksen PH, Holt RI (2009) IGF-I abuse in sport: current knowledge and future prospects for detection. Growth Horm IGF Res 19: 408-4011.

47. Lasne F, de Ceaurriz J (2000) Recombinant erythropoietin in urine. Nature 405: 635.

48. Birkeland KI, Stray-Gundersen J, Hemmersbach P, Hallen J, Haug E, et al. (2000) Effect of rhEPO administration on serum levels of sTfR and cycling performance. Med Sci Sports Exerc 32: 1238-1243.

49. Delanghe JR, Joyner MJ (2008) Testing for recombinant human erythropoietin. J Appl Physiol 105: 395-396.

50. Ashenden M, Varlet-Marie E, Lasne F, Audran M (2006) The effects of microdose recombinant human erythropoietin regimens in athletes. Haematologica 91: 1143-1144.

51. Lundby C, Achman-Andersen NJ, Thomsen JJ, Norgaard AM, Robach P (2008) Testing for recombinant human erythropoietin in urine: problems associated with current anti-doping testing. J Appl Physiol 105: 417-419.

52. Reichel C (2011) Recent developments in doping testing for erythropoietin. Anal Bioanal Chem 401: 463-481.

53. Beullens M, Delanghe JR, Bollen M (2006) False-positive detection of recombinant human erythropoietin in urine following strenuous physical exercise. Blood 107: 4711-4713.

54. Catlin D, Green G, Sekera M, Scott P, Starcevic B (2006) False-positive Epo test concerns unfounded. Blood 108: 1779-17780.

55. Ekblom B, Berglund B (1991) Effect of rhEPO admin on maximal aerobic power in man. Medicine & Science in Sports & Exercise 1: 125-130.

56. http://news.bbc.co.uk/sport1/hi/other_sports/cycling/8694452.stm

57. Berglund B, Ekblom B (1991) Effect of rhEPO treatment on BP and haematological parameters in healthy males. Journal of Internal Medicine 229: 125-130.

58. Bamberger M, Yaeger D (1997) Over the edge. Sports Illustrated 14: 62-70.

59. Piloto N, Teixeira HM, Teixeira-Lemos E, Parada B, Garrido P, et al. (2009) Erythropoietin promotes deleterious cardiovascular effects and mortality risk in a rat model of chronic sports doping. Cardiovasc Toxicol 9: 201-210.

60. Goldspink G (2005) Research on mechano growth factor: its potential for optimising physical training as well as misuse in doping. Br J Sports Med 39: 787-788.

61. Yang SY, Goldspink G (2002) Different roles of the IGF-I Ec peptide (MGF) and mature IGF-I in myoblast proliferation and differentiation. FEBS Lett 522: 156-160.

62. Matheny RW, Nindl BC, Adamo ML (2010) Minireview: Mechano-growth factor:

a putative product of IGF-I gene expression involved in tissue repair and regeneration. Endocrinology 151: 865-875.

63. Lee SJ, McPherron AC (2001) Regulation of myostatin activity and muscle growth. Proc Natl Acad Sci USA 98: 9306-9311.

64. 'Mighty mice' made mightier http://www.eurekalert.org/pub_releases/2007-08/jhmi-mm082407.php.

65. "Success Boosting Monkey Muscle Could Help Humans" http://www.npr.org/templates/story/story.php?storyId=120316010.

66. Graham MR, Ryan P, Davies B, Evans PJ, Baker JS (2009) Dope Opera! Is Nandrolone a Medicine or Doping Agent? Journal of Exercise Physiology 12: 40-43.

8

Phytoestrogenic Compounds and Their Synthetic Analogs, Contrary to Estradiol- 17β Stimulates Human Derived Female Cultured Bone Cells in Hyperglycemic Conditions

D. Somjen[1], S. Katzburg[1], S. Tamir[2], O. Sharon, D. Hendel[3] and Y. Vaya[2]

[1]Institute of Endocrinology, Metabolism and Hypertension, Tel-Aviv Sourasky Medical Center; Tel-Aviv 64239, and the Sackler Faculty of Medicine, Tel-Aviv University, Tel-Aviv, Israel

[2]Laboratory of Human Health and Nutrition Sciences, MIGAL-Galilee Technology Center, Kiryat- Shmona 11016

[3]Department of Orthopedic Surgery, Shaarei- Zedek Medical Center, Jerusalem, Israel

Abstract

Cultured female- derived human osteoblasts (hObs) responded by different parameters to the phytoestrogens: daidzein (D), glabrene (Gla) and glabridin (Glb), to their synthetic derivatives; carboxy-daidzein (cD) and to estradiol-17β (E_2). Since the skeletal protective effects of estrogens are not discernible in diabetic women, we tested the effects of these compounds on hObs grown in growth medium with high glucose (HG; 9.0g/L; 44mM) compared to normal glucose (NG; 4.5g/L; 22mM) using the stimulation of creatine kinase specific activity (CK) and ^{3}[H] thymidine incorporation into DNA (DNA) as hormonal responsiveness markers. HG slightly increased DNA and CK in hObs. Stimulations by E_2 was abolished and by cD and D was slightly decreased in HG, but not by Gla and Glb in both age groups. Growing hObs in HG upregulated the expression of mRNA of both ER and ERβ in cells from pre- but not from post-menopausal women. Cells from both age groups express also mRNA for 25 hydroxy vitamin D_3 1-α hydroxylase and showed enzymic activity which were down-regulated by HG in both age groups. Whether Gla and Glb act differentially via ERs and/or 1-α hydroxylase is not yet established. Since these compounds are active even in HG, they might be used for treating hyperglycemic/diabetic women.

Keywords: Human derived bone cells; Hyperglycemia; Estradiol-17β; Phytoestrogens; DNA synthesis; Creatine kinase

Introduction

We have previously studied the effects of estrogens on bone in a rat model [1-3] using the increase in the specific activity of creatine kinase as a response marker. The brain type (BB) isoenzyme of creatine kinase (CK) which is part of the "energy buffer" system, regulates the cellular concentration of ATP and ADP, is the major component of the "E_2-induced protein" of rat uterus [4] and is an efficient response marker to detect activity of E_2 as well as other estrogenic compounds, in bone cells *in vivo* and *in vitro* [1,5] which contain low concentrations of E_2 receptors [6,7]. Notably, the stimulation of CK in cultured bone cells, correlated with increased DNA synthesis in bone, requires the higher end of the physiological range of estrogen concentrations [1,5].

Estrogen is well known for its beneficial effect in osteoporosis [8]. Osteoporosis is characterized by reduction in bone mineral density, with the result of fracture after minimal trauma. The effect of estrogen in the different tissues is initiated by its binding to estrogen receptors (ERs). Two ERs have been identified, ER and ERβ, which differ in their structure and tissue distribution [9]. Estrogen deficiency is known to be involved in osteoporosis [10], which affects every third woman above the age of 65. Although estrogen treatment is efficient in preventing bone loss, it can also stimulate the growth of estrogen-dependent tumors. Hence, new compounds, which can replace current hormone replacement therapy treatments with no such deleterious effects, are highly desirable [11].

In human- derived cultured osteoblasts (hObs), we found that E_2 increased cell proliferation and CK specific activity in a gender specific manner [12] as a response marker for hormonal treatment beyond estrogen itself in cells containing the relevant receptors.

Phytoestrogens are heterogenous group of plant-derived compounds some of which are selective estrogen receptor modulators (SERMs). All phytoestrogens are polyphenolic compounds with structural similarities to natural and synthetic estrogens; however they bind to the estrogen receptors with much lower affinity than E_2 [13]. Soybeans and soy foods are the most significant dietary sources of the isoflavone class of phytoestrogens, which includes genistein, daidzein and biochainin A [14,15] and have estrogenic action on bone and the cardiovascular system but have anti-estrogenic action on breast cancer [16].

Diabetes has been associated with a net loss of bone [17,18], with reduction of new bone formation and decreased bone mineral density. In diabetic mice the up-regulation of specific transcription factors is attenuated, resulting in deficiency in conversion of mesenchymal cells to osteoblasts [17,18].

In the present study we analyzed the effects of high glucose on the response to phytoestrogens and their synthetic derivatives of human-derived cultured bone cells, which is relevant at least to some of the important factors existing in diabetes. The compounds we analyzed were the licorice derived compounds glabrene (Gla) and glabridin (Glb) [19], the carboxy-derivative of daidzein (cD) [20] and the phytoestrogen from soy the daidzein (D) [21] similar to the synthetic derivatives of D the DT56a (femarelle) [22].

*Corresponding author: Dalia Somjen PhD, Institute of Endocrinology, Metabolism and Hypertension, Tel-Aviv Sourasky Medical Center, 6 Weizman St. Tel-Aviv, 64239 Israel, E-mail: dalias@ tasmc.health.gov.il

Materials and Methods

Reagents

All reagents used were analytical grade. Estradiol-17β (E_2), daidzein (D) and the creatine kinase (CK) assay kit were purchased from Sigma Chemicals Co. (St. Louis, MO). Carboxy-D (cD) was synthesized by us [20], licorice products: Gla and Glb were produced by us [19].

Cell cultures

Human bones were obtained from biopsies of patients undergoing corrective surgery following accidental injury, hip or knee replacement. All patients (women and men) were healthy, non-osteoporotic and not receiving hormonal replacement treatment. Three groups were defined: Pre-menopausal women, ranging between 37- 55 years old, (n=5). Post-menopausal women, ranging between 60- 84 years old, (n=5). The non-enzymic method for isolation and culture of human bone cells and their characterization as osteoblasts was described previously [12]. Briefly, samples of the trabecular surface of the iliac crest or long bones were cut into $1mm^3$ pieces and extensively and repeatedly washed with phosphate buffered saline (PBS) to remove blood components. The explants, with no enzymatic digestion, were seeded in 100mm diameter tissue culture dishes and incubated in DMEM medium without Ca^{++} (to avoid fibroblastic growth [12], containing 10% fetal calf serum (FCS) and antibiotics. Cell outgrowth from the bone explants was apparent after 6-10 days. First passage cells were seeded at a density of $3x10^5$ cells per 35mm tissue culture dish in phenol red free DMEM with 10% charcoal stripped FCS and incubated at 37°C in 5% CO_2. To obtain "high glucose" (HG) conditions, the medium including the FCS, was supplemented with glucose up to a final concentration of 44nM (9.0gm/liter). Glucose concentration in the regular medium (NG) was 22nM (4.5gm/liter).

Hormonal treatment

At sub-confluence cells were treated with 30nM E_2, 300nM cD, Gla or Glb and D at 3µM for 24h, followed by harvesting for CK or for DNA synthesis assays.

Creatine kinase (CK) extraction and assay

Cells were scraped off the culture dishes and homogenized by freezing and thawing three times in cold isotonic extraction buffer [12]. Supernatant extracts were obtained by centrifugation at 14000xg for 5 min at 4°C in an Eppendorf micro- centrifuge. Creatine kinase specific activity (CK) was measured in a Kontron Model 922 Uvicon Spectrophotometer at 340nm using a Sigma coupled assay kit (procedure 47-UV). Protein was assayed by Coomassie brilliant blue dye binding, using BSA as the standard [12].

Assessment of DNA synthesis

Cells were grown until sub- confluence and then treated with various hormones as indicated for CK. Twenty-two hours later [³H] thymidine was added for 2h. Cells were then treated with 10% ice-cold trichloroacetic acid (TCA) for 5min and washed twice with 5% TCA and then with cold ethanol. The cellular layer was dissolved in 0.3ml of 0.3N NaOH, samples were aspirated and [³H] thymidine incorporation into DNA was determined [23].

Competitive binding assay for membrane estrogen binding activity

Cells were cultured in 24-well plates ($4x10^5$ cells/well) for 48h and washed once with ice-cold binding medium (DMEM + 0.1% BSA and 25mM HEPES, pH 7.4) using reaction conditions as described previously [21]. Subsequently, cells were incubated for 90min at 4°C with either of the steroid protein conjugates (estradiol 6-carboxymethyl-oxime; E_2-6-CMO-ovalbumin [26-29], 10µM/well, E_2-Ov conjugate labeled with Europium (1:1000, 200µl in binding medium) were then added and the incubation was continued for another 60 minutes at 4°C. Binding was terminated by four successive washes with ice-cold binding medium. Enhancement solution (300µl/well) was then added to the cells, and the samples (200µl) were collected for fluorescence determination using an Arcus time resolved fluorometer (Wallac, Turku, Finland) [21, 23, 24]. Specific binding was defined as total binding of Europium protein conjugates minus binding in the presence of a 500 folds excess of conjugated estrogenic compounds or E_2 where appropriate.

Competitive binding assay for intracellular estrogen binding activity

Cells grown, cultured and washed as described above, were incubated for 60min at 37°C with ³[H] E_2 with or without excess of different unlabelled estrogenic compounds. Binding was terminated by four successive washes with ice-cold binding medium, and cellular content of ³[H] E_2 was measured in a Packard tricarb scintillation counter [21]. Specific binding was defined as the total binding of ³[H] E_2 minus binding in the presence of a 500 folds excess of free estrogenic compounds.

Determination of mRNA for ERα and ER by real time PCR

RNA was extracted from cultured human bone cells, shown previously [28] to contain ERα and ERβ by western blot analysis [5], and subjected to reverse transcription as previously described [20]. For ERα, we used 5µl of cDNA in the reaction mixture with the primers 5' AATTCTGACAATCGACGCCAG 3' (forward) and 5' GTGCTTCAACATTCTCCCTCCTC 3' (reverse). For ERβ, the same amount of cDNA was used with the primers 5' TGCTTTGGTTTGGGTGATTGC 3' (forward) and 5' TTTGCTTTTACTGTCCTCTGC 3' (reverse). The reaction was carried out for 30 cycles at 94°C, for 30 sec at 58°C and at 72°C for 1 min; ERα and ERβ cDNA were used as standard controls and compared to RNAse P as internal control for mRNA.

Determination of mRNA for 25 hydroxy vitamin D_3 1-α hydroxylase (1-OHASe) by real time PCR

Total RNA from cultured hOB was extracted using the Trizol Reagent (Gibco). An aliquot of 1µg RNA from each sample was reverse transcribed (RT) using Advantage RT for PCR kit (Clonthec), as previously described [25]. 1-OHase mRNA levels were analyzed using the ABI 7700 sequence detection system. Amplification of its cDNA was performed in 25µl of the sample on 96 wells plates in a reaction buffer containing Taqman universal PCR master kit. The sequences of nucleotides were as follows; forward primers: CACCCGACACGGAGCCTT; reverse primers: TCAACAGTGGACACAAACA; Taqman probe: TCCGCGCTGTGGGCTCGG. RNAse P expression served as an internal control for each sample and was performed by an assay on demand gene expression products, which consists of a 20x mixture of unlabeled PCR primers and Taqman MGB probe labeled with 5' carboxy fluorescein (FAM) dye. Measurements were performed in triplicates. The PCR conditions were: 50°C for 2min, 95°C for 15sec and 60°C for 1min. The total volume of the reaction was 25µl ; 12.5µl universal master mix, 1.25µl 20x assay on demand mix and 11.25µl cDNA [25].

Assesment of 25 hydroxy vitamin D₃ 1-α hydroxylase activity

25 hydroxy vitamin D_3 1-α hydroxylase activity was assessed by the measurement of 1,25 $(OH)_2D_3$ (1,25D) generated in hObs within 60min after the addition of 25(OH)D_3 (200ng/ml) to culture, using 1,25D ^{125}I RIA kit from DiaSorin, Mn, USA [25]. Protein of the layer was assayed by the Bradford method.

Statistical significance

The significance of differences between experimental and control values P, was evaluated using a non-paired, two-tailed Student's *t*-test in which n=number of donors.

Results

Expression and modulation of ERα and ERβ in human female-derived osteoblasts by high glucose

Female- derived osteoblasts from both age groups expressed mRNA for both ERα and ERβ as measured by real time PCR (Figure 1). The ratio of ERα To ERβ was 121:1 in pre- and 77:1 in post-menopausal derived osteoblasts with no significant difference between the mRNA levels in both age groups. High glucose increased the expression of both ERα and ERβ, in female- derived cells from both age groups with higher effect in pre-menopausal Obs (Figure 1).

Modulation of creatine kinase specic activity in response to different phytoestrogens in human female-derived osteoblasts in high glucose medium

Female derived hObs treated with E_2, Gla, Glb, cD or D for 24 h, showed a significant increase in CK specific activity in both age groups (Figure 2). The response of pre-menopausal cells was higher with E_2 and D whereas Gla was more effective in post-menopausal osteoblasts, and no age dependent difference was observed in treatments with Glb or cD (Figure 2). Growing the cells in HG increased constitutive level of the specific activity of CK in pre-menopausal osteoblasts by 46±5% and in post- menopausal osteoblasts by 34±8%. Growth of the cells in high glucose led to abolishment of the response of CK specific activity

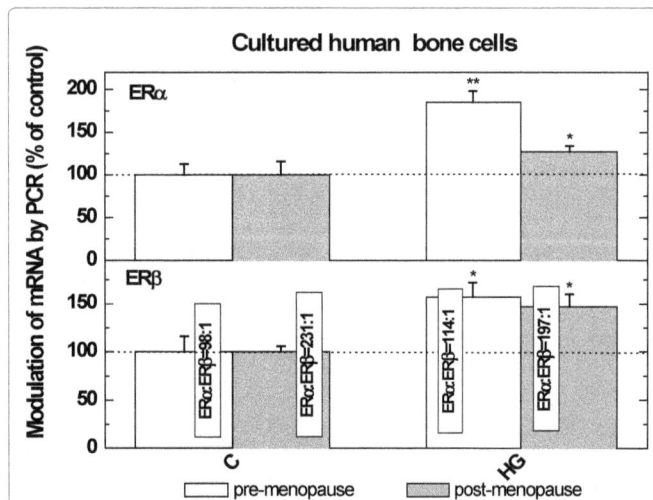

Figure 2: Stimulation of CK specific activity by different phytoestrogens and E_2 in primary bone-derived cells, from pre- and post- menopausal women, grown at different glucose concentrations; either normal (NG; 22mM) or high (HG; 44mM gray bars) glucose concentrations. Bone cells were cultured, treated and assayed for CK activity as described in Materials and Methods. Cells were treated for 24h with vehicle or 30nM E_2 or 300nM of cD, Gla or Glb or 3000nM of D. Results are means ± SEM for triplicate cultures from 5 women/group for each group. Control means of CK specific activity were 28.6±6.5 and 24.6±4.0nmol/min/mg protein, for pre- and post-menopausal women respectively. Experimental means compared to control means: *, $P < 0.05$; **, $P < 0.01$; ***, $P < 0.001$. Means of cells at HG+ estrogenic compounds vs. cells at NG+ estrogenic compound: #, $P < 0.05$; ##, $P < 0.01$.

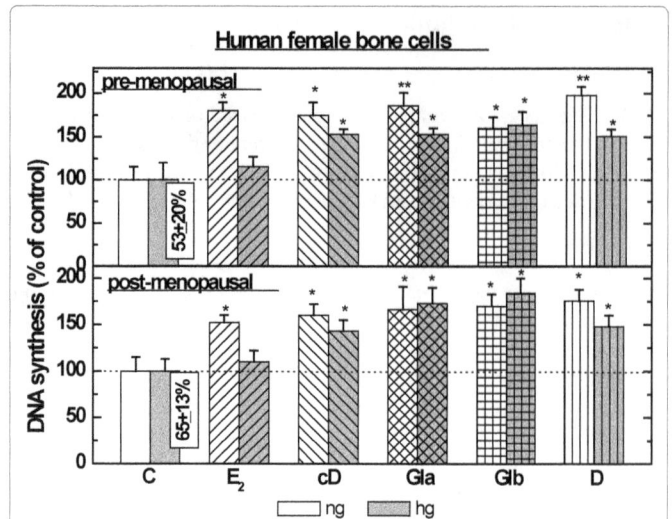

Figure 3: Stimulation of DNA synthesis by the different phytoestrogens and E_2 in primary bone-derived cells from pre- and post-menopausal women, grown at different glucose concentrations either normal (4.5g/L; 22mM light) or high (9.0g/L; 44mM gray bars) glucose concentrations. Bone cells were cultured, treated and assayed for CK activity as described in Materials and Methods. Cells were treated for 24h with vehicle or 30nM E_2 or 300nM of cD, Gla or Glb or 3000nM of D. Results are means ± SEM for triplicate cultures from 5 women/group for each group. Control means of CK specific activity were 3870± 350 and 3460± 400dpm/well, for pre- and post-menopausal women respectively. Experimental means compared to control means: *, $P < 0.05$; **, $P < 0.01$; ***, $P < 0.001$. Means of cells at HG+ estrogenic compounds vs. cells at NG+ estrogenic compound: #, $P < 0.05$; ##, $P < 0.01$.

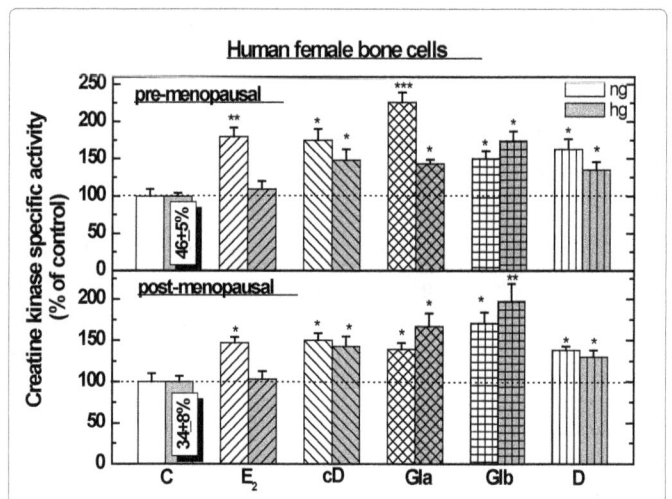

Figure 1: Modulation by hyperglycemia of the expression of mRNA for ERα and ERβ in primary human female- derived osteoblasts. Bone cells were obtained and cultured, and extracts prepared for real time PCR analysis as described in Materials and Methods. Results are means SEM for triplicate cultures from 5 donors for each group. Means of cells grown in high glucose (grey bars) were compared to cells grown in normal glucose (open bars): *, $P < 0.05$; **, $P < 0.01$.

to treatment with E_2, slightly reduction in the response to cD or D but did not change the response to Gla or Glb in cells from both age groups (Figure 2).

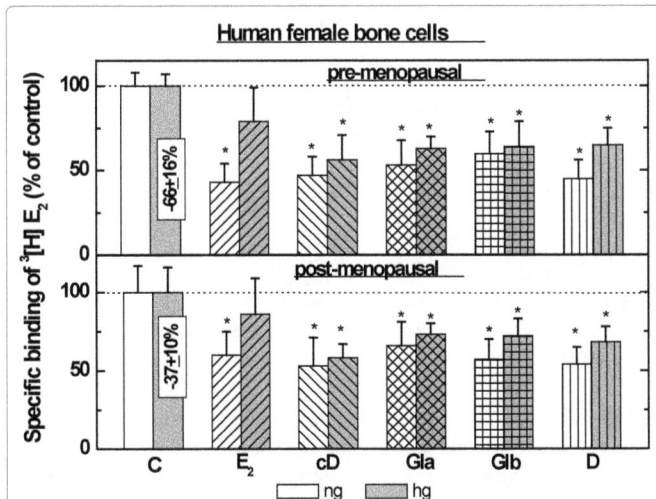

Figure 4: Modulation of the specific binding of estrogenic compounds to nuclear binding sites in primary bone-derived cells from pre- and post- menopausal women, grown at different glucose concentrations either normal (NG; 22mM) or high (HG; 44mM gray bars) glucose concentrations. Bone cells were cultured, treated and assayed for nuclear binding of ^{3}[H] E_2 as described in Materials and Methods. Results are means ± SEM for % of specific binding of triplicate cultures in the presence of 500 fold excess concentration of the different phytoestrogens as competitors. Experimental means compared to control means: *, $P < 0.05$.

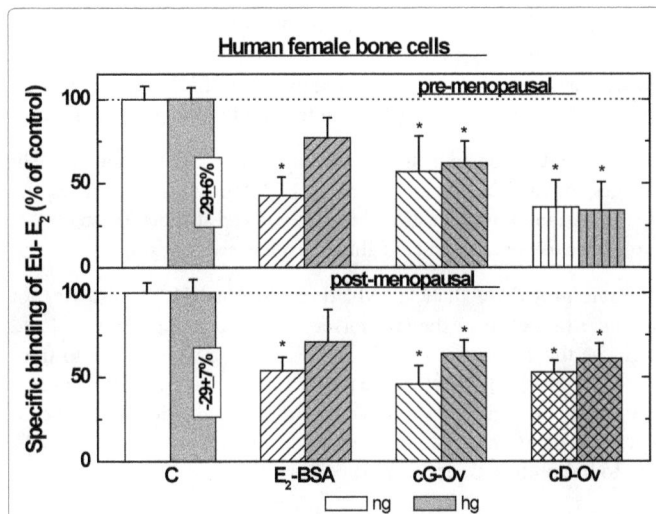

Figure 5: Modulation of the specific binding of estrogenic compounds to membranal binding sites in primary bone-derived cells from pre- and post-menopausal women, grown at different glucose concentrations either normal (NG; 22mM) or high (HG; 44mM gray bars) concentrations. Bone cells were cultured, treated and assayed for membranal binding of Eu- Ov- E_2 as described in Materials and Methods. Results are means ± SEM for % of specific binding of triplicate cultures in the presence of 500 fold concentration of the different phytoestrogenic-protein conjugates as competitors. Experimental means compared to control means: *, $P < 0.05$.

Modulation of DNA synthesis response to different phytoestrogens in human female-derived osteoblasts by high glucose

Female- derived hObs treated with E_2, Gla, Glb, cD and D for 24 h, showed a significant increase in DNA synthesis in both age groups (Figure 3). The response of pre-menopausal cells was higher with E_2 and D treatments whereas no age dependent difference with the other compounds (Figure 3). Growing the cells in HG increased basal level of DNA synthesis in pre-menopausal osteoblasts by 53±20% and in post-

menopausal osteoblasts by 65±13%. Growth of the cells in high glucose led to abolishment of the response of DNA synthesis to treatment with E_2, slightly reduction in the response to cD or D but did not change the response to Gla or Glb cells from both age groups (Figure 3).

Intracellular binding of the different phytoestrogens and its modulation in human female derived- osteoblasts in high glucose medium

Both pre- and post- menopausal human female-derived osteoblasts

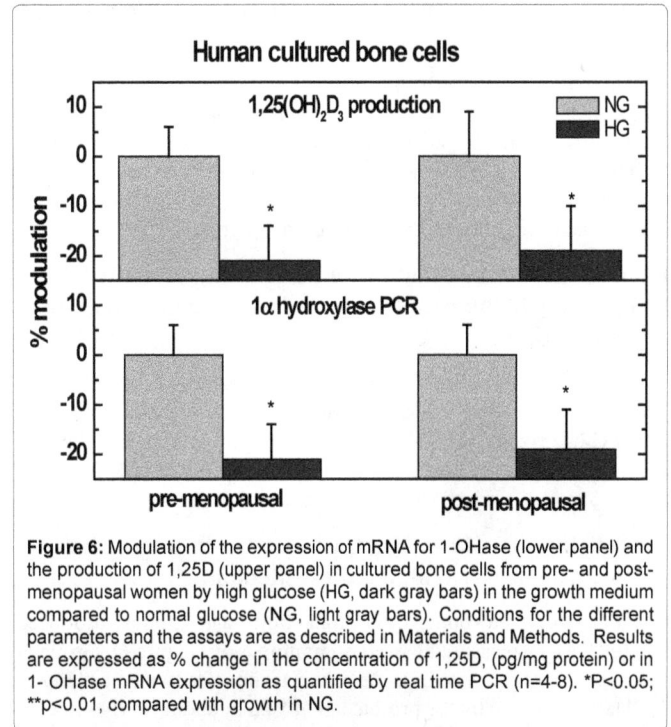

Figure 6: Modulation of the expression of mRNA for 1-OHase (lower panel) and the production of 1,25D (upper panel) in cultured bone cells from pre- and post-menopausal women by high glucose (HG, dark gray bars) in the growth medium compared to normal glucose (NG, light gray bars). Conditions for the different parameters and the assays are as described in Materials and Methods. Results are expressed as % change in the concentration of 1,25D, (pg/mg protein) or in 1- OHase mRNA expression as quantified by real time PCR (n=4-8). *P<0.05; **p<0.01, compared with growth in NG.

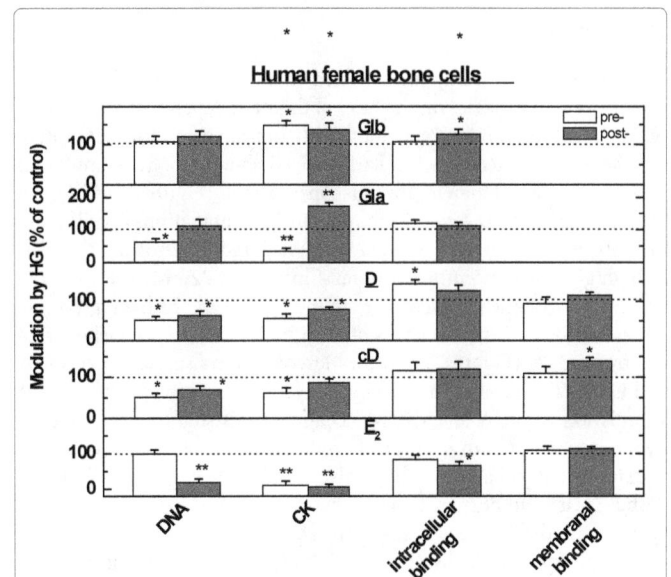

Figure 7a and 7b: Summary of the effects of HG on responses of cultured bone cells from pre- and post-menopausal women, to the different hormones on the different parameters as described in the legends to previous figs. *P<0.05; **p<0.01, compared with control incubates containing the vehicle for the active compound only.

(Obs) demonstrated specific binding of ^{3}[H] E$_2$ (Figure 4) which is competed for by the different phytoestrogens, presumably to predominantly nuclear under these conditions (37° for 60min). All phytoestrogens tested for competition with ^{3}[H] E$_2$, showed significant binding in both age groups. Growing the cells in HG decreased the specific binding of E$_2$ but not that of the other phytoestrogens in their competition of binding of ^{3}[H] E$_2$ in cells from both age groups (Figure 4). Also the total binding was increased by 57-66% at both age groups.

Modulation of specific membranal binding of the different phytoestrogens in human female- derived osteoblasts in high glucose medium

Growth of female derived osteoblasts from both age groups at high glucose concentration decreased total binding of Eu– Ov- E$_2$ in both age groups but did not affect the competition with E$_2$-BSA or cD-Ov in both age groups, but the competition with cD-Ov was decreased slightly but not statistically significant (Figure 5). Also the total binding was increased significantly by 29% at both age groups.

Expression and modulation of 25 hydroxy vitamin D$_3$ 1-α hydroxylase in human female-derived osteoblasts in high glucose medium

Female-derived bone cells from both ages expressed mRNA for 25 hydroxy vitamin D$_3$ 1-α hydroxylase (1-OHase) as measured by real time PCR, corrected for RNAse P mRNA (Figure 6). Growing the cells in high glucose in the medium decreased the expression of 1-OHase by about 35 to 65% respectively, in both age groups.

Modulation of 1, 25 (OH)$_2$D$_3$ production in human female-derived osteoblasts in high glucose medium

Female-derived bone cells from both age groups produced 1,25(OH)$_2$D$_3$ as measured by radio-immunoassay (Figure 6). Growing the cells in high glucose in the medium resulted decreased activity of 1-OHase measured by the production of 1,25 by about 80-70% in cells from both age groups (Figure 6).

Discussion

The estrogenic compounds tested in our studies can be divided roughly into two classes on the basis of their age dependent stimulation of DNA synthesis and CK specific activity in primary cultures of human female derived-osteoblast. Similarly to E$_2$, D showed higher stimulation in pre-menopausal than in post-menopausal cells (Figures 2 and 3). On the other hand cD, D, Gla, Glb showed similar stimulations in cells from pre- or post-menopausal women (Figures 2 and 3). Growing the cells in high glucose concentration (44mM instead of 22mM) sharpens the ability to distinguish between the groups. First of all, the hyperglycemia increased the constitutive levels of DNA by 53-65% respectively and of CK by 46-34% (Figures 2 and 3). Moreover, the stimulation of DNA and CK by E$_2$ was abolished by hyperglycemia in both age groups, the stimulation of DNA and CK by cD and D was slightly decreased by hyperglycemia in both age groups, while the effects of Gla and Glb were not significantly changed by hyperglycemia in either age group (Figures 2 and 3). It is important to note that the constitutive levels of DNA synthesis and CK specific activitybwere increased by hyperglycemia in age group bone cells (Figures 2 and 3).In order to understand the mechanism of the changes induced by hyperglycemia in the present study, we show that the abolition of estrogenic stimulation by hyperglycemia occurs in our non-transformed human-derived primary osteoblasts, was accompanied in contrast, by increases in mRNA levels of ERα and to less extent in ERβ in female cells at both ages (Figure 1).

We also analyzed total cellular (mainly nuclear) and membranal estrogen binding in the different cells. While in normal hObs, the phytoestrogens tested, were bound to both nuclear and membranal sites, with no age-dependent difference in the binding. This parallels our previous findings [21,23,24] using human vascular smooth muscle cells. Attempt to correlate estrogen receptors mRNAs with the changes in nuclear and/or membrane binding failed also in these vascular cells [21,23,24].

The high glucose abolished nuclear binding (Figure 4) of E$_2$ but not the phytoestrogenic compounds tested are parallel to the decreased responsiveness by growth in high glucose (Figures 2 and 3) but opposite to the increases in ERs mRNA (Figure 1). Also the membranal binding of E$_2$, as well as the other phytoestrogens tested was not affected by hyperglycemia (Figure 5). Membranal binding is therefore not correlated with the abolishment of DNA synthesis and CK specific activity stimulated by E$_2$ and the slight reduction of the stimulations by some of the phytoestrogens used in hyperglycemia (Figure 7a and b). This indicates that membranal mediated pathways are not involved in DNA and CK stimulation by estrogenic compounds tested in this study and others [24] as it is mainly nuclear receptor mediated. This finding is in accordance with our previous finding that impermeable protein-bound hormones were unable to stimulate CK in human vascular smooth muscle cells in the manner that E$_2$ and phytoestrogens do, but they bind to membranal binding sites [21,23,24].

When we assayed the changes in ERs mRNA expression by real time PCR, while ERα and ERβ mRNA were found in both ages of female-derived bone cells at higher abundance of ERα, hyperglycemia increased ERα and ERβ expression in female-derived cells (Figure 1).

The modulation of ERs is a recent addition to the spectrum of changes induced by hyperglycemia [21,23,24], which stimulates the differentiation of osteoblasts and osteoclasts and stimulates osteoblasts to produce osteocalcin and alkaline phosphatase.

Bone growth in diabetes which is disturbed [17,28] is also not enhanced to the same extent by hormone replacement therapy [26] and might be the result of lower hip BMD in young women due to their type 1 diabetes [27]; therefore the use of the specific phytoestrogens and their synthetic derivatives that we use in this study, might provide an alternative solution. Further studies in this direction in animal models have to be conducted for this purpose.

References

1. Somjen D, Weisman Y, Harell A, Berger E, Kaye AM (1989) Direct and sex specific stimulation by sex steroids of creatine kinase activity and DNA synthesis in rat bone. Proc Natl Acad Sci U S A 86: 3361- 3363.

2. Somjen D, Weisman Y, Mor Z, Harell A, Kaye AM (1991) Regulation of proliferation of rat cartilage and bone by sex steroid hormones. J Steroid Biochem Mol Biol 40: 717-723.

3. Kaye A M, Weisman Y, Harell A, Somjen D (1990) Hormonal stimulation of bone cell proliferation. J Steroid Biochem Mol Biol 37: 431- 435.

4. Reiss N, Kaye AM (1981) Identification of the major component of the estrogen induced protein of rat uterus as the BB isozyme of creatine kinase. J Biol Chem 256: 5741-5749.

5. Fournier B, Haring S, Kaye AM, Somjen D (1996) Stimulation of creatine kinase specific activity in human osteoblast and endometrial cells by estrogens and anti-estrogens and its modulation by calciotropic hormones. J Endocrinol 150: 275-285.

6. Eriksen EF, Colard DS, Berg NJ, Graham ML, Mann KG, et al. (1988) Evidence of estrogen receptors in normal human osteoblast- like cells. Science 241: 84-86.

7. Komm BS, Terpening CM, Benz DJ, Graeme KA, Kox M, et al. (1988) Estrogen binding, receptor mRNA, and biological response in osteoblast- like osteosarcoma cells. Science 241: 81-84.

8. Manolagas SC, Kousteni S, Jilka RL (2002) Sex steroids and bone. Recent Progr Horm Res 57: 385-409.

9. Enmark E, Gustafsson JA (1999) Oestrogen receptors - an overview. J Intern Med 246: 133-138.

10. Delmas PD (2000) Treatment of postmenopausal osteoporosis. Lancet 359: 2018- 2026.

11. Miksicek RJ (1994) Interaction of naturally occurring non-steroidal estrogens with expressed recombinant human estrogen receptor. J Steroid Biochem Mol Biol 49: 153-160.

12. Katzburg S, Ornoy A, Hendel D, Lieberherr M, Kaye AM, et al. (2001) Age and gender specific stimulation of creatine kinase specific activity by gonadal steroids in human bone-derived cells in culture. J Endocrin Invest 24: 166- 172.

13. Setchell KD, Lydeking-Olsen E (2003) Dietary phytoestrogens and their effect on bone: evidence from in vitro and in vivo, human observational, and dietary intervention studies. Amer J Clin Nutr 78: 593S-609S.

14. Brzezinski A, Debi A (1999) Phytoestrogens: the "natural" selective estrogen receptor modulators? J Obstet Gynecol Reprod Biol 85: 47-51.

15. Tham DM, Gardner CD, Haskell WL (1998) Potential health benefits of dietary Phyto-estrogens: A review of the clinical, epidemiological, and mechanistic evidence. J Clin Endocrinol Metab 83: 2223- 2235.

16. Morabito N, Crisafulli A, Vergara C, Gaudio A, Lasco A, et al. (2002) Effects of genistein and hormone-replacement therapy on bone loss in early postmenopausal women: a randomized double-blind placebo-controlled study. J Bone Miner Res 17: 1904-1912.

17. He H, Liu R, Desta T, Leon C, Gerstenfeld LC, et al. (2004) Diabetes causes decreased osteoclastogenesis, reduced bone formation and enhanced apoptosis of osteoblastic cells in bacteria stimulated bone loss. Endocrinology 145: 447-452.

18. Katzburg S, Lieberherr M, Ornoy A, Klein BY, Hendel D, et al. (1999) Isolation and hormonal responsiveness of primary cultures of human bone-derived cells: gender and age differences. Bone 25: 667-673.

19. Somjen D, Katzburg S, Vaya J, Kaye AM, Hendel D, et al. (2004) Estrogenic activity of glabridin and glabrene from licorice roots on human osteoblasts and prepubertal rat skeletal tissues. J Steroid Biochem Mol Biol 91: 241-246.

20. Somjen D, Zaltsman Y, Gayer B, Kulik T, Knoll E, et al. (2002) 6-Carboxymethyl genistein: A novel selective oestrogen receptor modulator (SERM) with unique differential effects on the vasculature, bone and uterus. J Endocrinol 173: 415-427.

21. Somjen D, Kohen F, Lieberherr M, Gayer B, Schejter E, et al. (2005) Membranal effects of phytoestrogens and carboxy derivatives of phytoestrogens on human vascular and bone cells: New insights based on studies with carboxy-biochanin A. J Steroid Biochem Mol Biol 93: 293- 303.

22. Somjen D, Katzburg S, Sharon O, Hendel D, Yoles I (2011) DT56a (Femarelle), contrary to estradiol-17β, is effective in human derived female osteobl asts in hyperglycemic condition. J Steroid Biochem Mol Biol 123: 25-29.

23. Somjen D, Kohen F, Gayer B, Sharon O, Limor R, et al. (2004) Role of putative membrane receptors in estradiol on human vascular cell growth. Amer J Hyperten 17: 462- 469.

24. Somjen D, Paller CJ, Gayer B, Kohen F, Knoll E, et al. (2004) High glucose blocks estradiol's effects on human vascular cell growth: differential interaction with estradiol and raloxifene. J Steroid Biochem Mol Biol 88: 101-110.

25. Somjen D, Katzburg S, Stern N, Kohen F, Sharon O, et al. (2007) 25 Hydroxy- vitamin D₃- 1α Hydroxylase expression and activity in cultured human osteoblasts and their modulation by parathyroid hormone, estrogenic compounds and dihydrotestosterone. J Steroid Biochem Mol Biol 107: 238-244.

26. Effects of menopause and estrogen replacement therapy or hormone replacement therapy in women with diabetes mellitus: Consensus opinion of The North American Menopause Society. (2000) Menopause 7: 87-95.

27. Liu EY, Wactawaski- Wende J, Donhaue RP, Dmochowski J, Hovey KM, et al. (2003) Does low bone mineral density start in post- teenage years in women with type 1 diabetes? Diabetes Care 26: 2365-2369.

28. Somjen D, Katzburg S, Sharon O, Kaye AM, Gayer B, et al. (2004) Modulation of response to estrogens in cultured human female bone cells by a non-calcemic Vitamin D analog: changes in nuclear and membranal binding. J Steroid Biochem Mol Biol 89-90: 393-395.

9

Rapid Action of Aldosterone on Protein Expressions of Protein Kinase C Alpha and Alpha1 Sodium Potassium Adenosine Triphosphatase in Rat Kidney

Somchit Eiam-Ong[1]*, Kittisak Sinphitukkul[1], Krissanapong Manotham[2] and Somchai Eiam-Ong[3]

[1]Department of Physiology, Faculty of Medicine, Chulalongkorn University, Bangkok, Thailand
[2]Department of Medicine, Lerdsin General Hospital, Bangkok, Thailand
[3]Deparment of Medicine (Division of Nephrology), Faculty of Medicine, Chulalongkorn University, Bangkok, Thailand

Abstract

Previous *in vitro* studies showed that aldosterone rapidly stimulates protein kinase C alpha (PKC α) that could activate alpha (α) 1 isoform of Na, K-ATPase and then enhances its activity. There are, however, no *in vivo* data that demonstrate the rapid effects of aldosterone on renal protein expressions of PKC α and α1-Na, K-ATPase simultaneously. The present study further investigates the expression of these proteins. Male Wistar rats were intraperitoneally injected with normal saline solution or aldosterone (150 µg/kg BW). After 30 minutes, abundances and localizations of PKC α and α1-Na, K-ATPase proteins were determined by Western blot analysis and immunohistochemistry, respectively. Aldosterone administration significantly increased plasma aldosterone levels from 1,251.95 ± 13.83 to 6,521.78 ± 209.92 pmol/L. By Western blot analysis, aldosterone enhanced renal protein abundances of PKC α (homogenate samples) and α1-Na, K-ATPase (plasma membrane) approximately 50% and 30%, respectively ($P<0.05$). From immunohistochemistry examination in sham group, the protein expression of PKC α was prominent in the medulla. Aldosterone stimulated the expression both in the cortex and medulla with the translocation from the basolateral to luminal side of the proximal convoluted tubule (PCT). As for α1-Na, K-ATPase protein expression, the sham rats showed a strong immunostaining in the distal convoluted tubules, collecting ducts, and thick ascending limbs. Aldosterone elevated the expression in the PCT and medullary collecting duct (MCD). This *in vivo* study is the first to demonstrate simultaneously that aldosterone rapidly elevates PKC α and α1-Na, K-ATPase protein abundances in rat kidney. Both immunoreactivities were stimulated in the cortex and medulla. The greater affected areas were noted for PKC α expression, whereas the alterations of α1-Na, K-ATPase were observed only in the PT and MCD. The stimulation of Na, K-ATPase protein expression by aldosterone, per se, may occur through PKC activation.

Keywords: Rapid action; Aldosterone; PKC α; α1-Na, K-ATPase; Protein abundance; Immunohistochemistry; Rat kidney

Introduction

The rapid nongenomic effect of aldosterone regulates wide varieties of cellular responses including the regulation of ion transport [1]. One of the key signaling mediators regulating this action is protein kinase C (PKC) [1]. The activation of PKC is a prominent aspect of the aldosterone-stimulated rapid signaling responses in epithelia [2]. In the kidney, PKC modulates several physiological functions of renal epithelial cells, including the transport of sodium, water, and organic anions and cations [3].

It has been shown that aldosterone administration of cortical collecting duct (CCD) cells results in the rapid activation of protein kinase C alpha (PKC α) [4]. PKC also stimulates the alpha (α) 1 isoform of Na, K-ATPase property [5]. Rapid responses of aldosterone-induced Na, K-ATPase function in renal cells have been reported [6-8]. *In vitro* studies showed that aldosterone rapidly induces Na, K-ATPase activity in rat microdissected CCD and in Madin-Darby canine kidney (MDCK) cells [9,10]. In animal investigation, after 30 minutes of intravenous injection of aldosterone in adrenalectomized rats, Na, K-ATPase activity was increased markedly in microdissected medullary thick ascending limb (mTAL) of Henle's loop and CCD but not in MCD [11].

At present, there are no available *in vivo* data regarding the rapid effects of aldosterone on protein abundance and localization of renal PKC α and α$_1$-Na, K-ATPase, simultaneously performed in the same study. Therefore, this study examined rat kidneys 30 minutes after normal saline solution or aldosterone injection with use of Western blot analysis and immunohistochemistry to determine protein abundance and localization of renal PKC α and α$_1$-Na, K-ATPase.

Materials and Methods

Experimental design

Male Wistar rats weighing 200-240 g (National Center of Scientific Use of Animals, Mahidol University, Nakornpathom, Thailand) were given conventional housing and diet. All animal protocols were approved by the Ethics Committee of Research, Chulalongkorn University. Serum creatinine of each rat should be <1 mg/dl [12,13]. The rats were divided into two groups (n=8/group): sham (normal saline solution; NSS: 0.5 ml/kg BW by intraperitoneal injection, i.p.); and Aldo (aldosterone 150 µg/kg BW, diluted in NSS, i.p.; Sigma, St. Louis, MO, USA). We used this dose as previously performed in the study of rapid action of aldosterone on the protein expressions of

*Corresponding author: Somchit Eiam-Ong, Associate Professor, Department of Physiology, Faculty of Medicine, Chulalongkorn University, Bangkok, Thailand 10330, E-mail: eiamong@yahoo.com

upstream mediators [12]. Therefore, in the present investigation, we further examine this dose on PKC α and α₁-Na, K-ATPase.

On the date of the experiment, after a 30-minute injection period of NSS or aldosterone, the rats were anesthetized with thiopental (100 mg/kg BW, i.p.). Kidneys were removed, and a half of each kidney was fixed in liquid nitrogen, and then stored at -80°C until use for measurement of PKC α and α1-Na, K-ATPase protein abundances by Western blot analysis. The other half of renal tissue was fixed in 10% paraformaldehyde for localization of these proteins by immunohistochemistry [12].

Western blot analysis

The renal tissue samples were homogenized on ice with a homogenizer (IKA, T25 Basic, Selangor, Malaysia) in homogenizing buffer [(20 mM Tris-HCl; pH 7.5, 2 mM $MgCl_2$, 0.2 M sucrose, and 5% (v/v) protease inhibitor cocktail (Sigma, MO, USA)]. To get rid of crude debris, the kidney homogenates were centrifuged at 12,000 g (Biofuge PrimoR, Heracus, Germany) for 20 minutes at 4°C. The supernatant was collected and used as homogenate sample. To harvest plasma membrane, this supernatant was centrifuged at 37,500 g for 20 minutes at 4°C [14]. The pellet was dissolved in buffer. Total protein concentration of both homogenate samples and plasma membrane were measured with Bradford protein assay reagent (Pierce, Rockford, IL, USA) following the manufacturer's protocol. The measurement of protein abundance was performed as previously described [12]. Proteins were resolved on 8% sodium dodecyl sulfate polyacrylamide gel eletrophoresis (SDS-PAGE) for PKC α, α1-Na, K-ATPase, or β-actin, and blotted onto nitrocellulose membrane (Bio-Rad, Hercules, CA, USA). The membranes were incubated with primary monoclonal antibody to PKC α (H-7: sc-8393; 1:1000; Santa Cruz Biotechnology, Santa Cruz, CA, USA), α1-Na, K-ATPase (C464.6; 1:2500; Millipore, Temecula, CA, USA), or to β-actin (Santa Cruz Biotechnology), followed by the respective horseradish peroxidase-linked secondary antibody (Bio-Rad). Immunoreactive proteins were detected by chemiluminescence detection (Super Signal West Pico kit; Pierce) and exposed to film (CL-XPosure™; Pierce). Relative protein levels of PKC α and α1-Na, K-ATPase in each sample were presented as a percentage of the control normalized to its β-actin content.

Immunohistochemical study

Detection of protein localization was performed as previously described [12]. Paraffin-embedded kidney sections were cut at 4 μm in thickness. The slides were deparaffinized and endogenous peroxidase was blocked by treatment with 3% H_2O_2. The sections were incubated with the primary antibody PKC α (1:400; Santa Cruz Biotechnology), or α1-Na, K-ATPase (1:2000; Millipore) at 4°C overnight, followed by the respective horseradish peroxidase-linked secondary antibody (Bio-Rad), then reacted with 3,3′-diaminobenzidine (DAB) solution (Sigma). Three pathologists independently scored the staining intensity on a semi-quantitative five-tiered grading scale from 0 to 4 (0 = negative; 1=trace; 2=weak; 3=moderate; 4=strong) as previously described [12].

Statistical analysis

Results of renal PKC α and α1-Na, K-ATPase protein abundances were expressed as mean ± SD. Statistical differences between the groups were assessed by ANOVA (analysis of variance) with post-hoc comparison by Tukey's test where appropriate. A P value of <0.05 was considered statistically significant. Statistical tests were analyzed using SPSS program version 15.0 (SPSS Inc., Chicago, IL, USA). Median staining intensity (score) of renal PKC α and α1-Na, K-ATPase protein expressions was presented as previously described [12].

Results

Effect of aldosterone on renal PKC α and α1-Na, K-ATPase protein abundances

The protein levels of PKC α (80 kDa) and α1-Na, K-ATPase (130 kDa) were assessed in the rat kidney with Western blot analysis. As shown in Figure 1, aldosterone significantly enhanced protein abundance of renal PKC α in homogenate samples (sham=100%; Aldo =152.5 ± 9.8%, $P<0.05$). Interestingly, aldosterone elevated protein abundance of α1-Na, K-ATPase only in the plasma membrane (sham= 100%; Aldo=131.9 ± 8.9%, $P<0.05$).

Effect of aldosterone on renal PKC α protein localization

The rapid action of aldosterone on PKC α expression in the rat kidney was examined by immunohistochemistry. As shown in Table 1, in the cortex of sham, immunoreactivity of renal PKC α protein distribution/ localization was moderate in the glomerulus, whereas trace staining was observed in the peritubular capillary (Pcap), basolateral side of proximal convoluted tubule (PCT) and of distal convoluted tubule (DCT; Figure 2a). In the cortical collecting duct (CCD), the expression was weak. Aldosterone increased the immunoreactivity from trace to be weak in PCT with the translocation from the basolateral to luminal side (Figure 2b). The intensity score in the glomeruli was elevated from 3 to 4, and in Pcap from 1 to 2 by aldosterone (Figure 2b). Of noted, no staining in the DCT and CCD was detected after aldosterone administration.

In the outer stripe of outer medulla (OM) of the Aldo group, immunoreactivity in the thick ascending limb of Henle's loop (TALH), medullary collecting duct (MCD), and proximal straight tubule (PTs) was enhanced (Figures 2c and 2d). In the inner stripe of OM (Figures 2e and 2f), aldosterone increased staining in both apical and basolateral sides of TALH (score=2) and MCD (score=3), whereas the strong expression was noted in the vasa recta (VR) and thin limb of

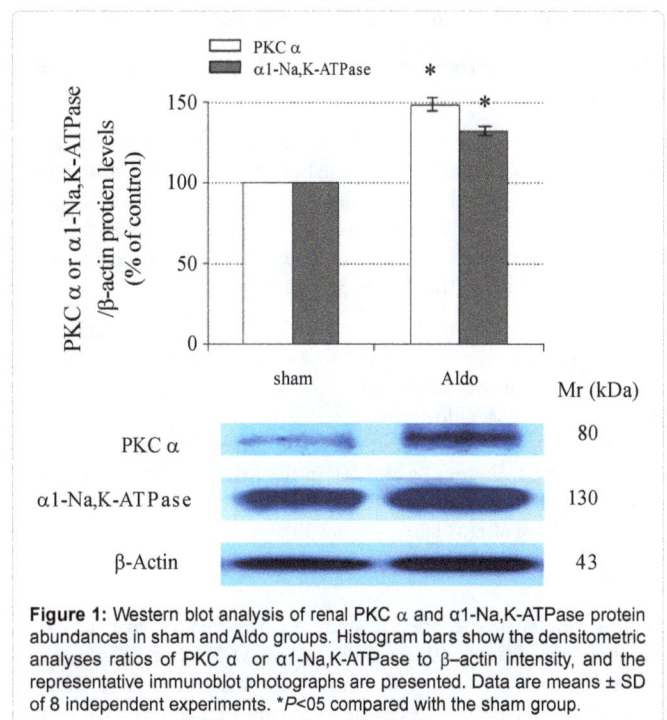

Figure 1: Western blot analysis of renal PKC α and α1-Na,K-ATPase protein abundances in sham and Aldo groups. Histogram bars show the densitometric analyses ratios of PKC α or α1-Na,K-ATPase to β–actin intensity, and the representative immunoblot photographs are presented. Data are means ± SD of 8 independent experiments. *P<05 compared with the sham group.

	Median staining intensity (score)			
	PKC α		α1-Na,K-ATPase	
	sham	Aldo	sham	Aldo
Cortex				
Glomerulus	3	4	0	0
PCT	1	3	2	3
DCT	1	0	4	4
CCD	2	0	4	4
Pcap	1	2	1	1
Outer medulla				
Outer stripe				
TALH	3	4	4	4
MCD	3	4	4	4
PTs	1	2	3	2
Inner stripe				
TALH	1	2	4	4
MCD	1	3	2	3
VR	3	4	1	1
tLH	3	4	1	1
Inner medulla				
MCD	4	2	3	4
VR	4	4	1	1
tLH	3	4	1	1

Staining intensity: 0: negative, no reactivity; 1: trace, faint, or pale brown staining with less membrane reactivity; 2: weak, light brown staining with incomplete membrane reactivity; 3: moderate, shaded of brown staining of intermediate darkness with usually almost complete membrane reactivity; 4: strong, dark brown to black staining with usually complete membrane pattern, producing a thick outline of the cell [10].
PCT: Proximal Convoluted Tubule; DCT: Distal Convoluted Tubule; CCD: Cortical Collecting Duct; Pcap: Peritubular capillary; TALH: Thick Ascending Limb of Henle's Loop; MCD: Medullary Collecting Duct; PTs: Proximal Straight Tubule; VR=Vasa Recta; tLH: thin limb of Henle's loop.

Table 1: Median staining intensity (score) of renal PKC α and α$_1$-Na,K-ATPase protein expressions.

Henle's loop (tLH). In the inner medulla (IM), immunoreactivity in VR remained strong, whereas the expression was elevated in tLH but declined in MCD by aldosterone (Figures 2g and 2h) (Table 1).

Effect of aldosterone on renal α1-Na, K-ATPase protein localization

The immunostaining of α1-Na, K-ATPase protein expression was obvious at the basolateral membrane both in the cortex and medulla. In sham (Figure 3a and Table 1), the expression was strong in the DCT and CCD, whereas the staining was weak in the PCT and trace in Pcap. No staining was noted in the glomerulus. Aldosterone increased the intensity score only in the PCT to 3 (Figure 3b).

In the outer stripe of OM, aldosterone slightly suppressed the intensity score in the PTs from 3 to 2 (Figures 3c and 3d), whereas the strong immunoreactivity in the TALH and MCD remained. In the inner stripe of OM, aldosterone elevated the intensity score from 2 to 3 in the MCD, whereas the staining in the TALH, VR and tLH did not change (Table 1, Figures 3e and 3f). In the IM, immunoreactivity was enhanced to be strong in the MCD, while the intensity score in the VR and tLH did not alter (Figures 3g and 3h).

Discussion

The results in the present study are the first *in vivo* data that simultaneously show both renal PKC α and α1-Na, K-ATPase protein expressions after 30-min aldosterone administration. According to Western blot analysis, aldosterone significantly enhanced renal PKC α

protein level from homogenate samples by approximately 50% (Figure 1). A previous *in vitro* study in rat cortical collecting duct cells showed that aldosterone administration for 15 min could enhance activity as well as protein abundance of PKC α with time- and dose-dependent manners [4]. Moreover, aldosterone promotes the activation of PKC α in MR-independent pathway [15]. The mechanism that aldosterone could activate PKC α has been clarified. One outstanding *in vitro* examination demonstrated the direct interaction between aldosterone with PKC α that has the specific binding site within the C$_2$ domain, resulting in activation and auto phosphorylation of the kinase [16]. Therefore, PKC α serves as a receptor for aldosterone inducing the rapid effects [16,17]. Our present data provide the evidence that aldosterone rapidly activates PKC α protein expression *in vivo*.

For protein localization in the sham group, the immunoreactivity of PKC α was expressed in both cortex and medulla (Table 1 and Figure 2). In the cortex, the expression was abundant in the glomerulus with a lesser extent in PCT, DCT, and CCD. The more intense immunoreactivity of PKC α was observed in the TALH and MCD (outer stripe), VR and tLH (inner stripe) of the outer medulla. The reactivity was strong in the inner medulla. The baseline regional distribution of PKC α protein in the present study is in agreement with a previous study in normal rat kidney [18]. The present study shows that aldosterone had a greater activation on PKC α in the medulla area, especially at both membrane sides of TALH and MCD (Table 1 and Figures 2c-f). Furthermore, aldosterone stimulated the translocation of PKC α expression from basolateral to apical membrane of PCT

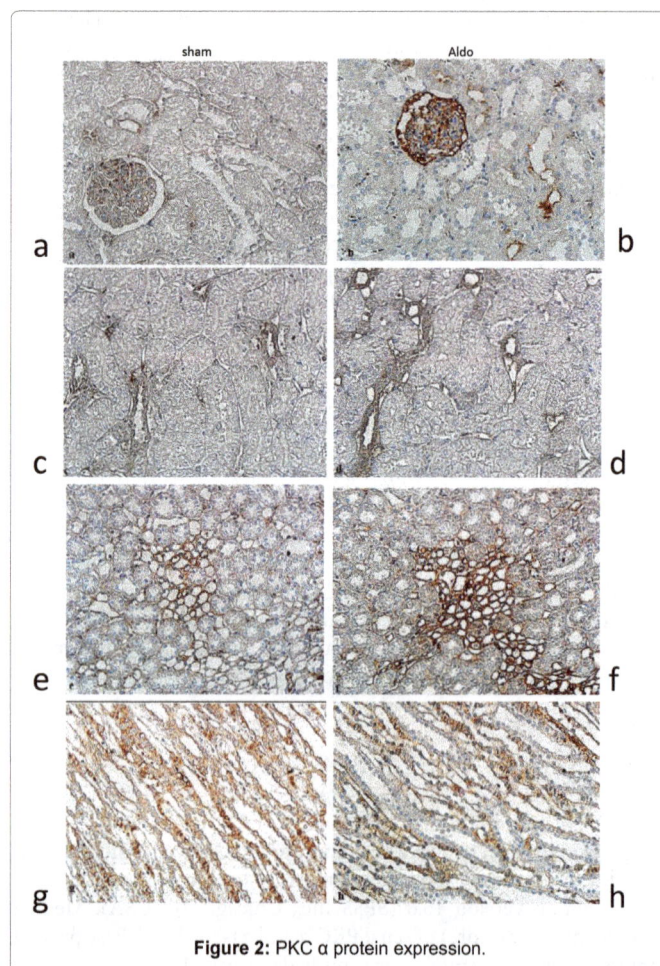

Figure 2: PKC α protein expression.

(Figure 2b). This suggests a significant action of aldosterone on tubular transport via PKC in this segment.

The PKC signaling cascades that are rapidly activated in response to aldosterone are emerging as important modulators of the functional changes in several cell types [2]. *In vitro* investigations related to the kidney have demonstrated that PKC could regulate renal cell function. PKC activation by phorbol myristate acetate for 4 minutes increased sodium hydrogen exchanger 3 activity in luminal membrane vesicle isolated from rat kidney cortical tubules [19]. Previous studies demonstrated that PKC plays an important role to maintain normal cellular functions and to mediate repair of mitochondrial and transport functions after toxicant-induced injury [20] as well as regulation of cell survival in renal proximal tubular cells [3]. Further *in vivo* study is required to clarify this circumstance. However, a recent study in mice kidney revealed that PKC α protects against angiotensin II-induced decreases in urine concentrating ability by maintaining aquaporin 2 water channels [21].

As for Na, K-ATPase, this ubiquitous membrane-bound enzyme composes of at least two subunits: the α subunit carrying the catalytic and ion transport properties and the β subunit involving in enzyme maturation and modulation of transport activity [22]. The fundamental function of Na, K-ATPase is to regulate and maintain high sodium and potassium gradient across the plasma membrane of animal cells [22]. In renal tubular epithelial cells, Na, K-ATPase provides the driving force for active sodium reabsorption and its activity is modulated by multihormonal control, including aldosterone [8,23]. For protein localization in the sham group, the immunoreactivity of α1-Na, K-ATPase was expressed abundantly in both cortex and medulla (Table 1 and Figure 3). In the cortex, the tubular areas had prominent staining in DCT and CCD, whereas the reactivity in TALH and MCD was obvious in the medulla. The baseline regional distribution of this protein in the present study is in agreement with a previous study in normal rat kidney [24]. The present results show that aldosterone enhanced immunoreactivity in the PCT to be moderate, and in the inner MCD to be strong (Table 1 and Figures 3a,3b,3e-3h).

Since the collecting duct is the major site of aldosterone action for regulating Na, K-ATPase, many investigations in rapid action of aldosterone have provided the data from this segment. Previous *in vitro* examinations demonstrated that aldosterone produces a rapid stimulation of Na, K-ATPase activity in microdissected CCD and MDCK epithelial cells [9,10]. An intravenous infusion of aldosterone, for 30 minutes into the rat, also stimulated the Na, K-ATPase activity in microdissected CCD but reduced sodium excretion [11]. The authors revealed that aldosterone produces this rapid stimulation of pump activity via increased transporting rate assessed by ouabain-sensitive ^{86}Rb uptake assay [9]. Therefore, further investigation is needed to delineate whether aldosterone could affect this Na, K-ATPase property in the PCT.

For protein abundance, a previous examination showed that aldosterone administration for 15 minutes in renal collecting duct cells did not alter α1-Na, K-ATPase protein abundance [4]. However, in the present study, aldosterone injection for 30 minutes could enhance α1-Na, K-ATPase protein abundance from plasma membrane by 30%, whereas no changes were observed from homogenate samples (data not shown). Since this time course (30 minutes) is not enough for processes of transcription or translation the protein. Some investigations have provided explanations regarding to this alteration. In MDCK cells, the ^{3}H-ouabain binding assay indicated that aldosterone increased in pump numbers due to insertion of preexisting units [10]. Moreover, a previous

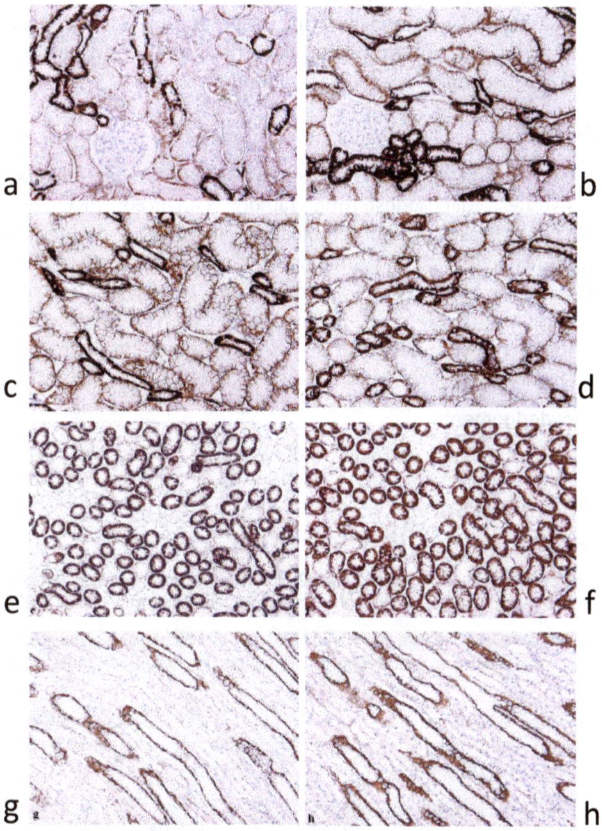

Figure 3: α1-Na, K-ATPase protein expression.

in vitro study demonstrated that, in the presence of aldosterone, a rise in cell sodium induces the recruitment and activation of latent pump at the basolateral membrane of rabbit CCD cells within 2-3 seconds [25]. Therefore, we suggest that the elevation of α1-Na, K-ATPase protein abundance in the present study may occur by the recruitment of the pump protein preexisting in the tubular cell which inserted to the plasma membrane.

Our present study demonstrates that both PKC α and α1-Na, K-ATPase were activated simultaneously by aldosterone. The influences of PKC on Na, K-ATPase property have been extensively examined. Several studies indicated that PKC activation could stimulate Na, K-ATPase. For example, a previous *in vitro* study in rat PCT provided clear evidences that direct activation of PKC by phorbol esters increases the affinity of Na, K-ATPase for sodium and thereby stimulates its transport activity [26]. Moreover, PKC activation induced phosphorylation of the catalytic α1-subunit of Na, K-ATPase and stimulated the ouabain-sensitive ^{86}Rb uptake by 47% and 42%, respectively in time- and dose-dependent fashions in the PCT [5]. Furthermore, in rat microdissected mTAL, the stimulation of Na, K-ATPase activity was associated with an increase in Na, K-ATPase α-subunit phophorylation through PKC-α activation [27]. In addition, it has been shown that aldosterone could rapidly stimulate another adenosine triphosphatase. A recent study demonstrated that aldosterone enhances vacuolar H-ATPase activity in renal acid-secretory intercalated cells mainly via a protein kinase C-dependent pathway [28]. Therefore, we propose that the increase in PKC activation in the present *in vivo* study may be accountable for Na, K-ATPase stimulation. However, additional *in vivo* investigations are needed to clarify whether this aldosterone action is MR-mediated process and dose-dependent manners. For further studies, we aim to unveil the rapid effects of aldosterone on the other sodium transporters and related PKC isoenzymes, such as β subunits.

Conclusion

In conclusion, this is the first *in vivo* study which simultaneously demonstrates that aldosterone rapidly enhanced PKC α and α1-Na, K-ATPase protein abundances in the rat kidney. Both immunoreactivities were stimulated in the cortex and medulla. The greater affected areas were noted for PKC α expression, whereas the alterations of α1-Na, K-ATPase were observed only in the PT and MCD. The stimulation of Na, K-ATPase protein expression by aldosterone, per se, may occur through PKC activation.

Acknowledgements

This study was supported by Grant no. RA 57/007 from the Ratchadapiseksompoth Research Fund, Faculty of Medicine, Chulalongkorn University.

References

1. Dooley R, Harvey BJ, Thomas W (2012) Non-genomic actions of aldosterone: from receptors and signals to membrane targets. Mol Cell Endocrinol 350: 223-234.

2. Thomas W, McEneaney V, Harvey BJ (2007) Aldosterone-stimulated PKC signalling cascades: from receptor to effector. Biochem Soc Trans 35: 1049-1051.

3. Dempsey EC, Newton AC, Mochly-Rosen D, Fields AP, Reyland ME, et al. (2000) Protein kinase C isozymes and the regulation of diverse cell responses. Am J Physiol Lung Cell Mol Physiol 279: L429-438.

4. Le Moëllic C, Ouvrard-Pascaud A, Capurro C, Cluzeaud F, Fay M, et al. (2004) Early nongenomic events in aldosterone action in renal collecting duct cells: PKCα activation, mineralocorticoid receptor phosphorylation, and cross-talk with the genomic response. J Am Soc Nephrol 15: 1145-1160.

5. Carranza ML, Féraille E, Favre H (1996) Protein kinase C-dependent phosphorylation of Na(+)-K(+)-ATPase alpha-subunit in rat kidney cortical tubules. Am J Physiol 271: C136-143.

6. Good DW (2007) Nongenomic actions of aldosterone on the renal tubule. Hypertension 49: 728-739.

7. Harvey BJ, Alzamora R, Stubbs AK, Irnaten M, McEneaney V, et al. (2008) Rapid responses to aldosterone in the kidney and colon. J Steroid Biochem Mol Biol 108: 310-317.

8. Thomas W, Harvey BJ (2011) Mechanisms underlying rapid aldosterone effects in the kidney. Annu Rev Physiol 73: 335-357.

9. Fujii Y, Takemoto F, Katz AI (1990) Early effects of aldosterone on Na-K pump in rat cortical collecting tubules. Am J Physiol 259: F40-45.

10. Shahedi M, Laborde K, Bussières L, Sachs C (1993) Acute and early effects of aldosterone on Na-K-ATPase activity in Madin-Darby canine kidney epithelial cells. Am J Physiol 264: F1021-1026.

11. El Mernissi G, Doucet A (1983) Short-term effect of aldosterone on renal sodium transport and tubular Na-K-ATPase in the rat. Pflugers Arch 399: 139-146.

12. Eiam-Ong S, Sinphitukkul K, Manotham K, Eiam-Ong S (2013) Rapid nongenomic action of aldosterone on protein expressions of Hsp90(α± and β) and pc-Src in rat kidney. Biomed Res Int 2013: 346480.

13. Sinphitukkul K, Eiam-Ong S, Manotham K, Eiam-Ong S (2011) Nongenomic effects of aldosterone on renal protein expressions of pEGFR and pERK1/2 in rat kidney. Am J Nephrol 33: 111-120.

14. Fernández-Llama P, Jimenez W, Bosch-Marcé M, Arroyo V, Nielsen S, et al.

(2000) Dysregulation of renal aquaporins and Na-Cl cotransporter in CCl4-induced cirrhosis. Kidney Int 58: 216-228.

15. Markos F, Healy V, Harvey BJ (2005) Aldosterone rapidly activates Na+/H+ exchange in M-1 cortical collecting duct cells via a PKC-MAPK pathway. Nephron Physiol 99: 1-9.

16. Alzamora R, Brown LR, Harvey BJ (2007) Direct binding and activation of protein kinase C isoforms by aldosterone and 17beta-estradiol. Mol Endocrinol 21: 2637-2650.

17. Alzamora R, Harvey BJ (2008) Direct binding and activation of protein kinase C isoforms by steroid hormones. Steroids 73: 885-888.

18. Pfaff IL, Wagner HJ, Vallon V (1999) Immunolocalization of protein kinase C isoenzymes alpha, beta1 and betaII in rat kidney. J Am Soc Nephrol 10: 1861-1873.

19. Karim ZG, Chambrey R, Chalumeau C, Defontaine N, Warnock DG, et al. (1999) Regulation by PKC isoforms of Na(+)/H(+) exchanger in luminal membrane vesicles isolated from cortical tubules. Am J Physiol 277: F773-778.

20. Nowak G (2003) Protein kinase C mediates repair of mitochondrial and transport functions after toxicant-induced injury in renal cells. J Pharmacol Exp Ther 306: 157-165.

21. Thai TL, Blount MA, Klein JD, Sands JM (2012) Lack of protein kinase C-α leads to impaired urine concentrating ability and decreased aquaporin-2 in angiotensin II-induced hypertension. Am J Physiol Renal Physiol 303: F37-44.

22. Pearce D, Bhalla V, Funder JW (2012) Aldosterone regulation of ion transport: Brenner & Rector's the kidney. (9th edn) W.B. Saunders Company, Philadelphia, USA.

23. Féraille E, Doucet A (2001) Sodium-potassium-adenosinetriphosphatase-dependent sodium transport in the kidney: hormonal control. Physiol Rev 81: 345-418.

24. Wetzel RK, Sweadner KJ (2001) Immunocytochemical localization of Na-K-ATPase alpha- and gamma-subunits in rat kidney. Am J Physiol Renal Physiol 281: F531-F545.

25. Blot-Chabaud M, Wanstok F, Bonvalet JP, Farman N (1990) Cell sodium-induced recruitment of Na(+)-K(+)-ATPase pumps in rabbit cortical collecting tubules is aldosterone dependent. J Biol Chem 265: 11676-11681.

26. Féraille E, Carranza ML, Buffin-Meyer B, Rousselot M, Doucet A, et al. (1995) Protein kinase C-dependent stimulation of Na(+)-K(+)-ATP epsilon in rat proximal convoluted tubules. Am J Physiol 268: C1277-1283.

27. Tsimaratos M, Roger F, Chabardès D, Mordasini D, Hasler U, et al. (2003) C-peptide stimulates Na+,K+-ATPase activity via PKC alpha in rat medullary thick ascending limb. Diabetologia 46: 124-131.

28. Winter C, Kampik NB, Vedovelli L, Rothenberger F, Paunescu TG, et al. (2011) Aldosterone stimulates vacuolar H(+)-ATPase activity in renal acid-secretory intercalated cells mainly via a protein kinase C-dependent pathway. Am J Physiol Cell Physiol 301: C1251-1261.

10

Testicular Changes in Male Albino Rat Pups Exposed to Medroxy-Progesterone Acetate during Lactational Period

Ahmed SI[1]*, Ali TO[2], Elsheikh AS[3], Attia GA[1], Abdalla AM[4] and Mohamed MH[5]

[1]*Department of Anatomy, Faculty of Medicine, Najran University, Saudi Arabia*
[2]*Faculty of Graduate Studies & Scientific Research, National Ribat University, Sudan*
[3]*Department of Applied Medical Sciences, Community faculty Najran, Saudi Arabia*
[4]*Department of Anatomy, Faculty of Medicine, King Khalid University, Saudi Arabia*
[5]*Department of Anatomy, Faculty of Medicine, Jazan University, Saudi Arabia*

Abstract

There are great concerns regarding the use of synthetic progesterone during breastfeeding due to probable negative effects on future fecundity of male infants. Therefore the present study was conducted to evaluate the effects of exposing male rat pups to depot medroxyprogesterone acetate (DMPA) during lactational period on pubertal testicular histology, morphometry and cells quantitation. Twenty male Wistar rat pups reared to dams treated with DMPA (10 mg/kg BW) every other day during their early lactation period; were employed to achieve the objectives of this study. Other 20 male rat pups reared to untreated dams served as control. The pups were allowed to reach 90 days old, sacrificed, their testes were dissected and weighed and histological sections were prepared.

The results showed that exposing male rat pups to DMPA during the lactational period significantly (P<0.001) affected their testicular histology, morphometry and the quantities of testicular cells. The thickness of the germinal epithelium (GE) and the diameter of the seminiferous tubules (ST) were reduced; while the interstitial space (IS) thicknesses were increased. The testicular cells of the rats reared on dams treated with DMPA experienced varying degrees of apoptosis and count reduction. The ST appeared with unusual configuration with detached and/or folded basal lamina, it has few germinal layers, decreased Sertoli cells (SC) and their lumen contained cells debris and very few sperms; while the wide IS contained few Leydig cells (LC). Exposure to DMPA during the lactational period adversely affects the testicular structure. Thus foretells a negative impact on future fertility.

Keywords: Medroxyprogesterone acetate; Testicular structure; Fertility; Lactational period; Morphometry

Introduction

The synthetic progesterone is widely used in human reproductive clinics for many therapeutic purposes such as a contraceptive especially during lactation period [1,2] to reduce the risk of recurrent preterm birth, to treat endometrial hyperplasia, heavy menstrual bleeding, endometriosis, pelvic pain syndromes, breast and uterine cancer, loss of appetite and weight related to AIDS and cancer and topically in certain skin diseases [3-5]. This situation entails that male infants kept on breastfeeding will be exposed to these synthetic hormones; suggesting disorder of their reproductive health at puberty [6-8].

The effects of these synthetic hormones on the reproductive functions of the male human and animal cause considerable concerns among researchers who care to improve the male reproductive health [9-12]. Abnormal changes in the male reproductive health such as abnormal sexual development, alteration in testicular functions and increment of infertility rates were suggested by current studies [10,12-14]. Although, there is minimum evidences that exposure of male infants to exogenous hormones is harmful to their reproductive health, the concern of the use of DMPA during lactation remains [15,16].

Although many studies have asserted that exposure to synthetic progesterone hormone during pregnancy has critical effects on testicular structure and function [4,12-16], great controversies and doubts exist concerning its adverse effects on the male reproduction following their exposure to synthetic progesterone during suckling period. Thus, the aim of the current study is to evaluate the effects of exposing male rat pups during early suckling period to DMPA on pubertal testicular histology, morphometry and cells quantitation.

Materials and Methods

Materials

Experimental animals: Ten weeks old 8 pregnant female Wistar albino rats were grouped into two groups (4 rats each) and kept separate away from any stress in sterilized polypropylene cages (90 cm × 45 cm × 15 cm) lined with woody husk. They were kept at 28 ± 7°C temperature in light/dark cycle (12:12 h), fed on commercial pellet and offered water ad libitum. After delivery 4 dams with 20 male pups (Group I) were injected with a placebo to serve as controls; while 4 dams with 20 male pups (Group II) were subcutaneously injected with 10 mg/kg BW of depot medroxy-progesterone acetate (DMPA; Depo-Provera®) every other day (on the first fifteen days) of lactational period. The dam body weights were taken on each day of injection to adjust the dose. The 40 male rat pups were allowed to grow for 90 days where they reach maturity [2,4,10-12].

Study design: This one factorial experiment study was designed to investigate the effects of lactational exposure to DMPA on suckling male rat's pups' testis histological structure, morphometry, cells quantities at

*Corresponding author: Ahmed SI, Department of Anatomy, faculty of Medicine, Najran University. P.O. Box 1988. Najran, Saudi Arabia,
E-mail: samyanatomist@yahoo.com

puberty. Twenty male rat pups born to the experiment group and 20 pups born to the control group were allowed to grow for 90 day where they reached maturity. The testes were collected and prepared as above. Morphometry and cell quantitation were carried as described above.

Methods

Tissue collection and preparation: Animals were anesthetized with chloroform and sacrificed with cervical dislocation [12,13,17]. The testis was dissected and separated from its adjacent epididymis and connective tissue and its relative weight was then calculated. Then the testes were immediately fixed in aqueous Bouin's solution for 18 h, dehydrated with 70%, 90% and 100% ascending grades of alcohol. The fixed testes were cleared with xylene and embedded in paraffin wax and micro-sections of 5 μm thickness were made by an American Optical microtome (A0-821. USA). Then the micro-sections were mounted onto glass slides, deparaffinized and stained with H&E stain [18].

Histomorphometry: Longitudinal sections of each rat's testis were prepared and stained with H&E as described elsewhere [19,20]. Then 10 round or nearly round STs were chosen randomly to measure their diameters, the height of GE, the thickness of IS and the number of GE cells using Olympus BX-40 light microscope supported with an image Pro Plus program ×100 [12]. Two tubular diameters for each seminiferous tubule were mapped and their mean recorded. The thicknesses of IS were measured by measuring three dimensions of each interstitial space from the space centre to the basement membrane of the surrounding ST. The mean of the three dimensions was calculated and multiplied by 2 to obtain the whole thickness of the interstitial space. The GE height was obtained for the same tubules used to determine tubular diameter. The GE height was assumed from the basement membrane to the latest stage of GE (spermatids).

Cells quantitation: After animal sacrifice, testes were fixed by perfusion with Bouin's fixative for 30 min as above. They were then cut into 3 vertical longitudinal slices where middle slices include

the mediastinum. After immersion and fixation in Bouin's fixative for another 1.5 h, the slices were dehydrated in ethanol, cleared with xylene and embedded in paraffin wax. From each slice 5 sections of 5 μm were cut, thus 15 sections were obtained and mounted individually onto slides. The testicular cells (spermatogonia type A & B, primary spermatocytes cells, LC and SC) of each rat testis were counted under Olympus BX-40 microscope supported with an Image Pro Plus program. The mean counts of each cell type were recorded per section for each group [12,21,22].

Statistical analysis: Data were subjected to one way ANOVA using SPSS-16.020 (Chicago, USA). The means that have been expressed as mean ± SD were compared with Dunnett's test. The level of significance was set at $P<0.05$.

Results

Testis histological observations

The cross sections of the control rats' testes showed compactly arranged, semi-round or oval ST with intact normal basement membrane, normal GE, and normal IS (Figure 1A and 1C). The different stages of spermatogenesis were observed in all the ST. The SCs were normal resting on a normal basement membrane and their lumens are contained masses of spermatozoa (Figure 2A). The IS is normal and contained normal clusters of LC (Figure 3A). The sections of testes of rats reared on dams treated with DMPA showed marked degenerative changes. The ST appear smaller disperse and lost its normal arrangement. The basement membrane of the ST are detached and/or folded and the GE were extremely reduced (Figure 1B). Obvious intercellular cavitations appeared in-between the GE lining the ST as a result of degenerative changes. The GE cells are few and the lumen of the ST is wider with few scattered spermatozoa and necrotic cells' debris (Figure 1D and Figure 2B). The SCs are few, lost their integration with the surrounding GE (Figure 1D and Figure 2B). The IS are wide due to

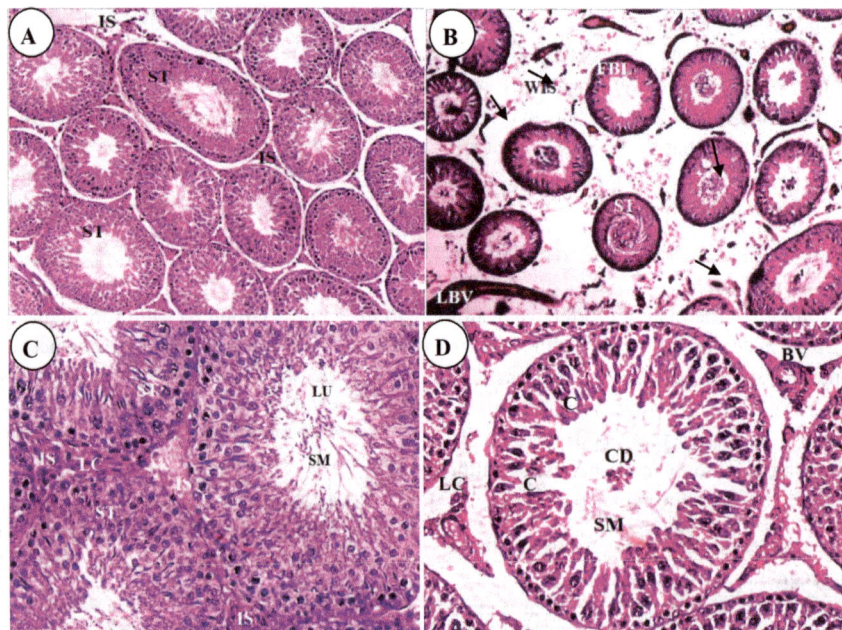

Figure 1: Light photomicrographs of rat's testes parenchyma. Control rat testis (A) and experimental rat testis (B) (H&E ×100). Control rat testis (C) and experimental rat testis (D) (H&E × 400). Seminiferous tubules (ST), interstitial spaces (IS), detached and folded basal laminae (arrowed; FBL) wide interstitial space (WIS), Lumen (LU), sperm mass (SM), Leydig cell (LC), cell debris in the lumen (CD) and large blood vessels (LBV).

ST hypoplasia and the LCs are very few and there are some vacuoles in the ISs (Figure 3B).

Histomorphometry

Relative testicular weights: The mean relative testicular weights of male rats reared on dams treated with DMPA were significantly (P<0.001) reduced compared to those of the control (Table 1 and Figure 4). The mean relative testicular weights of the control and experimental groups were (0.011 ± 0.001) and (0.008 ± 0.001) gm, respectively.

Measurements of Sts diameters, Ge And Iss thicknesses: The diameter of the ST, GE height and the thicknesses of the IS of the control and male rats reared on dams treated with DMPA varied significantly (P<0.001). The mean diameters of ST of the control and the treatment rats were 281.5 ± 17.2 and 253.2 ± 13.7 μm, respectively. The heights of the GE were 93.7 ± 9.6 and 71.4 ± 7.2 μm, in the same respective as above. The mean thickness of the IS of the control was 110.5 ± 11.3 μm and that of the treatment rats was 133.1 ± 5.5 μm (Table 1 and Figure 5).

Testicular cells quantitation: The counts of the different testicular cells per cross section varied significantly (P<0.01) with treatment. As in (Table 2 and Figure 6), the mean counts of spermatogonia type A of the control and male rats reared on dams treated with DMPA were 38.55 ± 3.47 and 27.00 ± 3.73 and type B mean counts were 36.50 ± 3.07 and 21.35 ± 4.11, respectively. The primary spermatocytes mean counts were 37.50 ± 4.02 and 28.10 ± 4.08, SC means were 17.65 ± 2.32 and 9.65 ± 2.50 and LC means were 12.35 ± 2.32 and 6.95 ± 2.35 in the same order as above.

Discussion

This study clearly demonstrates the negative effects of DMPA hormone on the testes of male rats that were breastfed on dams treated with this hormone during lactation period.

The marked abnormalities found in this study are comparable to the findings of Goyal et al. [2] who reported similar effects in neonatal male exposure to steroid hormones. One of the most serious effects of DMPA on the testis observed in this study is the reduction in the number of SC. The SC provide structural support and nutrition to the developing germ cells, produce proteins that regulate and/or stimulate pituitary hormones release and are responsible of phagocytosis of

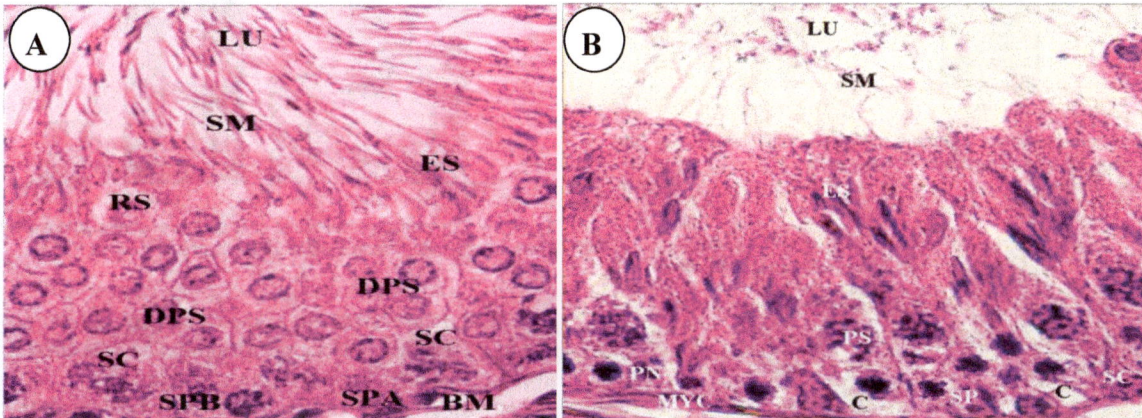

Figure 2: Light photomicrographs of rats Sertoli cells with germinal epithelium. Control rat (A) and experimental rat (B). Basement membrane (BM), myoid cell (MYC), Sertoli cell (SC), cytoplasmic vacuole (C), spermatogonia type A (SPA), spermatogonia type B (SPB), primary spermatocyte (PS), elongated spermatids (ES), rounded spermatids (RS), dividing primary spermatocyte (DPS), tubular lumen (LU) and SM: sperm mass (H&E × 1000).

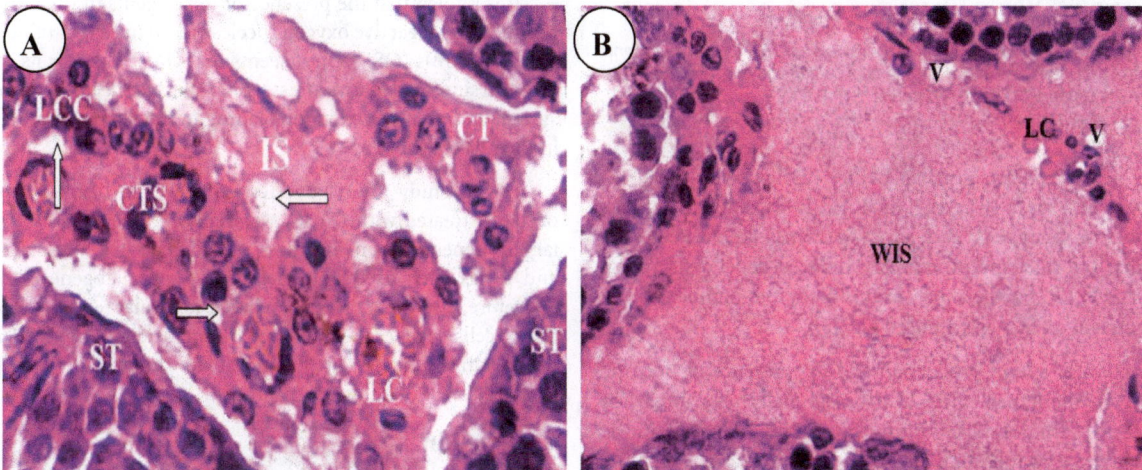

Figure 3: Micrographs of rat's testes interstitial space (IS) of the control (A) and experimental (B). Wider interstitial spaces with few cells (WIS), single Leydig cell (LC), Leydig cell clusters (LCC), vacuoles (arrowed and V), connective tissue (CT) with connective tissue cells (CTS) and surrounding seminiferous tubules (ST) (H&E × 1000).

Parameter	Synthetic medroxyprogesterone Injected(10 mg/kg body weight)	
	Control	Experiment
Relative Testicular Weight/gm	(0.011 ± 0.001)[a]	(0.008 ± 0.001)[b]
Seminiferous tubule diameter/µm	(281.5 ± 17.2)[a]	(253.2 ± 13.7)[b]
Height of germinal epithelium/µm	(93.7 ± 9.6)[a]	(71.4 ± 7.2)[b]
Thickness of interstitial space/µm	(110.5 ± 11.3)[a]	(133.1 ± 5.5)[b]

Data are presented as mean ± SD. Experiment: denotes male rats reared by females dams injected with medroxyprogesterone during lactation. [a, b] Values with different superscripts in the same raw significantly different (P<0.001).

Table 1: Effects of synthetic medroxyprogesterone on the relative testicular weights, ST diameter, height of GE and thickness of IS.

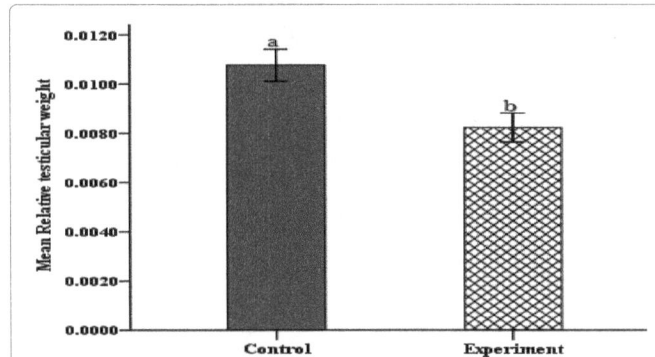

Figure 4: Mean relative testicular weights of control and experimental rats. Bars represent the mean ± SD of 20 replicates. [a,b] differ at P<0.01.

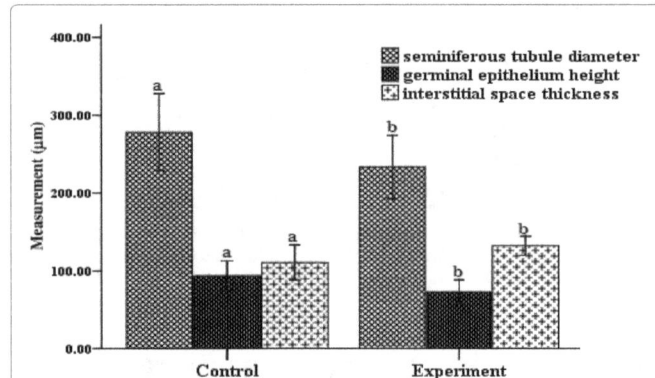

Figure 5: Compares the measurements of seminiferous tubule diameter, germinal epithelium height and interstitial space thickness of control and experimental rats. Bars represent the mean ± SD of 20 replicates. [a,b] P<0.01.

Parameter	Synthetic Progesterone Injected (10 mg/kg body weight)	
	Control	Experiment
Spermatogonia Type (A)	(38.55 ± 3.47)[a]	(27.00 ± 3.73)[b]
Spermatogonia Type (B)	(36.50 ± 3.07)[a]	(21.35 ± 4.11)[b]
Primary Spermatocyte	(37.50 ± 4.02)[a]	(28.10 ± 4.08)[b]
Sertoli	(17.65 ± 2.32)[a]	(9.65 ± 2.50)[b]
Leydig cells	(12.35.77 ± 2.32)[a]	(6.95 ± 2.35)[b]

Data are presented as mean ± SD. Experiment: denotes male rats reared by females dams injected with medroxyprogesterone during lactation. [a, b] Values with different superscripts in the same raw significantly different (P<0.01).

Table 2: Effects of synthetic medroxyprogesterone on the testicular cells count.

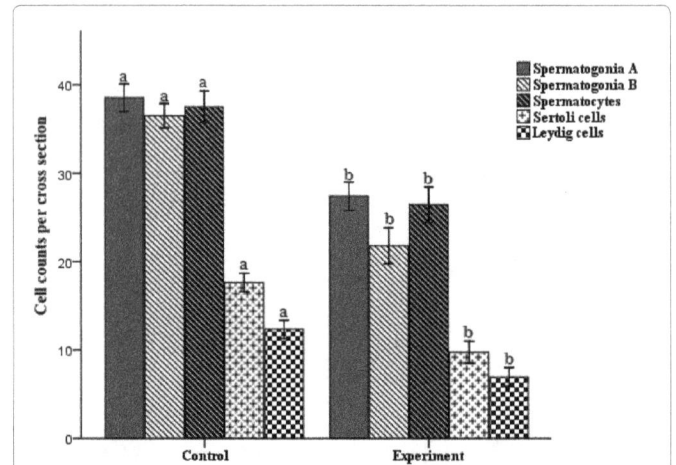

Figure 6: Comparison of testicular cells counts of control and experimental rats. Bars represent the mean ± SD of 20 replicates. [a,b] differ at P<0.01.

present study provides clear evidence that exposure of neonatal male rats to DMPA during lactation period has adverse effect on testicular structure that foretells poor fertility. This finding is in accordance with that of Patel et al. [28] and Truit et al. [29] who thought that newborns cannot metabolize and excrete the steroid hormones ingested during breastfeeding because of their immature liver and kidneys. Additionally they suggested a low plasma-binding capacity which leads to high levels of free biologically active hormones in their bodies.

It is known that the presence of toxic agents in the body enhances production of reactive oxygen species (ROS) in cells & tissues and exert oxidative stress (OS) [30]. It seems that DMPA and/or its metabolites; induced similar oxidative stress which affected the testicular antioxidant system and lipid peroxidation leading to the observed cellular changes in the rats testes [31].

In this study the relative testicular weight of male rats breastfed on dams treated with DMPA was reduced. The weight of the testis is largely dependent on the mass of differentiated spermatogenic cells and it has been used as a measure of spermatogenesis in rats [32]. Therefore, the decrement in relative testicular weight is presumably due to cells degeneration and low sperm production [4,12,16]. Also the degenerative processes are behind the low number of GE cells reported in this study.

Conclusion

Exposing male rat's pups to DMPA hormone have serious adverse effects on pubertal testis structures, morphometry and sperm production which in turn may affect male reproductivity.

degenerating germ cells and residual bodies [23]. Also in male, SC maintain spermatogenesis whereby each SC is capable to support certain number of germ cells; such function makes the entire sperm production and the total sperm number produced dependent on the total number SC [23]. Furthermore, in this study the number of LC; which is dependent on SCs was reduced [24,25].

The reduction of sperm production and the presence of necrotic cellular debris in the lumen of ST of neonatal male rats exposed to DMPA is a clear indication for SC dysfunction [26]. Reduction in the SC and LC observed in this study indicates that exposure of suckling male to DMPA might affect the gonadal-pituitary hormonal axis and/or it impeded the processes of differentiation and maturation of LC and SC. Thus it might have potential hazardous effects on the testis [27]. The

Recommendations

Animals in this study were only observed till 90 days of age, and it is possible that other testicular disorders /recovery may become evident with ageing. Therefore, longer term studies may be necessary to identify the full effect of this synthetic drug.

More studies should also be conducted to help identify safety profile of medroxyprogesterone use as a contraceptive during lactation particularly in the presence of any testicular abnormality.

Acknowledgements

The authors would like to acknowledge all members of the anatomy department of Najran University for many useful discussions and support. The authors apologize to all colleagues whose work could not be cited due to space limitations.

References

1. Palmlund I, Apfel R, Buitendijk S, Cabau A, Forsberg JG (1993) Effect of diethylstilbestrol (DES) medication during pregnancy. J Psychosom Obstet Gynaecol 14: 71-89.

2. Goyal HO, Robateau A, Braden TD, Williams CS, Srivastava KK, et al. (2003) Neonatal estrogen exposure of male rats alters reproductive functions at adulthood. Biol Reprod 68: 2081-2091.

3. Marianowski P, Radwańska E (2000) Intramuscular vs vaginal progesterone for luteal support in cycles of in vitro fertilization. Ginekol Pol 71: 1064-1070.

4. Harini C, Sainath SB, Sreenivasula Reddy P (2009) Recovery of suppressed male reproduction in mice exposed to progesterone during embryonic development by testosterone. Reprod 137: 439-448.

5. Vidaeff AC, Belfort MA (2013) Critical appraisal of the efficacy, safety, and patient acceptability of hydroxyprogesterone caproate injection to reduce the risk of preterm birth. Pat Prefer Adher 7: 683-691.

6. Fielden MR, Halgren RG, Fong CJ, Staub C, Johnson L, et al. (2002) Gestational and lactational exposure of male mice to diethylstilbestrol causes long-term effects on the testis sperm fertilizing ability in vitro and testicular gene expression. Endocrinol 143: 3044-3059.

7. Storgaard L, Bonde JP, Olsen J (2006) Male reproductive disorders in humans and prenatal indicators of estrogen exposure. A review of published epidemiological studies. Reprod Toxicol 21: 4-15.

8. Delbès G, Levacher C, Habert R (2006) Estrogen effects on fetal and neonatal testicular development. Reproduction 132: 527-538.

9. Carlsen E, Giwercman A, Keiding N, Skakkebaek NE (1992) Evidence for decreasing quality of semen during past 50 years. Br Med J 304: 609-613.

10. Pushpalatha T, Ramachandra Reddy P, Sreenivasula Reddy P (2002) Effect of prenatal exposure to hydroxyprogesterone on steroidogenic enzymes in male rats. Naturwissenschaften 90: 40-43.

11. Ahmed SI, Elsheikh AS, Attia GA, Ali TO (2016) Prenatal progesterone exposure of male rats induces morphometric and histological changes in testes. Asian Pacific J Reprod 5: 204-209.

12. Ahmed SI, Elsheikh AS, Attia GA, Ali TO (2016) Ultra-structure of testes of rats born to dams treated with hydroxy-progesterone hexanoate. Asian Pacific J Reprod 5: 510-513.

13. Knez J (2013) Endocrine-disrupting chemicals and male reproductive health. Reprod Biomed 26: 440-448.

14. Halderman LD, Nelson AL (2002) Impact of early postpartum administration of progestin-only hormonal contraceptives compared with nonhormonal contraceptives on short-term breast-feeding patterns. Am J Obstet Gynecol 186: 1250-1258.

15. Brownell EA, Fernandez ID, Howard CR, Fisher SG, Ternullo SR, et al. (2012) A systematic review of early postpartum medroxyprogesterone receipt and early breastfeeding cessation: evaluating the methodological rigor of the evidence. Breastfeed Med 7: 10-8.

16. Pushpalatha T, Ramachandra Reddy P, Sreenivasula Reddy P (2004) Impairment of male reproduction in adult rats exposed to hydroxyl-progesterone caproate in utero. Naturwissenschaften 91: 242-244.

17. Elsheikh AS, Takahashi Y, Hishinuma M, Kanagawa H (1997) Effect of encapsulation on development of mouse pronuclear stage embryos in vitro. Anim. Reprod Sci 48: 317-324.

18. Bancroft JD (2008) Fixation and fixatives. In: Theory and practice of histological techniques. 5th Ed. New York, London, San Francisco, Tokyo: Churchill Livingstone 31: 725.

19. Thienpot D, Rochelle F, Vanpariis OFJ (1986) Diagnosing Helmin-thiasis by Corprological Examination. 2nd Ed. Beerse: Janssen Foundation p205.

20. Batra N, Nehru B, Bansal MP (2001) Influence of lead and zinc on rat male reproduction at biochemical and histopathological levels. J Appl Toxicol 21: 507-512.

21. Heller G, Leach DR (1971) Quantitation of Leydig cells and measurement of Leydig cell size following administration of human chorionic gonadotrophin to normal men. J Reprod Fertil 25: 185-192.

22. Dykes JRW (2001) Histometric assessment of human testicular biopsies. J Pathol Bacteriol 97: 429-440.

23. Russell LD, Griswold MD (1993) The sertoli cell. Cache River Press, Clearwater, FL.

24. Baker PJ, Sha JA, McBride MW, Peng L, Payne AH, et al. (1999) Expression of 3b-hydroxysteriod dehydrogenase type I and VI isoforms in the mouse testis during development. Eur J Biochem 260: 911-916.

25. Nef S, Shipman T, Parada LF (2000) A molecular basis for estrogeninduced cryptorchidism. Dev Biol 224: 354-361.

26. Johnson L (1991b) In: Cupps P (Ed.) Spermatogenesis. Reproduction in Domestic Animals, fourth ed. Academic Press Inc., San Diego, CA p.173-219.

27. Sharpe RM, Rivas A, Walker M, McKinnell C, Fisher JS (2003) Effect of neonatal treatment of rats with potent or weak (environmental) oestrogens, or with a GnRH antagonist, on Leydig cell development and function through puberty into adulthood. Int J Androl 26: 26-36.

28. Patel SB, Toddywalla VS, Betrabet SS, Kulkarni RD, Patel ZM, et al. (1994) At what „infant-age" can levonorgestrel contraceptives be recommended to nursing mothers? Adv Contracept 10: 249-255.

29. Truitt ST, Fraser AB, Grimes DA, Gallo MF, Schulz KF (2003) Combined hormonal versus nonhormonal versus progestin-only contraception in lactation. Cochrane Database Syst Rev 2.

30. Davies KJ, Quintanilha AT, Brooks GA, Packer L (1982) Free radicals and tissue damage produced by exercise. Biochem Biophys Res Commun 107: 1198-1205.

31. Husain K, Somani SM (1998) Interaction of exercise training and chronic ethanol ingestion on testicular antioxidant system in rat. J Appl Toxicol 18: 421-429.

32. Kavlock RJ, Daston GP, De Rosa C, Fenner CP, GrayKattari LE, et al. (1996) Research needs for the risk assessment of health and environmental effect of endocrine disruptors: A report of the USEPA sponsored workshop. Env Hlth Perspect 104: 714-740.

11

A Short Review of Methods for the Allylic Oxidation of Δ^5 Steroidal Compounds to Enones

Wendell SG and Edward JP*

Department of Chemistry and Biochemistry, College of Science and Mathematics,Auburn University, Auburn, Alabama 36849-5319, USA

Abstract

Introduction of α, β-unsaturated ketones to Δ^5 steroidal olefins changes the characteristics and biological function of those compounds. Several synthetic methods have been reported to accomplish carbonyl introduction to Δ^5 steroidal olefins. Herein, this short review will catalogue many of those oxidative methods, particularly those proceeding through a peroxide intermediate and/or use chromium complexes as reagents.

Keywords: Allylic oxidation; TBHP; Chromium; Steroids

Introduction

The oxidation of the B ring in steroidal compounds leads to products exhibiting numerous biological functionalities. Ring B oxidized sterols and steroids have shown anti-cancer activity [1-3]. 7-Ketodehydroepiandrosterone has been shown to improve the memory of mice [4] and 3-acetyl-7-oxo-DHEA increases the resting metabolism of persons on calorie restrictive diets [5]. 7-Ketopregnenolone's has shown anti-cortisone properties [6]. 7-Ketocholesterol has shown some regulatory function in the biosynthesis of cholesterol [7]. Furthermore, B ring oxidized steroidal compounds may be used as synthetic reagents to make other steroidal products, such as a steroidal pyrazoline [8].

Several Δ^5 allylic oxidation methods leading to enone formation have been reported and are catalogued in this review. The Δ^5 steroidal olefins are very common. Other steroidal olefins, with the exception of Δ^4 olefins perhaps, are much less common. As the precursor of steroids, cholesterol's Δ^5 moiety is retained until the steroids are enzymatically isomerized [9]. Thus, methods stated in this review have many potential steroidal substrates.

There are three allylic carbons (C4, C7 and C10) to the C5 double bond in a typical steroidal nucleus before isomerization to Δ^4. The C10 carbon is a stable quaternary carbon. Thus, allylic oxidation occurs only at C4 and C7, albeit not equally. The C4 carbon is located on the sterically hindered β side with its axial hydrogen extending also in the β direction. On the other hand, the C7 carbon is located on the exposed α side with its axial hydrogen extending further in the α direction [10]. There is also an energetic advantage for C7 oxidation. Resonance originating from C7 oxidation is more energetically favored than resonance originating from C4 oxidation due to delocalization to the tertiary C5 carbon rather than to the secondary C6 carbon. It was calculated that radical oxidation at C7 is favored by -4.65 kcal/mol over C4 on a two ring system containing the A and B ring moiety of cholesterol [11] (Figure 1). It should be noted as an exception that selenium complexes have been reported to oxidize C4 rather than C7 [12,13].

Steroidal compounds can be fairly resistant to deprotonation, especially within the B ring. Ring strain, that is incurred from the sp^3 to sp^2 hybridization change (bond angle distortion), is higher than that of non-fused ring systems due to "conformational transmission" [14].

Perhaps this explains why the oxidative methods surveyed in Tables 1-5 occur exclusively through a radical mechanism. With respect to the radical mechanism, it is important to note that tertiary carbons are present on steroidal compounds that can be radically oxidized leading

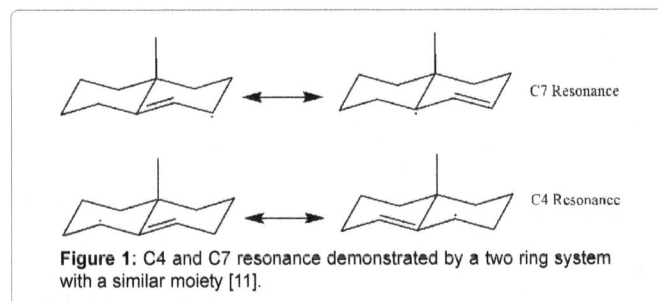

Figure 1: C4 and C7 resonance demonstrated by a two ring system with a similar moiety [11].

to undesired side products, one in particular being C25 for steroids with side chains [15]. Furthermore, cleavage of the side chain can occur concurrent with allylic oxidation [16].

Protecting the C3 hydroxy group is commonly accomplish by esterification using acetic anhydride to make cholesteryl acetate. The authors of this review prefer esterification with benzoyl chloride since cholesteryl benzoate products can be more easily isolated with recrystallization in acetone and water than the steroidal acetates. This esterification is necessary because many oxidants and catalysts will convert the C3 hydroxyl group to a ketone [17].

Due to interest in "green" or environmentally benign chemistry, chemists have questioned the ethics of earlier catalysts. Environmental and health concerns have motivated the search for new oxidants and catalysts [18]. From chromium based catalysts, the next phase in steroidal allylic oxidation manifested through more environmentally friendly metallic catalysts that use TBHP as an oxygen donor. Meanwhile, several methods have been reported to give steroidal oxidation without any metal catalysts using as sodium chlorite and sodium hypochlorite [19,20]. Additionally, recoverable heterogeneous catalysts, clay

*Corresponding author: Edward JP, Department of Chemistry and Biochemistry, College of Science and Mathematics, Auburn University, Auburn, Alabama 36849-5319, USA, 179 Chemistry Bldg, E-mail: parisej@auburn.edu

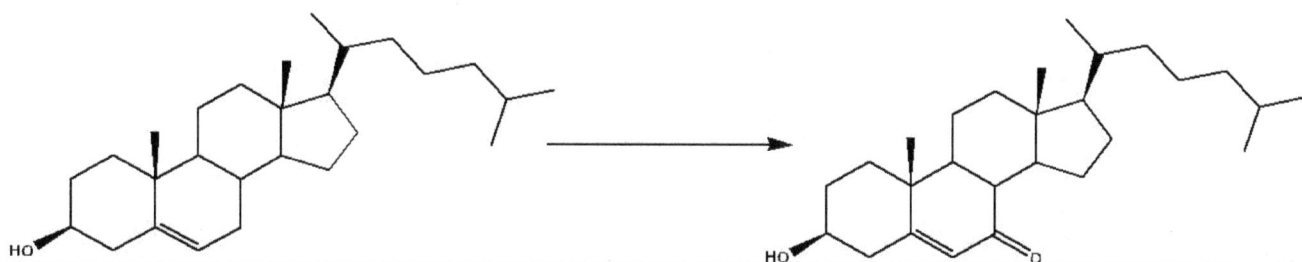

Substrate: Cholesterol				
Catalysts, Reagents, Solvents and Conditions	TBHP used as Oxidant (Yes/No)	Date Reported	% Yield Reported	Reference #
Rh$_2$(cap)$_4$, DCM (DCE), r.t, 15 h	Yes	2009	30	[26]
Rh$_2$(cap)$_4$, DCM (DCE), r.t, 20 h	Yes	2007	63	[27]
NaOCl, DCE, 4°C, 10 h	Yes	2004	68	[20]
CrO$_3$/NHPI-activated clay, DCM, r.t, 58 h	No	2009	52	[21]
2-quinoxalinol salen Cu(II) complex catalyst, Acetonitrile, 70°C, 12 h	Yes	2010	69	[11]
RuCl$_3$, Cyclohexane, r.t, 24 h	Yes	1996	51	[28]
VOCl$_3$, r.t, 5 days	Yes	2015	45	[29]

Table 1: Cholesterol to 7-ketocholesterol.

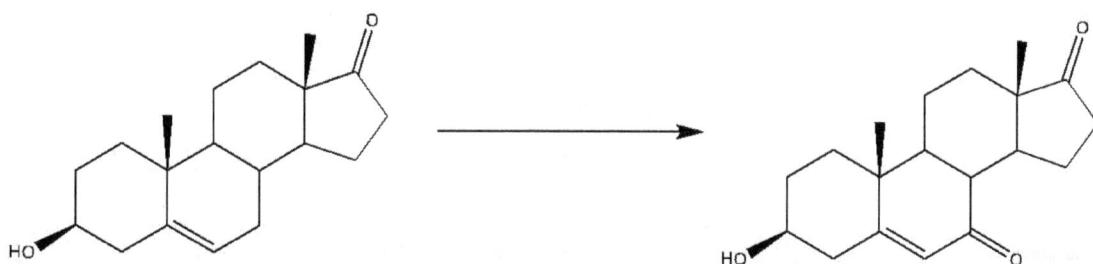

Substrate: DHEA				
Catalysts, Reagents, Solvents and Conditions	TBHP used as Oxidant (Yes/No)	Date Reported	% Yield Reported	Reference #
Rh$_2$(cap)$_4$, DCE, 40°C, 20 h	Yes	2007	74	[27]
NaOCl, Ethylacetate/Tert-butanol (8:2), 4°C, 10 h	Yes	2004	70	[20]
CrO$_3$/NHPI-activated clay, DCM, r.t, 58 h	No	2009	67	[21]
BiCl$_3$, Acetonitrile, 70°C, 28 h	Yes	2005	80	[30]
BiCl$_3$/K-10, Acetonitrile, 70°C, 11 h	Yes	2005	77	[30]
NaClO$_2$, Acetonitrile/Water (2:1), 50°C, 20 h	Yes	2007	65	[19]
NaClO$_2$/NHPI, Acetonitrile/Water (2:1), 50°C, 11 h	No	2007	50	[19]
VOCl$_3$, r.t, 5 days	Yes	2015	19	[29]

Table 2: DHEA to 7-keto DHEA.

supported and organometallic polymer catalysts, have been reported to yield allylic oxidation products of steroidal compounds [21–23].

Reported Methods

The following Tables 1-5 are divided by substrates used in our allylic oxidation reaction with TBHP and vanadium complexes. Reagents, conditions, dates, and isolated yields reported for various steroidal allylic oxidation reactions are displayed. All reagents are listed, with TBHP given a special column (TBHP was mainly, if not exclusively used).

Caution must be taken when comparing the reported yields because there were various methods used to identify "isolated" yields (using HPLC instead of obtaining mass for example) [20], differing standards on purity of the isolated product (i.e., reporting an isolated yield that is 67% pure) [19], differing sampling sizes, and an overall lack

of supporting information. Several reported steroidal allylic oxidation reactions have not been included in the tables due to low yields of 7-keto product, such as oxygen irradiation with and without photosensitizer [24] and Gif chemistry [25].

The importance of identifying TBHP usage in allylic oxidation reactions is that those reactions share a similar intermediate. It has been noted, "that different catalysts produce essentially the same mixture of products with the same relative yields suggests that the catalyst is not involved in product-forming steps" [26]. Indeed, tert-butoxide and tert-butyl peroxy radicals are formed through degradation of TBHP by catalysts. Those radicals then oxidize steroidal compounds [19,20,26-33,36].

All of the reactions in Table 1-5 can be funneled, generally speaking, into two mechanisms. The first mechanism, oxidation through formation of a C7 peroxide, is shared by auto-oxidation, TBHP-metal

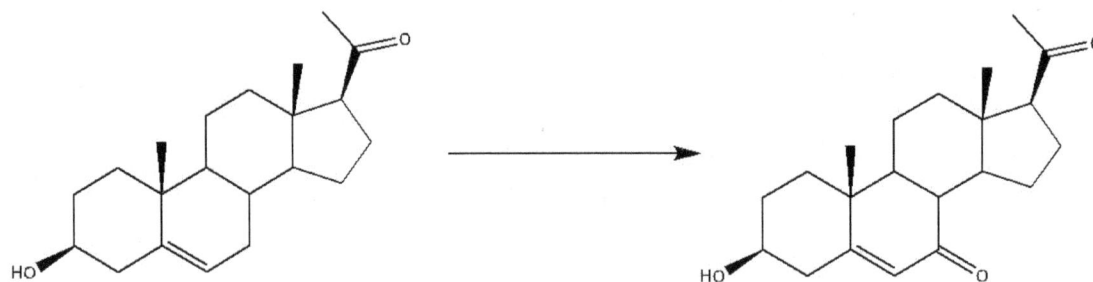

Substrate: Pregnenolone				
Catalysts, Reagents, Solvents and Conditions	TBHP used as Oxidant (Yes/No)	Date Reported	% Yield Reported	Reference #
Rh$_2$(cap)$_4$, DCE, 40°C, 20 h	Yes	2007	40	[27]
CrO$_3$/NHPI-activated clay, DCM, r.t, 58 h	No	2009	54	[21]
2-Quinoxalinol salen Cu(II) complex catalyst, Acetonitrile, 0°C, 12 h	Yes	2010	53	[11]
VOCl$_3$, r.t., 5 days		Yes	2015	24	[29]

Table 3: Pregnenolone to 7-ketopregnenolone.

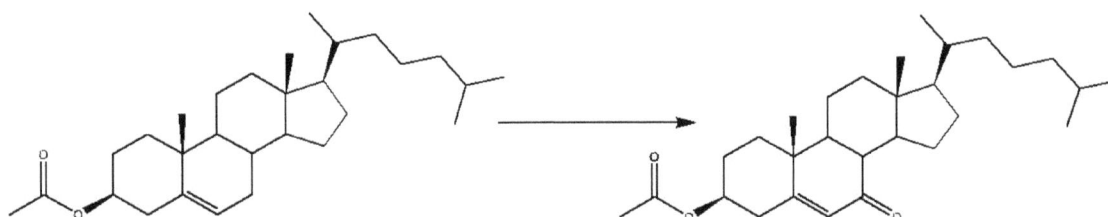

Substrate: Cholesteryl Acetate				
Catalysts, Reagents, Solvents and Conditions	TBHP used as Oxidant (Yes/No)	Date Reported	% Yield Reported	Reference #
Co(OAc)$_2$/SiO$_2$, Benzene, 50°C, 24 h, N$_2$	Yes	2001	70	[22]
ZrO$_2$/SiO$_2$/Cr(VI), Benzene, r.t, pH 3	Yes	1999	48	[31]
RuCl$_3$, Cyclohexane, r.t, 24 h	Yes	1996	51	[28]
Rh$_2$(cap)$_4$, DCE, 40°C, 20 h	Yes	2007	80	[27]
TiO(acac)$_2$, Benzene, 80°C, 24 h, Ar	Yes	1981	25	[32]
98 VO(acac)$_2$, Benzene, 80°C, 24 h, Ar	Yes	1981	26	[32]
Cr(acac)$_3$, Benzene, 80°C, 24 h, Ar	Yes	1981	52	[32]
Mn(acac)$_2$, Benzene, 80°C, 24 h, Ar	Yes	1981	11	[32]
Mn(acac)$_3$, Benzene, 80°C, 24 h, Ar	Yes	1981	10	[32]
Fe(acac)$_3$, Benzene, reflux, 24 h, Ar	Yes	1979	74	[32]
Co(acac)$_2$, Benzene, 80°C, 24 h, Ar	Yes	1981	12	[32]
Co(acac)$_3$, Benzene, 80°C, 24 h, Ar	Yes	1981	43	[32]
Ni(acac)$_2$, Benzene, 80°C, 24 h, Ar	Yes	1981	38	[32]
Cu(acac)$_2$, Benzene, 80°C, 24 h, Ar	Yes	1981	83	[32]
Ce(acac)$_2$, Benzene, 80°C, 24 h, Ar	Yes	1981	24	[32]
Cu(Oac)$_2$/SiO$_2$, Benzene, 70°C, 48 h, N$_2$	Yes	2002	72	[23]
CuI, Acetonitrile, reflux, 4 h	Yes	2003	79	[33]
CuI/TBAB, DCM, reflux, 4 h	Yes	2003	76	[33]
CrO$_3$/Py$_2$, Triflourotoluene, r.t, 31 h, N$_2$	Yes	2006	76	[34]
CrO$_3$/Py$_2$, DCM, r.t, 24 h, N$_2$	No	1969	74	[10]
PCC, DCM, 40°C, 66 h	Yes	2006	41	[34]
CrO$_2$, Acetonitrile/Benzene (9:1), reflux, 72 h, N$_2$	No	Note	48	
Cr(CO)$_6$, Acetonitrile, reflux, 15 h	Yes	1985	80	[35]
Mn$_3$O(Oac)$_9$, Ethyl Acetate, 40°C, 48 h, N$_2$	Yes	2006	87	[36]
NaOCl, DCE, 4°C, 10 h	No	2004	68	[20]
2-QuinoxalinolsalenCu(II) complex catalyst, Acetonitrile, 70°C, 12 h	Yes	2010	97	[11]
BiCl$_3$, Acetonitrile, 70°C, 22 h	Yes	2005	82	[30]

NaClO₂, Acetonitrile, 60°C, 80 h	Yes	2007	66	[19]
NaClO₂/NHPI, 1,4-dioxane/water (3:1), 50°C, 25 h	No	2007	60	[19]
VOCl₃, r.t, 5 days	Yes	2015	83	[29]

Table 4: Cholesteryl acetate to 7-ketocholesteryl acetate.

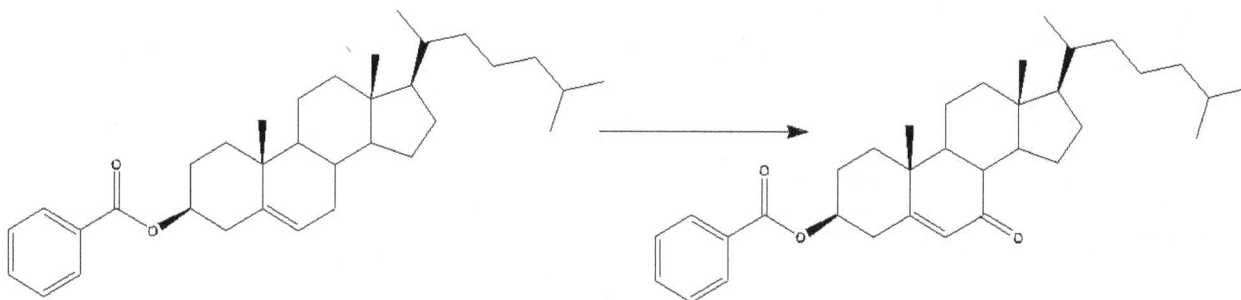

Substrate: Cholesteryl Benzoate'				
Catalysts, Reagents, Solvents and Conditions	TBHP used as Oxidant (Yes/No)	Date Reported	% Yield Reported	Reference #
PFC, Benzene, reflux, 48 h, N₂	No	1996	88	[37]
CrO₂, Acetonitrile/benzene (9:1), reflux, 72 h, N₂	No	Note	52	[35]
CrO₃/DMP, DCM, -10°C to -20°C, 4 h	No	1978	75	[38]
PCC, Benzene, refluxed, 24 h, N₂	No	1987	87	[39]
VOCl₃, r.t, 5 days	Yes	2015	98	[29]

Table 5: Cholestryl benzoate to 7-ketocholesteryl benzoate.

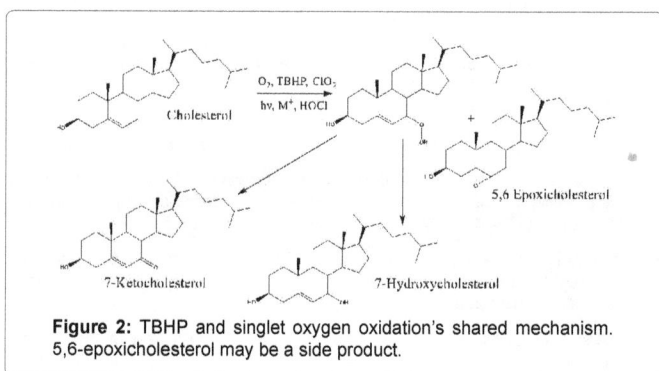

Figure 2: TBHP and singlet oxygen oxidation's shared mechanism. 5,6-epoxicholesterol may be a side product.

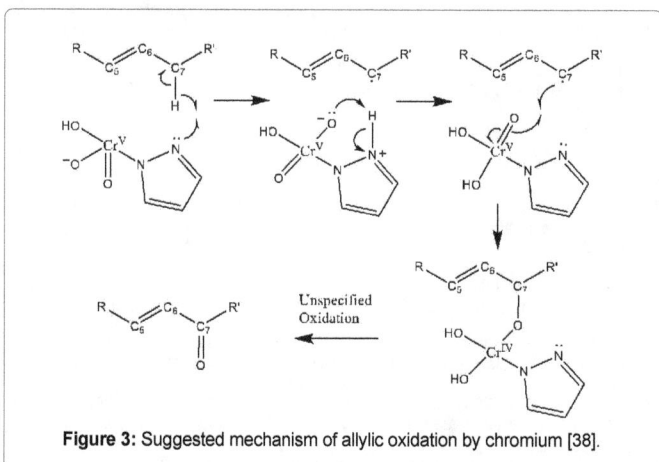

Figure 4: Hydrogen abstraction in benzophenoneaminocholestene [43].

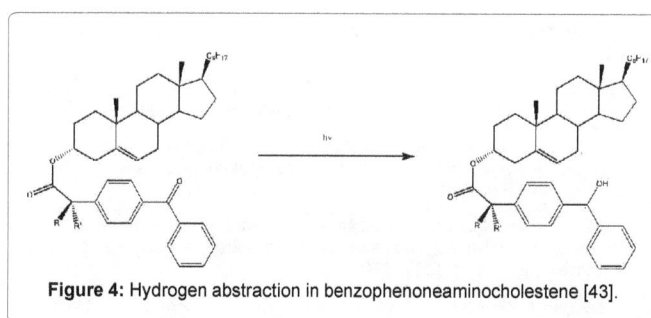

Figure 3: Suggested mechanism of allylic oxidation by chromium [38].

metal leads to radicals that form a C7 peroxide. Bleach initiates radical formation from TBHP, similar to the metal catalysts [20]. When only sodium chlorite and NHPI are used, NHPI becomes phthalimide N-oxyl (PINO), a radical initiator of molecular oxygen [19]. Those radicals in addition to radicals formed from ClO₂ lead to a C7 peroxide. The C7 peroxide degrades to form a ketone or hydroxyl group [40-42] (Figure 2).

The second mechanism is that of oxidation via chromium reagent. During the first step of the suggested mechanism (Figure 3), there is complexation of chromium and a ligand containing a functional group, imine preferably, such as DMP or pyridine. After complexation, the ligand abstracts the C7 hydrogen leaving a resonating steroidal radical. An oxo group on the chromium complex will terminate the radical, reducing the chromium. Oxidation of the steroid then proceeds in an unspecified manner. It is important to note that the chromium complex may be monomeric [38].

Acetonitrile, benzene, pyridine, DCM, DCE, trifluorotoluene, 1,4-dioxane/water, and cyclohexane were used as solvents in Tables 1-5. Using laser flash photolysis and benzophenoneaminocholestene, it has been shown that the C7 hydrogens are abstracted at a much greater rate (more than double) in DCM than in acetonitrile, dioxane, and

oxidation, and hypochlorite oxidation. In auto-oxidation, a peroxide is formed via singlet oxygen (ene reaction) at the C5 carbon [24], which rearranges to the C7 position [40,41]. Likewise, TBHP degradation by

methanol [43] (Figure 4). Thus, the least polar solvents appear to work best for allylic oxidation. This is, however, limited by the solubility of the steroidal substrate.

Conclusion

Converting Δ^5 steroidal compounds to their corresponding enones is an endeavor that has spanned several decades. The authors of this review suggest that all of the oxidative methods found within this review utilize one of two general mechanisms. One mechanism involves formation of a peroxide at the allylic position and the other achieves oxidation through reduction of a chromium complex. Both mechanisms occur via radical formation. Various solvents were used in the reported methods, but flash photolysis experiments from at least one article indicate that nonpolar solvents may be more affective.

References

1. Carvalho JF, Silva MM, Moreira JN, Simões S, Sá e Melo ML (2010) Sterols as anticancer agents: synthesis of ring-B oxygenated steroids, cytotoxic profile, and comprehensive SAR analysis. J Med Chem 53: 7632-7638.

2. Parish EJ, Chitrakorn S, Luu B, Schmidt G, Ourisson G (1989) Studies of the oxysterol inhibition of tumor cell growth. Steroids 53: 579-596.

3. de Medina P, Paillasse MR, Ségala G, Khallouki F, Brillouet S, et al. (2011) Importance of cholesterol and oxysterols metabolism in the pharmacology of tamoxifen and other AEBS ligands. Chem Phys Lipids 164: 432-437.

4. Shi J, Schulze S, Lardy HA (2000) The effect of 7-oxo-DHEA acetate on memory in young and old C57BL/6 mice. Steroids 65: 124-129.

5. Zenk JL, Frestedt JL, Kuskowski MA (2007) HUM5007, a novel combination of thermogenic compounds, and 3-acetyl-7-oxo-dehydroepiandrosterone: each increases the resting metabolic rate of overweight adults. J Nutr Biochem 18: 629-634.

6. Marshall CW, Ray RE, Laos I, Riegel B (1957) 7-Keto Steroids. II. Steroidal 3ß-Hydroxy- 5-7-ones and 3,5-7-ones. J Am Chem Soc 79: 6308-6313.

7. Kandutsch AA, Chen HW (1973) Inhibition of sterol synthesis in cultured mouse cells by 7alpha-hydroxycholesterol, 7beta-hydroxycholesterol, and 7-ketocholesterol. J Biol Chem 248: 8408-8417.

8. Shamsuzzaman, Khanam H, Mashrai A, Sherwani A, Owais M, et al. (2013) Synthesis and anti-tumor evaluation of B-ring substituted steroidal pyrazoline derivatives. Steroids 78: 1263-1272.

9. Ghayee HK, Auchus RJ (2007) Basic concepts and recent developments in human steroid hormone biosynthesis. Rev Endocr Metab Disord 8: 289-300.

10. Dauben WG, Lorber ME, Fullerton DS (1969) Allylic Oxidation of Olefins with Chromium Trioxide-Pyridine Complex. J Org Chem 34: 3587-3592.

11. Li Y, Wu X, Lee TB, Isbell EK, Parish EJ, et al. (2010) An effective method for allylic oxidation of Delta5-steroids using tert-butyl hydroperoxide. J Org Chem 75: 1807-1810.

12. Barton DHR, Crich D (1985) Oxidation of Olefins with 2-Pyridineseleninic Anhydride. Tetrahedron 41: 4359-4364.

13. Crich D, Zou Y (2004) Catalytic allylic oxidation with a recyclable, fluorous seleninic acid. Org Lett 6: 775-777.

14. Barton DHR, Head AJ, May PJ (1957) Long-range Effects in Alicyclic Systems. Part II. The Rates of Condensation of Some Triterpenoid Ketones with Benzaldehyde. J Chem Soc (Resumed) pp: 935-944.

15. Parish E, Aksara N, Boos T, Kizito S (1998) Methodology and Synthetic Studies on the Remote Functionalization of Steroid Side Chains. Rec Res Devel Org Chem 2: 95-105.

16. Takano S, Sato S, Ogasawara K (1985) Simple Synthesis of 3ß, 24-Dihydroxychol-5-en-7one by Oxidative Cleavage of the Side Chain of Cholesterol. Chem Lett 14: 1265-1266.

17. Parish EJ, Kizito SA, Qiu Z (2004) Review of chemical syntheses of 7-keto-delta5-sterols. Lipids 39: 801-804.

18. Salvador JAR, Silvestre SM, Moreira VM (2006) Catalytic Oxidative Processes in Steroid Chemistry: Allylic Oxidation, ß-Selective Epoxidation, Alcohol Oxidation and Remote Functionalization Reactions Current Organic. Curr Org Chem 10: 2227-2257.

19. Silvestre SM, Salvador JAR (2007) Allylic and Benzylic Oxidation Reactions with Sodium Chlorite. Tetrahedron 63: 2439-2445.

20. Marwah P, Marwah A, Lardy HA (2004) An Economical and Green Approach for the Oxidation of Olefins to Enones. Green Chem 6: 570-577.

21. Liu J, Zhu HY, Cheng XH (2009) CrO3/NHPI Adsorbed on Activated Clay: A New Supported Reagent for Allylic Selective Oxidation of 5-Sterols. Synthetic Communications 39: 1076-1083.

22. Salvador JAR, Clark JH (2001) The Allylic Oxidation of Unsaturated Steroids by tert-Butyl Hydroperoxide Using Homogenous and Heterogenous Cobalt Acetate. Chem Commun pp: 33-34.

23. Salvador JAR, Clark JH (2002) The Allylic Oxidation of Unsaturated Steroids by tert-Butyl Hydroperoxide Using Surface Functionalised Silica Supported Metal Catalysts. Green Chem 4: 352-356.

24. Kulig MJ, Smith LL (1973) Sterol metabolism. XXV. Cholesterol oxidation by singlet molecular oxygen. J Org Chem 38: 3639-3642.

25. Barton DHR, Boivin J, Hill CH (1986) Functionalisation of Saturated Hydrocarbons. Part 6. Selective Oxidation of Steroids and Related Compounds. J Chem Soc Perkin Trans pp: 1797-1804.

26. McLaughlin EC, Choi H, Wang K, Chiou G, Doyle MP (2009) Allylic oxidations catalyzed by dirhodium caprolactamate via aqueous tert-butyl hydroperoxide: the role of the tert-butylperoxy radical. J Org Chem 74: 730-738.

27. Choi H, Doyle MP (2007) Optimal TBHP allylic oxidation of Delta5-steroids catalyzed by dirhodium caprolactamate. Org Lett 9: 5349-5352.

28. Miller RA, Li W, Humphrey GR (1996) A Ruthenium Catalyzed Oxidation of Steroidal Alkenes to Enones. Tetrahedron Lett 37: 3429-3432.

29. Grainger WS, Parish EJ (2015) Allylic oxidation of steroidal olefins by vanadyl acetylacetonate and tert-butyl hydroperoxide. Steroids 101: 103-109.

30. Salvador JAR, Silvestre SM (2005) Bismuth-Catalyzed Allylic Oxidation Using t-Butyl Hydroperoxide. Tetrahedron Lett 46: 2581-2584.

31. Baptistella LHB, Sousa IMO, Gushikem Y, Aleixo AM (1999) Chromium (VI) Adsorbed on SiO$_2$/ZrO$_2$, a New Supported Reagent for Allylic Oxidations. Tetrahedron Lett 40: 2695-2698.

32. Kimura M, Muto T (1981) The Reactions of Cholesteryl Acetate with tert-Butyl Hydroperoxide and Molybdenum Complexes. Chem Pharm Bull 29: 35-42.

33. Arsenou ES, Koutsourea AI, Fousteris MA, Nikolaropoulos SS (2003) Optimization of the allylic oxidation in the synthesis of 7-keto-delta5-steroidal substrates. Steroids 68: 407-414.

34. Fousteris MA, Koutsourea AI, Nikolaropoulos SS, Riahi A, Muzart J (2006) Improved Chromium-Catalyzed Allylic Oxidation of 5-Steroids with t-Butyl Hydroperoxide. J Mol Catal A: Chem 250: 70-74.

35. Pearson AJ, Chen YS, Han GR, Hsu SY, Ray T (1985) A New Method for the Oxidation of Alkenes to Enones. An Efficient Synthesis of 5-7-Oxo Steroids. J Chem Soc, Perkin Trans pp: 267-273.

36. Shing TK, Yeung YY, Su PL (2006) Mild manganese(III) acetate catalyzed allylic oxidation: application to simple and complex alkenes. Org Lett 8: 3149-3151.

37. Parish EJ, Sun H, Kizito SA (1996) Allylic Oxidation of 5-Steroids with Pyridinium Fluorochromate. J Chem Res pp: 544.

38. Salmond WG, Barta MA, Havens JL (1978) Allylic Oxidation with 3,5-Dimethylpyrazole. Chromium Trioxide Complex. Steroidal 5-7-Ketones. J Org Chem 43: 2057-2059.

39. Parish EJ, Wei TY, Livant P (1987) A facile synthesis and carbon-13 nuclear magnetic resonance spectral properties of 7-ketocholesteryl benzoate. Lipids 22: 760-763.

40. Smith LL, Teng JI, Kulig MJ, Hill FL (1973) Sterol metabolism. 23. Cholesterol oxidation by radiation-induced processes. J Org Chem 38: 1763-1765.

41. Tai CY, Chen YC, Chen BH (1999) Analysis, Formation, and Inhibition of Cholesterol Oxidation Products in Foods: An Overview (Part 1). J Food Drug Anal 7: 243-257.

42. Kimura M, Muto Toshiki (1979) On the Reaction of Cholesteryl Acetate with tert-Butyl Hydroperoxide in the Presence of Tris(acetylacetonato)iron(III). Chem Pharm Bull 27: 109-112.

43. Andreu I, Palumbo F, Tilocca F, Morera IM, Boscá F, et al. (2011) Solvent effects in hydrogen abstraction from cholesterol by benzophenone triplet excited state. Org Lett 13: 4096-4099.

12

Clomiphene Stimulation Test in Men Abusing Anabolic-Androgenic Steroids for Long Time

Medras M[1,2], Jozkow P[2*], Terpilowski L[3] and Zagocka E[4]

[1]Department of Endocrinology, Diabetology and Isotope Treatment, Wroclaw Medical University, ul. Pasteura 4, 50-367 Wroclaw, Poland
[2]Department of Sports Medicine, University School of Physical Education, ul, Paderewskiego 35, 51-612 Wroclaw, Poland
[3]Department of Emergency Medical Services, Wroclaw Medical University, ul. Pasteura 4, 50-367 Wroclaw, Poland
[4]Laboratory of Male Infertility, ul. Kosciuszki 108A/18, 50-441 Wroclaw, Poland

Abstract

Objective: Androgenic-anabolic steroids (AAS) are commonly used by athletes and recreational athletes. In some cases they induce persistent anabolic steroid-induced hypogonadism (ASIH).

Design: In an observational study we assessed the function of the pituitary-gonadal axis in a series of men with suspected ASIH.

Methods: Clomiphene stimulation test (CST) was performed in 13 hypogonadal adult men with previous, prolonged exposure to AAS. We evaluated the response of luteinizing hormone (LH), follicle-stimulating hormone (FSH) and total testosterone (T) to 50 mg of clomiphene daily administered for a week.

Results: Mean concentrations of hormones before and after clomiphene administration were respectively (mean ± SD): 3 ± 1.2 and 8.3 ± 2 mIU/ml for LH; 3 ± 1.1 and 10 ± 14.6 mIU/ml for FSH; and 2.3 ± 0.6 and 7.2 ± 1.7 ng/ml for T (p<0.001).

Conclusions: Men with ASIH, after a long-time withdrawal of AAS, present an intact reaction of gonadotropins and testosterone to clomiphene stimulation.

Keywords: Anabolic agents; Hypogonadism; Clomiphene; Diagnostic tests; Gonadotropins; Testosterone

Introduction

Illicit use of AAS is widespread in many parts of the world. Recent surveys show that 2.4% of Australian students report lifetime AAS use [1], while in Sweden between 10 000 and 100 000 subjects may be exposed to AAS every year [2]. In Poland 6.2% of young males and 2.9% of young females admit that they use anabolic agents. Data from other countries and continents suggest that AAS users can be counted in millions [3-5]. The situation is emerging as a public health concern [6].

Side effects of AAS are common and involve diverse body organs and systems [7-9]. One of the most prominent AAS effects is suppression of the hypothalamo-pituitary-gonadal (HPG) axis leading to decreased production of testosterone and spermatozoa. Although the gonadal function usually recovers after withdrawal of AAS, in a growing number of cases there is observed a secondary, functional, often hypogonadotropic, anabolic steroid- induced hypogonadism (ASIH) [10]. Low concentration of testosterone may persist even after several months-long cessations of AAS.

Hypogonadism understood as testosterone deficiency is associated with a broad range of somatic, sexual and psychological symptoms [10-12]. Acquired, hypogonadotropic hypogonadism (AHH) is a consequence of anatomical and functional alterations of the hypothalamus and/or the pituitary. It is found in tumors, infiltrative and vascular disorders of the sellar region. It may be also observed after brain injury, neurosurgery, in the course of anemia, uremia, alcoholism or as a side effect of gonadotropin suppression during endocrinological, psychiatric or urological treatments [13,14]. Data on clinical aspects of ASIH is scarce.

Our aim was to assess the HPG axis with use of the clomiphene stimulation test in adult men with a history of long-term exposure to AAS.

Subjects and Methods

The study had an observational character. It was performed in thirteen adult men (aged 25 ± 4), former AAS users, who were referred to an andrological outpatient clinic because of low testosterone concentration. Studied subjects were informed on the aim of the investigation and the diagnostic procedure to which a written consent was given.

Each athlete had a medical interview with a full andrological checkup. None of the studied cases presented disturbances of sexual differentiation and maturity or physical symptoms of hypogonadism. They did not suffer from any chronic medical conditions and did not receive medications for at least 3 months prior the investigation.

All of the investigated men had total testosterone (T) concentration ≤3.2 ng/ml. Their clinical status was good (normal: body mass index, blood pressure, testicular volume). Four of the studied men fathered children before starting AAS, one – during AAS use.

Our cases derived from the same sport environment and received AAS in a similar manner (3-4 cycles of several weeks duration eg. Deca Durabolin 4000 mg, Omnadren 7000 mg, Metanabol 1200 mg and/or Oxandrolone 5000 mg during a year). They used AAS for 3.9 ± 1.6 years. The drug-free interval before the investigation was 2.1 ± 1.0 years.

***Corresponding author:** Pawel Jozkow, Department of Sports Medicine, University School of Physical Education, ul. Paderewskiego 35, 51-612 Wroclaw, Poland, E-mail: jozkow@gmail.com

Laboratory evaluation consisted of fasting measurements of: luteinizing hormone (LH), follicle-stimulating hormone (FSH), total testosterone (T), estradiol (E2), sex-horrmone binding globulin (SHBG), prolactin (PRL), sperm count assessed after 7-days sexual abstinence. In 7 cases magnetic resonance imaging of the pituitary was performed showing intact anatomy of the sellar region.

After confirmation of hypogonadism a week-long test with 50 mg clomiphene citrate/day, (clomiphene stimulation test, CST) was performed [15,16]. We compared basal and stimulated concentrations of LH, FSH and T.

Blood samples were obtained from the ulnar vein between 7.00 and 9.00 AM. Serum was stored at − 20°C until being used in the certified laboratory. Radioimmunoassay kits were used for measurements of T and E2 (Diagnostic Products Corporation, USA). The intra- and inter-assay coefficients of variation (CV) were 5.5 % and 5.9% for T and 5.8% and 7.4% for E2. SHBG, FSH and LH were measured using immunoradiometric assay-IRMA kits (Immunotech, Czech Republic). The intra- and interassay CV were 3.8 and 7.0% for SHBG; 5.0% and 3.8% for FSH; 6.7% and 3.7% for LH.

The statistical analysis was performed using the PQ Stat version 1.4.4.126. Concentrations of hormones in the CST test were assessed with the Wilcoxon signed-rank test. Associations among: age, duration of AAS use, duration from AAS withdrawal and results of the CST test were evaluated with U Mann-Whitney test and Spearman's rank correlation coefficient (fold changes of hormones' concentrations). A p-value less than 0.05 were considered significant.

Results

The raw results of the clomiphene stimulation test in the investigated men are presented in table (Table 1).

S.No	Age (years)	Length of AAS use (years)	Length of AAS withdrawal (years)	LH (mIU/ml)	FSH (mIU/ml)	T (nmol/l)
1	22	3	1.5	1.9	2.7	2.43
				8.1	6.52	7.3
2	31	5	3	2.8	3.46	2.5
				6.7	58	6.92
3	19	3.5	1	1.1	4.1	1.37
				9.9	6.2	7.12
4	24	4	2.2	3.72	3.5	2.91
				9.6	7.46	7.61
5	22	5	1.2	4.1	3.53	3.01
				9.5	8.2	9.9
6	28	7	4	4.48	3.15	2.33
				7.58	4.2	7.13
7	27	6	2	1.6	2.7	3.2
				9.1	7.5	8.7
8	30	4	3.2	2.2	1.9	2.3
				3.7	3.0	10.0
9	32	4.4	2.2	2.1	0.9	1.64
				11.8	3.2	6.1
10	29	3.0	1.5	2.68	1.8	1.61
				8.7	4.1	6.56
11	25	1.9	1.3	3.2	2.1	1.83
				6.7	3.3	3.61
12	21	2	3	4.45	3.97	2.2
				8.8	7.78	5.61
13	27	2	1	4.46	4.73	2.18
				7.66	9.49	6.74

Table 1: Raw results of the clomiphene stimulation test in the studied subjects. Hormone concentrations before and after (lines below) administration of clomiphene.

Mean concentrations of LH, FSH and T before and after clomiphene administration were respectively (mean±SD): 3 ± 1.2 and 8.3 ± 2 mIU/ml; 3 ± 1.1 and 10 ± 14.6 mIU/ml; 2.3 ± 0.6 and 7.2 ± 1.7 ng/ml (p<0.001) (Table 2).

	Descriptive statistics							Wilcoxon signed-rank test P
	Mean	SD	Min	Lower Quartile	Median	Upper Quartile	Max	
LH(mIU/ml)	2.08	1.17	1.10	2.10	2.80	4 10	4.48	0.0015
	8.30	1.96	3.70	7.58	8.70	9.50	11.80	
FSH(mIU/ml)	2.96	1.08	0.90	2.10	3.15	3.53	4.73	0.0015
	9.92	14.61	3.00	4.10	6.52	7.78	58.00	
T(ng/ml)	2.27	0.56	1.37	1.83	2.30	2.50	3.20	0.0015
	7.18	1.71	3.61	6.56	7.12	7.61	10.00	

Table 2: Changes of hormones concentrations in the clomiphene stimulation test. Hormone concentrations before and after clomiphene citrate (lines below).

Neither age of athletes, length of AAS use or length of AAS withdrawal influenced the CST outcomes in our study (Table 3).

	Age (years)	Duration of AAS use(years)	Duration of AAS withdrawal (years)
LH	-0.1735	0.1215	-0.3950
FSH	0.3691	0.2928	0.0083
T	0.2121	0.1768	-0.1878

Table 3: Spearman's rank correlation coefficient between: age of subjects, duration of AAS use and duration of withdrawal and changes of concentration of LH, FSH and T.

Discussion

There is little data on persistent pituitary dysfunction after AAS exposure. Laboratory findings in ASIH usually comprise low/normal levels of gonadotropins and low testosterone. Subjective symptoms do not appear until sometime after the onset of the disorder. Disruption of spermatogenesis may lead to infertility with structural and genetic sperm damage [17,18].

ASIH tends to be temporal. In most cases the androgenic milieu restores within a year after cessation of AAS, however in a number of male athletes low testosterone and sperm production disturbances may persist [19].

ASIH that arises a long time after AAS withdrawal is a poorly recognized condition. The occurrence of ASIH in AAS users is unknown and mechanism leading to hypogonadism and sperm count disturbances remains unexplained. To our knowledge associations between this specific forms of ASIH (eg. duration of AAS abuse, type of AAS used) and alterations of the sperm count have not been addressed in the literature. There is no information on its reversibility as well.

In our experience AAS-induced secondary hypogonadism emerges as an important form of the central nervous system dysfunction. The classical pathways of AAS effects in the brain comprise androgen and estrogen receptors (α, β) which are present in highest concentrations in basal telencephalon and diencephalon. Several enzymes play an important role here: 5α-reductase, aromatase, 3α-HSD, 3β-HSD, and 17β-HSD. AAS are thought to induce transcription and synthesis of new proteins. They may permanently modify activity of sex steroids receptors [20]. Apart from genomic effects, AAS modulate kinase activity, ion channels, and G-protein second-messenger systems. Some of these actions are much quicker than those induced through transcription factors [20]. Testosterone derivatives may act as partial opioid agonists. They may increase beta-endorphin levels in the ventral tegmental area and the thalamus, decrease levels of kappa receptors in the nucleus accumbens and increase: mu, delta and kappa receptor binding in the hypothalamus, striatum and midbrain periaqueductal gray [21,22]. AAS reduce the expression of serotonin receptors in the anterior hypothalamus (1A), globus pallidus (1B) or hippocampus [23,24]. They decrease serotonin concentration in basal forebrain and dorsal striatum [25], but increase in the cerebral cortex [26]. AAS are also likely to influence the brain GABA system and modify the mesolimbic dopamine system by stimulation of dopamine release and synthesis [26].

Clinical application of the clomiphene stimulation test (CST) has a long history with well-understood physiological basis [27]. It is a simple and widely accepted tool to evaluate the hypothalamo- pituitary-gonadal axis in men [15,16]. The CST in healthy subjects leads to doubling of LH, 20-50% increase of FSH and 30-220% increase of testosterone concentration [12]. A similar situation is observed in men with hyperprolactinemia [28] or during aging [29].

In turn organic damage to the CNS or the testicular feminization syndrome are associated with impaired results of the CST [30].

We have to admit that we had no data on the hormonal status of our study cases from before starting AAS doping. However our findings confirm that deregulation of the hypothalamus/the pituitary in men suspected of having ASIH (low LH, FSH and T) is reversible by application of an antiestrogen. Clomiphene stimulation in the studied men induced the same results as in healthy subjects. The mean rise of LH, FSH and T was respectively: 178%, 237% and 215%. Further research is

needed to establish the effects of antiestrogens used for longer periods and the influence of this treatment on sperm count. At the moment we have no information on permanence of the antiestrogen effects. There is no doubt that such a pharmacological regimen is more comfortable than gonadotropin therapy. Unlike androgens it has no detrimental effects on gonadal function [31].

We have not observed any differences of gonadotropins or testosterone reactions that would associate with doping course parameters (types of compounds, duration of use, time from withdrawal).

Lack of information on hormonal status (and sperm count) of the investigated subjects before initiation of AAS, missing information on sperm parameters and a small number of cases are major limitations of our observation. All of the studied men declared that clinical symptoms developed after withdrawal of AAS. We can add that five of our cases (38%) fathered children. None of them presented clinical features of congenital hypogonadal hypogonadism.

Future research on antiestrogens application in ASIH should involve monitoring of both: hormonal balance and sperm count.

Conclusions

Long-term AAS users who develop secondary, steroid- induced hypogonadism present an intact reaction of the HPG axis to clomiphene stimulation. Our data support rationale for an antiestrogen application to restore testosterone concentration in such cases.

References

1. Dunn M, White V (2011) The epidemiology of anabolic-androgenic steroid use among Australian secondary school students. J Sci Med Sport 14: 10-14.

2. Lood Y, Eklund A, Garle M, Ahlner J (2012) Anabolic androgenic steroids in police cases in Sweden 1999-2009. Forensic Sci Int 219: 199-204.

3. Galduróz JC, Noto AR, Nappo SA, Carlini EA (2005) Household survey on drug abuse in Brazil: study involving the 107 major cities of the country--2001. Addict Behav 30: 545-556.

4. RachoÅ D, Pokrywka L, Suchecka-RachoÅ„ K (2006) Prevalence and risk factors of anabolic-androgenic steroids (AAS) abuse among adolescents and young adults in Poland. Soz Praventivmed 51: 392-398.

5. Harmer PA (2010) Anabolic-androgenic steroid use among young male and female athletes: is the game to blame? Br J Sports Med 44: 26-31.

6. Kanayama G, Hudson JI, Pope HG Jr (2008) Long-term psychiatric and medical consequences of anabolic-androgenic steroid abuse: a looming public health concern? Drug Alcohol Depend 98: 1-12.

7. Angell P, Chester N, Green D, Somauroo J, Whyte G, et al. (2012) Anabolic steroids and cardiovascular risk. Sports Med 42: 119-134.

8. Turillazzi E, Perilli G, Di Paolo M, Neri M, Riezzo I, et al. (2011) Side effects of AAS abuse: an overview. Mini Rev Med Chem 11: 374-389.

9. Quaglio G, Fornasiero A, Mezzelani P, Moreschini S, Lugoboni F, et al. (2009) Anabolic steroids: dependence and complications of chronic use. Intern Emerg Med 4: 289-296.

10. Tan RS, Scally MC (2009) Anabolic steroid-induced hypogonadism-- towards a unified hypothesis of anabolic steroid action. Med Hypotheses 72: 723-728.

11. Traish AM, Miner MM, Morgentaler A, Zitzmann M (2011) Testosterone deficiency. Am J Med 124: 578-587.

12. Brower KJ (2009) Anabolic steroid abuse and dependence in clinical practice. Phys Sportsmed 37: 131-140.

13. Salenave S, Trabado S, Maione L, Brailly-Tabard S, Young J (2012) Male acquired hypogonadotropic hypogonadism: diagnosis and treatment. Ann Endocrinol (Paris) 73: 141-146.

14. Kanayama G, Brower KJ, Wood RI, Hudson JI, Pope HG Jr (2010) Treatment of anabolic-androgenic steroid dependence: Emerging evidence and its implications. Drug Alcohol Depend 109: 6-13.

15. Petak SM, Nankin HR, Spark RF, Swerdloff RS, Rodriguez-Rigau LJ (2002) American Association of Clinical Endocrinologists Medical Guidelines for clin-

ical practice for the evaluation and treatment of hypogonadism in adult male patients--2002 update. Endocr Pract 8: 440-456.

16. Rabijewski M, ZgliczyÅ„ski W (2009) [Pathogenesis, evaluation and treatment of hypogonadism in men]. Endokrynol Pol 60: 222-233.

17. Pope HG, Kanayama G, Ionescu-Pioggia M, Hudson JI (2004) Anabolic steroid users' attitudes towards physicians. Addiction 99: 1189-1194.

18. de Souza GL, Hallak J (2011) Anabolic steroids and male infertility: a comprehensive review. BJU Int 108: 1860-1865.

19. van Breda E, Keizer HA, Kuipers H, Wolffenbuttel BH (2003) Androgenic anabolic steroid use and severe hypothalamic-pituitary dysfunction: a case study. Int J Sports Med 24: 195-196.

20. Wood RI (2008) Anabolic-androgenic steroid dependence? Insights from animals and humans. Front Neuroendocrinol 29: 490-506.

21. Johansson P, Hallberg M, Kindlundh A, Nyberg F (2000) The effect on opioid peptides in the rat brain, after chronic treatment with the anabolic androgenic steroid, nandrolone decanoate. Brain Res Bull 51: 413-418.

22. Johansson P, Lindqvist A, Nyberg F, Fahlke C (2000) Anabolic androgenic steroids affects alcohol intake, defensive behaviors and brain opioid peptides in the rat. Pharmacol Biochem Behav 67: 271-279.

23. Ricci LA, Rasakham K, Grimes JM, Melloni RH, Jr. (2006) Serotonin-1A receptor activity and expression modulate adolescent anabolic/ androgenic steroid-induced aggression in hamsters. Pharmacol Biochem Behav 85: 1-11.

24. Kindlundh AM, Lindblom J, Bergström L, Nyberg F (2003) The anabolic- androgenic steroid nandrolone induces alterations in the density of serotonergic 5HT1B and 5HT2 receptors in the male rat brain. Neuroscience 119: 113-120.

25. Lindqvist AS, Johansson-Steensland P, Nyberg F, Fahlke C (2002) Anabolic androgenic steroid affects competitive behaviour, behavioural response to ethanol and brain serotonin levels. Behav Brain Res 133: 21-29.

26. Kurling S, Kankaanpää A, Ellermaa S, Karila T, Seppälä T (2005) The effect of sub-chronic nandrolone decanoate treatment on dopaminergic and serotonergic neuronal systems in the brains of rats. Brain Res 1044: 67-75.

27. Santen RJ, Leonard JM, Sherins RJ, Gandy HM, Paulsen CA (1971) Short- and long-term effects of clomiphene citrate on the pituitary- testicular axis. J Clin Endocrinol Metab 33: 970-979.

28. Ribeiro RS, Abucham J (2009) Recovery of persistent hypogonadism by clomiphene in males with prolactinomas under dopamine agonist treatment. Eur J Endocrinol 161: 163-169.

29. Da Ros CT, Averbeck MA (2012) Twenty-five milligrams of clomiphene citrate presents positive effect on treatment of male testosterone deficiency - a prospective study. Int Braz J Urol 38: 512-518.

30. Medina M, Ulloa-Aguirre A, Fernández MA, Pérez-Palacios G (1980) The role of oestrogens on gonadotrophin secretion in the testicular feminization syndrome. Acta Endocrinol (Copenh) 95: 314-318.

31. MedraÅ› M, Tworowska U (2001) [Treatment strategies of withdrawal from long-term use of anabolic-androgenic steroids]. Pol Merkur Lekarski 11: 535-538.

13

Early Experience with Diode Laser Combined with Systemic Steroid Therapy for Severe Stages of Retinopathy of Prematurity

Monika Modrzejewska[1]*, Ewelina Lachowicz[1], Joanna Kot D[1], Wojciech Lubiński[1], Jacek Rudnicki[2], Beata Czeszyńska[3], Anna Modrzejewska[1] and Jacek Patalan[4]

[1]Department of Ophthalmology, Pomeranian Medical University, Powst, Wlkp. Str. 72, 70 111 Szczecin, Poland
[2]Department of Neonatal Pathology, Pomeranian Medical University, Powst, Wlkp. Str. 72, 70 111 Szczecin, Poland
[3]Departament of Neonatology Pomeranian Medical University, Siedlecka Str. 2, Police, Poland
[4]Department of Neonatal Intensive Care Sp SZOZ-Zdroje, Mączna Str. 4, Szczecin, Poland

Abstract

Aims: To study the efficacy of diode laser-systemic steroid therapy in extremely and very-low-birth-weight prematures with severe Retinopathy of Prematurity (ROP).

Methods: 36 eyes of 18 prematures, mean gestational age 25.67 weeks (SD ± 1.28) and 811, 83 g birth weight (SD ± 299.08) with aggressive-posterior ROP (AP-ROP) and threshold 3 ROP with plus sign and Extraretinal Fibrovascular Proliferation (EFP) were enrolled. Indirect diode laser combined with intravenous course of Dexamethason was applied. Analyzed risk factors were correlated with the same ones received in cohort treated only with laser. Shapiro-Wilk, t-Student, U Mann-Whitney tests were involved in the statistical analysis (significance levels at p<0.05).

Results: Favorable anatomical results after mean 11.29 (SD ± 2.29) days of therapy were noted in 32 eyes (88.88%), ROP 5 developed in four eyes, but this difference was statistically non-significant (p=0.0612). Transient cortisol decreasing, hyperglycemia and partial adrenal fatigue were noted in some babies. During therapy, arterial systolic and diastolic pressures rose (p<0.05; p<0.01), significantly, which were related with severity of ROP, such as, C-reactive protein, erythrocyte and hematocrit, ventilation duration and number of transfusion (p<0.01).

Conclusion: Laser-steroid treatment might be additional effective alternative for severe ROP. Short- and long-term complications should be taken into account when starting this type of therapy.

Keywords: Retinopathy of prematurity; Systemic steroids application; Diode laser panfotocoagulation; Proinflammatory agents; Vasoproliferative factors

Abbreviations: ROP: Retinopathy of Prematurity; IL-6: Interleukin 6; CRP: C-Reactive Protein; IL-17: Interleukin 17; IL-8: Interleukin 8; TGF-α: Transforming Growth Factor-α; BDNF: Brain Derived Neurotrophin Factor; NT4: Neurotrophin-4; PDGF: Platelet-Derived Growth Factor; IGF-I: Insulin-Like Growth Factor; EGF: Epidermal Growth Factor; FGF: Fibroblast Growth Factor I; HIF-1 α: Hypoxia Inducible Factor; PKC: Protein Kinase C; SIMV: Synchronized Intermittent Mandatory Ventilation; IMV: Intermittent Mandatory Ventilation; IPPV: Intermittent Positive Pressure Ventilation; nCPAP: nasal Continuous Positive Airway Pressure; HFOV: High Frequency Oscillatory Ventilation

Introduction

Retinopathy of prematurity (ROP) is a vasoproliferative disease of the developing retina, complications of which might be the major cause of vision deterioration and blindness in infancy. This pathology is a biphasic process consisting of an initial phase of blunted vascular growth followed by a second phase of vasoproliferation that may be recognized by ophthalmoscopy 6 to 8 wks after birth [1]. Fundamental initiating process involved in retinal vascular development is angiogenesis which is regulated by growth factors, extracellular matrix components and complex of anti-and pro-inflammatory cytokines, among which IL-6, CRP, IL-17, IL-18, TNFα, TGF-β, BDNF, NT4, PDGF, IGF-I, EGF, FGF, PKC - protein kinase C- and HIF-1 α are recognized as key factors in the development of ROP. They have ability to modulate angiogenesis in ROP and are involved in dysregulation of this pathological phenomenon

mainly through up-regulating VEGF messenger RNA synthesis, in response to tissue hypoxia or inflammation [2-4]. Additionally, it has been revealed that the so-called Fetal Inflammatory Response (FIRS) is the result of chorioamnionitis, antenatal intrauterine as well as Candida infections which are important agents in pathogenesis of prematurity complications such as sepsis, Periventricular Leukomalacia (PVL), Intraventricular Hemorrhage (IVH), Necrotizing Enterocolitis (NEC) or bronchopulmonary dysplasia [2,3,5,6]. There are also studies which state that the abovementioned factors intensify frequency and severity of ROP, however neonatal noninfectious inflammation might further increase the inflammatory burden [5-7].

Dexamethasone is one of the mostly applied corticosteroids, both in different ophthalmological as well as in perinatal and neonatal disorders, where in the latter it is commonly used to limit the severity of chronic lung disease with severe respiratory distress syndrome [8]. It is the most potent anti-inflammatory agent, although the mode of its action has been poorly understood to this date. Some results of clinical and experimental studies have confirmed the decrease of the severity of retinopathy before and during oxygen exposure after intravenous administration of Dexamethasone in the mouse model and in broncho-pulmonary dysplasia [8-13]. Moreover, by modulating

*Corresponding author: Monika Modrzejewska MD PhD, Pomeranian Medical University, Powst. Wlkp. 72, 70 111 Szczecin, Poland, E-mail: monika_modrzej@op.pl

TNF-α, it simultaneously changes expression of the mentioned factor, which is important in reduction of inflammation and angiogenesis processes [14]. The purpose of this study was to present the preliminary outcomes for application of diode laser panfotocoagulation supported by systemic intravenous Dexamethasone course for selected severe stages of retinopathy of prematurity.

Subjects and Methods

A retrospective, comparative study was performed. Screening ophthalmic examinations were performed in 657 prematurely born babies. The examined subjects were under systematic, periodical supervision of Ophthalmic and Neonatal Clinical Departments and the follow-up period in this group was 3-years. Among that group, diode laser panfotocoagulation was undertaken in 48 infants (7.30%), however laser-steroid therapy was performed in 18 (2.73%) out of this treated group as a result of severe stages of ROP and rapid progression of the disease. Information on the course of ROP and the therapeutic management during the ophthalmologic care was collected from the medical records, computer images and what should be underlined, ophthalmic examinations were performed by one and the same experienced ophthalmologist and included: the funduscopy visualized by Ret-Cam II method (Clarity Medical Systems), ultrasonography (US–3300 Echo-Scan ultrasonic B-scan with 10-MHz sector probe equipment -Nidek Co. Japan) and intraocular pressure assessed by I-care PRO

Tonometer (Icare Finland Oy). Diode laser panfotocoagulation (Iris Medical, Ocu- Light S) of peripheral avascular retina was undertaken in general inhalatory anesthesia, with the mean parameters: power 200-500 mW, application time 50 ms, number of foci for one eye about 2454 ± 1525. Schedule of follow-up ophthalmic examinations was conducted individually for each baby, every 5-7 days in first weeks of observation until regression of the retinal lesions connected with the disease, next every 7-14 days in the first two months of post-operational period and subsequently it was prolonged to every 3-4 weeks for next two months. Prior to inclusion of laser-steroids therapy, prematures' parents had acknowledged the details of the disease course and the possibilities of its treatment on present day. They had also been informed about the option of Dexamethasone management as nonstandard therapy in ROP, taking into account mostly benefits but also likelihood of complications connected with steroids known from its use in various ophthalmic and multiorgan pathologies. Special emphasis was put on the side effects connected with steroids therapy, about which the parents were informed in much detail. After the written consent, systemic steroids course started being included. The study was approved by local ethics committee (approval No. KB-0012/52/12/10).

Data Collection

Detailed demographic, intrapartum, gestational, neonatal data were collected from patients' medical charts. Analyzed parameters were

Case #	Sex	Gestational age (weeks)	Birth Weight (g)	Delivery type	Causes for preterm birth	Pregnancy	Pregnancy/Delivery	Apgar score
1	F	25	650	N	preterm amniorrhexis, intrauterine infection	S	PIII DIII	2,3,4
2	M	27	1105	C	preterm amniorrhexis, intrauterine infection	S	PIII DII	1,1,1
3	F	24	600	C	Intrauterine infection	S	PV DII	4,4,5
4	M	28	1750	C	Intrauterine infection	S	PIII DII	6,4,7
5	F	25	530	N	preterm amniorrhexis, intrauterine infection	S	PI DI	2,2,3
6	F	25	530	C	placental abruption, threatening haemorrhage	S	PV DIII	0,6,6
7	M	25	850	C	placental abruption	M (2)	PIII DIII	4,7,8
8	M	24	700	C	hernia of foetal membranes, cross-birth, intrauterine infection	S	PIV DII	1,1,1
9	M	28	1200	C	preterm amniorrhexis.	M (2)	PII DII	6,6,7
10	F	27	900	C	placental abruption, intrauterine infection	S	PIII DIII	5,5,6
11	F	25	600	N	placental abruption, intrauterine infection	S	PI DI	2,2,2
12	F	25	720	C	placental abruption	M (2)	PIII DIII	5,5,8
13	M	26	650	C	preterm amniorrhexis, intrauterine infection	S	PI DI	2,2,2
14	M	26	760	C	preterm amniorrhexis	S	PIV DIII	5,6,6
15	M	24	560	N	preterm amniorrhexis	S	PV DV	6,6,6
16	M	27	790	C	intauterine infection	S	PIII DI	4,4,7
17	F	26	830	N	intrauterine infection	S	PIII DII	5,5,6
18	M	25	888	N	intrauterine infection	S	PI DI	5,6,6

Table 1: Characteristics of demographic, intrapartum, gestational and neonatological factors in studied group of premature babies.
Case #- patient's number, Sex: M- male, F- female, Delivery type: N- natural delivery, C-cesarean section, Pregnancy: S- single pregnancy, M- multiple pregnancy, P-pregnancy, D-delivery, SD- standard deviation.

showed in Table 1. Prior to inclusion of diode laser-steroid treatment, diagnosis of advanced stages of ROP had been done on the basis of ophthalmic RET-Cam II visualization and according to International Classification of Retinopathy of Prematurity (ICROP) criteria [15]. Eighteen extremely and very low birth weight prematures (ELBW and VLBW) born to multiparas (n=13; 72.22%) and primiparas (n=5; 27.77%), singleton pregnancy (15 neonates) and multiple pregnancy (3 newborns) among which 8 females and 10 males were enrolled. The average age was 25.67 weeks (SD ± 1.28) and mean birth weight was 811.83g (SD ± 299.08). For comparison, a control group comprised of eighteen volunteer-babies treated for ROP with diode laser panfotocoagulation only (9 females and 9 males) whose mean weight, age- and sex distributions were similar to those from the study group (Table 5).

Diode Laser Treatment, Systemic Steroid Administration and Local Treatment

Inclusion criteria

Among pediatric patients, the reason for general steroids therapy (Dexamethason sodium phosphate, Krka d.d., Novo mesto) inclusion was the presence of severe and rapidly progressing stages of threshold ROP: both ROP 3B and plus sign with Extraretinal Fibrovascular Proliferation (EFP) as well as agressive-posterior ROP (AP-ROP) which were confirmed in 6 (33.34%) and 12 (66.66%) prematures, respectively (Table 2). The abovementioned lesions were accompanied in some cases by pre-retinal hemorrhages located just in front of and on the ridge or extending in posterior pole of retina and posterior vitreous. Intravenous corticosteroids were used within 65.05 (SD ± 1.25) days of life; that is 34.69 (SD ± 1.06) postmenstrual week, Table 2. It was being administered twice a day to eighteen babies for the period of 9–16 days,

11.29 (SD ± 2.29) on average. The starting dose was 0.3 mg/kg/ day for consecutive 3 days and then gradually decreasing by half every 3 days until reaching 0.08 mg/kg/day as a final dose. In the basic schedule, 9 days of the therapy was suggested. Prolonging the drug application that is 12 days in nine babies and 16 days in three newborns was caused by aggressive course of the retinopathy coexisting with diseases of inflammatory origin. In case of no intravenous access, final drug dose was applied orally in two newborns. Duble blind trial was not used due to the knowledge about steroids action and their beneficial application in ophthalmic diseases of inflammatory origin both in adults as well as in children. Presuming the adverse effects of steroids, the mean values of the following parameters were evaluated: systolic and diastolic arterial blood pressures, blood glucose levels, tyreotropin, C-reactive protein, total bilirubin, as well as hematocrit, hemoglobin and erythrocyte titers (Table 3). In local treatment, Dexamethasone 0.1%, and Diclofenac in eye drops was used. Additionally, antihemorrhagic, absorbent, anti-permeability and anti-inflammatory drugs were included at the presence of multi-organ complications coexisting with subretinal hemorrhages. All infants from the analyzed group received single dose of surfactant because of Respiratory Distress Syndrome (RDS). Moreover, inhalatory steroids treatment was applied in 7 infants (38.88%) due to bronchopulmonary dysplasia (BPD), Table 3.

Exclusion criteria

Confirmation of viral infections in laboratory tests might be the exclusion criteria for the combined therapy, however it has not been noticed in the studied group.

Statistical tests

The normality of the distribution of individual traits was analyzed with the Shapiro-Wilk test. The differences in parameters between

Case #	ROP right eye	ROP left eye	Postmenstrual age when course started	Duration of therapy (days)	Therapy effect	Cortisol-1 ng/ml	Cortisol- 2 ng/ml	Cortisol -3 ng/ml
1	AP	AP	36	12	Y	0	0	0
2	3B+ EFP	3B+ EFP	35	9	Y	13.17	1.89	50.87
3	AP	AP	34	16	Y	26.04	3.08	56.11
4	3B+ EFP	3B+ EFP	34	9	Y	0	0	0
5	AP	AP	34	12	Y	0	0	0
6	AP	AP	33	16	Y	19.6	6.78	59.22
7	3B+ EFP	3B+ EFP	35	12	Y	0	0	0
8	AP	AP	36	14	Y	18.55	7.65	78.98
9	3B/4A+	3B+ EFP	34	12	Y	0	0	0
10	3B+EFP	3B+ EFP	35	9	Y	0	0	0
11	3B+EFP	3B+ EFP	34	9	Y	0	0	0
12	AP	AP	35	12	Y	0	0	0
13	AP	AP	34	12	Y	27.88	5.47	66.68
14	AP	AP	36	9	N	24.78	4.06	75.34
15	AP	AP	35	12	Y	0	0	0
16	AP	AP	35	9	N	0	0	0
17	AP	AP	34	12	Y	28.64	5.40	69.88
18	AP	AP	34	12	Y	0	0	0

Table 2: Data of the applied therapy and the advanced stage of ROP in consecutively studied prematures in whom combined therapy was applied
Case # - consecutive patients number, ROP–retinopathy of prematurity, AP–aggressive-posterior ROP, EFP–extraretinal fibrovascular proliferation; ROP3B+ EFP – ROP 3B and ridge, fibrous component in EFP and Plus Disease, therapy effect: Y–confirmed beneficial effect of treatment, N–No beneficial effect of treatment, Cortisol-1–Cortisol titer in 1-st day of course, Cortisol-2–Cortisol titer after 14 days of completed therapy, Cortisol-3–Cortisol titer after 3 months of completed therapy, (0- no measure).

Case #	SBP/DBP mmHg	GL mmol/l	TSH IU/mL	CRP mg/l	Total BIL mg/dl	Ht %	Hb g/dl	E T/L
1	75/54	3.66	2.56	24.32	6.16	25.4	8.4 0	2.65
2	77/46	5.22	3.75	2.36	9.05	29.6	10.5 0	3.5 0
3	70/56	5.49	0.847	3.15	7.54	28.6 8	10.54	3.40
4	75/55	5.55	0.67	4.89	9.76	26.97	9.69	2.97
5	82/54	5.49	3.74	92.02	11.79	22.38	7.70	2.45
6	80/67	6.60	3.87	17.43	9.54	28.44	6.50	2.47
7	76/47	6.22	4.80	10,79	5.13	25.11	7.70	2.93
8	79/52	5.44	2.56	11.98	6.71	27.01	6.98	2.77
9	70/55	7.55	6,15	34.89	4.9	30.50	10.6	3.59
10	81/54	6.55	5.54	2.78	7.7	28.54	9.54	3.21
11	78/60	5.16	3.44	27.50	6.96	29.41	10.42	2.83
12	78/59	6.16	4.44	4.37	7.05	24.10	8.99	2.83
13	80/63	5.11	3.12	9.08	6.98	27.01	7.75	2.76
14	77/50	4.33	0.41	29.88	23.98	32.00	7.91	3.55
15	79/40	4.99	0.77	8.56	5.36	23.01	9.42	2.76
16	70/59	6.38	9,14	42.98	4.89	23.33	8.37	2.84
17	77/45	5.72	0.86	69.54	7.65	24.01	9.65	2.44
18	74/50	5.38	3.18	77.09	5.34	24.77	8.20	2.52

Table 3: Mean values of selected laboratory factors in consecutively studied pre-matures with severe ROP in whom combined therapy was applied.
Case #- consecutive patient's number, APs- systolic arterial pressure, APd- diastolic arterial pressure, GL-mean glucose (normal babies' level 2.78-4.44mmol), TSH-mean tyreotropin (normal values from 2 weeks of life to 2 years old 0.8-9.1 IU/ml), CRP-mean C-reactive protein (normal 0-5mg/l), Total BIL-total bilirubin (normal<5.0 mg/dl), Ht-mean hematocrit (Normal 34-41%), Hb-mean hemoglobin, Er-mean erythrocyte (normal 4.3-5.5 mln/ul)

Case #	RDS	BPD	IVH	Hydrocephalus	Transfusion No.	Ventilation/days	Pneumonia	NEC	Osteopenia	PDA
1	III	+	III	+	3	56	+	+	0	0
2	II	0	III	0	6	33	+	0	0	+
3	IV	+	III	+	7	57	+	0	+	+
4	II	0	II	0	5	13	0	0	0	0
5	IV	+	III	+	15	64	+	+	0	+
6	I/II	0	II	0	14	52	+	+	0	+
7	IV	+	III	+	11	64	+	+	0	+
8	III	0	II	0	8	40	0	0	0	0
9	II	0	II	0	5	25	+	0	0	0
10	I	0	III	0	4	16	+	0	0	+
11	II	0	III	+	6	50	+	0	+	+
12	IV	0	III	+	13	50	+	+	0	+
13	II	0	III	0	7	44	0	+	0	+
14	II	+	IV	0	5	12	0	0	0	0
15	I	0	III	+	13	40	0	0	0	+
16	III	+	IV	+	9	60	+	+	+	+
17	II	0	II	+	3	65	+	+	0	0
18	II	+	III		2	56	+	+	+	+

Table 4: Characteristics of clinical features in consecutively studied prematures with severe ROP in whom combined therapy was applied.
Case # - consecutive patients number, RDS-respiratory distress syndrome (I,II,III,IV RDS-stages of RDS), BPD-bronchopulmonary dysplasia, (+/0 – presence or absence of examined feature), IVH-intraventricular hemorrhage, Transfusion No.-number of transfusions, Ventilation-mechanical ventilation (number of days), NEC-enterocolitis necroticans, PDA-patent ductus arteriosus, L-DPA patent ductus arteriosus surgical ligation.

groups were determined with the t-Student test, whereas the Mann-Whitney U test was used in the case of deviations from the normal distribution. The differences describing the number of retina attachments in the laser steroid group and the controls were measured with accurate Fisher test. Value probability was put in the table from the results of each test. Statistical significance of the parameters and the differences between them were tested at the significance levels of $p<0.01$ and p $p<0.05$.

Results

Premature spontaneous delivery was confirmed in 6 babies (33.33%), caesarian section was noted in 12 newborns (66.66%). The risk factors in a course of pregnancy for premature childbirth were

as follows: preterm amniorrhexis, intrauterine infection, premature placental abruption with threatening hemorrhages and hernia of membranes and cross-birth (Table 1). The abovementioned values were not statistically different in relation to the controls. Retina attachment was observed in 16 newborns (32 eyes; 88.88%) and varied in comparison to diode-laser alone preterms (12 eyes; 33.33%). However, this beneficial effect was not statistically significant (p=0.0612). In 2 babies (4 eyes; 11.11%) intravenous steroid application was interrupted after 9 days due to partial adrenal fatigue of iatrogenic origin. In them retina detachment was noticed (Table 2). Unfortunately, cortisol titer was evaluated only in some patients (n=7) because there was no constant scheme of its assessment on different neonatology units where the babies were hospitalized. In this group of patients, in the day of starting and ending the treatment, cortisol morning titers were 22.66 ng/ml (SD ± 5.07) and 4.90 ng/ml (SD ± 2.03) on average, respectively. Three months after the course completion, cortisol level increased to 65.29ng/ml (SD ± 10.33), Table 2. The averaged outcomes of laboratory tests turned out to be statistically insignificant and included: tyreotropin, bilirubin, glucose and hemoglobin levels (Table 3). Additionally, the incidence of following coexisting diseases was confirmed: bronchopulmonary dysplasia, osteopenia, intraventricular hemorrhage and hydrocephalus, pneumonia, enterocolitis necroticans, patent ductus arteriosus with its surgical closure, Table 4. Moreover, leucopenia, leukocytosis, thrombocytopenia, electrolyte dysregulation, metabolic acidosis, hypofibrinogenemia and parenteral alimentation were confirmed being without statistical significance in comparison to control group. The noticed increase of CRP (mean 37.39 mg/l) turned out to be statistically relevant (p=0.0000) (Table 5). Elevation of this factor was also significantly related to progression of ROP, being the highest in AP-ROP (r=0.5515) v.s. 3 ROP (r=0.3986; p<0.01). Decreased Ht 26.68% (SD ± 2.88) and Er 2.95T/L (SD ± 0.38), were statistically relevant (p<0.01), and together with lowering Hb 7.82 g/l (SD ± 1.27) were the reason for multiple transfusions of packed red blood cells (PRBCs) in all studied babies (n=18), average 9.75 (SD ± 3.34), (Tables 3 and 5). Association between high number of transfusion remained statistically significant (p=0.0000). This amount was significantly connected with progression of ROP, being the highest in AP-ROP v.s.3 ROP (r=0.5053; r=0.4010). Mechanical ventilation: SIMV, IMV, IPPV and nCPAP were applied in all babies; however additional HFOV was used in 2 of them, in whom retina detachment was observed in follow-up period. Duration of ventilation was 57.83 days, average (SD ± 15.89) and was significantly higher in laser-steroid patients (p=0.0000). It was prolonged in severe stages of ROP (r=0.5579 in AP-ROP and r=0.3908 in 3ROP).

Discussion

Retinopathy of prematurity (ROP) develops mostly in very low- and in extremely-low birth weight babies (VLBW and ELBW).

Examined factors	ROP (n=18)		Controls (n+18)		p
	Mean	sd	Mean	sd	
GA	25.66	1.21	25.83	1.72	0.7344
BW	811.83	156.9	819.44	134.39	0.8764
GL	5.61	0.84	5.07	1.00	0.0899
SBP	76.38	3.96	80.94	7.73	0.0330
DBP	53.67	6.61	58.50	1.36	0.0046
TSH	3.32	0.60	3.35	1.01	0.9429
CRP	37.39	5.69	0.86	0.98	0.0000
Total BIL	7.47	2.86	6.67	2.30	0.3616
Ht	26.68	2.88	33.70	2.87	0.0000
Hb	7.82	1.27	8.43	1.73	0.2451
Er	2.95	0.38	3.89	0.42	0.0000
Transfusion No.	9.75	3.34	1.33	0.50	0.0000
Ventilation/days	57.83	15.89	8.67	6.44	0.0000

Table 5: Characteristics of the mean value of examined factors in newborns with retinopathy of prematurity treated with diode-laser and steroids in comparison to only laser-diode group.
ROP – Examined Group of Pre-matures with ROP3B+ EFP (Ridge, Fibrous Component in EFP and Plus Disease) and AP-ROP, Controls – Only Laser-treated Premature Group, sd–Standard Deviation, GA – Gestational Age, BW – Birth Weight, GL– Glucose, SBP – Systolic Arterial Pressure, DBP - Diastolic Arterial Pressure, TSH – Tyreotropin, CRP – C-Reactive Protein, Total BIL – Total Bilirubin, Ht – Hematocrit, Hb – Hemoglobin, Er – Erythrocyte, Transfusion No.–Number of Transfusions, Ventilation – Mechanical Ventilation Duration (Number of Days), p- significance level.

Apart from diode laser panfotocoagulation, cryotherapy and trials of antiangiogenic therapy, there is no knowledge so far about efficient and new methods of treatment for both aggressive posterior ROP (AP-ROP) as well as rapidly appearing, severe stages of threshold ROP with plus disease and EFP [16-18].

After familiarizing with the action mechanisms of corticosteroids as potent anti-inflammatory drugs as well as their therapeutic possibilities in treatment and preventing the premature complications such as Chronic Lung Disease (CLD), the authors of this study have tried to apply systemic steroid combined with typical diode laser use in cases of suddenly progressing severe ROP [12-14,19,20]. According to the schemes of postnatal steroid treatment of premature CLD in the selected group of ELBW and VLBW newborns with ROP, Dexamethasone has been implemented intravenously [8]. During Dexamethasone treatment, hypothyreosis was observed only in 3 babies (16.66%). Moreover, cortisol titer remained in the lower range of laboratory norm already before the starting therapy, decreasing significantly on about 14th day of the course and returning to normal level on third month after the completed therapy. In accordance with other authors, levels of these hormones remain low in early postnatal period especially in VLBW and ELBW prematures which is connected with multi-organ immaturity simultaneously with the lack of the other adverse effects of iatrogenic drug application [19,21-28]. Moreover, important is that the newborns who develop BPD have low cortisol levels following ACTH stimulation during the first week of life, therefore the use of steroids in early postnatal period in case of BPD, seems to be justified [19,26,27,29,30]. The steroid therapy amounted to 11.29 days on average, which proved the procedure to be in compliance with steroids administered by other authors for BPD treatment. They applied the same or approximate dose of the drug, the administration of which started much earlier that is even below 8 day of life with continuation of the course even until 21-28 following days [8]. It should be noted on the basis of 3-year follow-up that the general condition of the analyzed newborns, did not show the presence of significant short and long distance cardiologic, gastrointestinal and neurologic complications, which could have been induced by steroids. However, it can not be excluded that clinical symptoms of significant transient rise of arterial pressures might be connected with implied steroids. Transient partial adrenal fatigue in the form of lack of appetite, weight loss, apathy and weakness on approximately 14-th day of the therapy were observed in two prematures. This was the reason for steroids termination. Such state might probably be related with coexistence of severe developmental immaturity, intrauterine growth retardation, congenital intestinal obstruction treated surgically, and metabolic bone disease. It could be hypothesized that the HFOV (High-Frequency Oscillatory Ventilation) used in those two most severe babies, through oscillating movement, might also have indirect influence on progressing retina deterioration in further step until its detachment, similarly to intraventricular haemorrhage which has been described in the literature [31].

Transient, nonsignificant increase of glycemia observed in laser-treated ROP prematures both with and without steroid course could possibly be the result of parenteral alimentation. Moreover, outcomes of neurological examination including 3-year follow-up period, did not confirm any additional features of any abnormalities in neurosensory development in connection to the application of the discussed drug. Nevertheless, the observed psychomotor retardation in most of the babies might be connected with general immaturity, intracranial hemorrhages' or the resulting hydrocephalus diagnosed in the first period of life [32]. The mentioned cranial lesions probably influenced eye movement disturbances such as nystagmus and squint

[21,32]. Most recent reports point out the presence of normal cerebral development in only 23.5% of VLBW newborns, confirming global, mental and psychomotor retardation in the remaining group with the lack of systemic steroids application [17]. Contrary to that, other data in the literature also underline that the majority of prematures exposed to Dexamethasone in BPD do not develop cerebral palsy or global developmental disability, nevertheless one cannot exclude other more subtle adverse effects after steroids in further periods of childhood [1,8,29,30,33-35].

In experimental studies, it has been revealed that the prolonged exposure to Dexamethasone in the neonatal rats leads to alterations in behavior, corticosteron response to stress and changes in Limbic-Hypothalamic Pituitary Adrenal (LHPA) axis circuitry, nevertheless it is not known if similar dysregulatory changes in this system appear in the human [29]. It might not be precluded that post-steroids complications could be associated with sulfite preservatives contained in the drug [36]. Relating to the data from available literature, it is worth mentioning that there are no clinical observations in connection to steroids application due to retinopathy of prematurity, although their use is commonly known in different retinal or retino-vitreous diseases even in early childhood, so it appears to be impossible to rely on an opinion of other authors in this field [37-44]. Three-year follow-up of combined laser-steroid course indicate beneficial effect of such therapy in the form of retina attachment which has been confirmed in 88.8 % selected cases. Validity of Dexamethasone use in advanced and severe ROP seems to be confirmed by hypothesis including the presence of proinflammatory agents in the development of retinal abnormalities. It is proved by the increased level of CRP in the analyzed laser-steroids group (p<0.01), being the highest in the most advanced ROP stages, coexisting with intrauterine infection, enterocolitis necroticans and pneumonia [2 5,7]. Moreover, in this group the significant increase of transfusion number, prolonged duration of ventilation and anemia was noticed (p<0.01), which is in accordance with data in the literature [45].

The inflammatory hypothesis has been acknowledged by most recent reviews in literature in extensive meta-analysis (35 studies and 4971 participants) among others, in which application of steroids in BPD led to significant decreasing of inflammatory process as well as lowering incidence of severe ROP [8,30]. The explanation of this phenomenon might be the TNF-α expression regulation secreted as a response to hyperoxia and hypoxia, which is an important factor in inflammation and angiogenesis in the mouse model of oxygen-induced retinopathy [45]. Some authors present a lot of evidence that Dexamethasone provides a protective action mechanism against the development of severe retinopathy and extraretinal neovascularization [8,11,14,30,41]. There exists a similarity to inhibitory effects of dexamethasone on TNF-α expression in the retina, as in endotoxin-induced uveitis with the use of local delivery steroid system in experimental model [11-14], what has been applied in many ophthalmic diseases in children and adults [38,40-43]. In the mentioned processes rapid nongenomic effects on cell metabolism and cell membrane functions such as altering intracellular signal transduction pathways, limiting tissular inflammatory reactions by inhibiting migration and aggregation of macrophages with enzyme release and growth factors, fibroblastic activity suppression, reducing vascular permeability and also regulating endothelial nitric oxide synthase by non-nuclear effects are used [9,11-13, 29,36].

We are aware of some limitations of our study: (a) the relatively small sample size of the study groups which did not allow to obtain statistical differences in analysis of retina attachment; (b) there was no possibility of comparing the effects of administering different doses of Dexamethasone; (c) we did not examine the effects of severe ROP improvement by application of other steroids used by the neonatologists (hydrocortisone, bethamethasone); (d) limited follow-up duration; (e) lack of routine schemes for cortisol evaluation during the steroid application which made it difficult to supervise the task

Conclusions

The benefits of the applied therapy in premature at risk of developing threshold 3 ROP and plus disease with extraretinal fibrovascular proliferation or aggressive-posterior ROP might appear to outweigh the real or potential adverse effects of this course. Short- and long-term steroid complications should be taken into account when starting the therapy. Despite some negative opinions on systemic steroids application in early postnatal period, it appears that the risk of severe decrease of vision or blindness in low-birth weight prematures with lack of possibility for anti-angiogenic treatment, allows applying the nonstandard steroids therapy as an additional, alternative option in selected ROP [45]. Although our primary experience with Dexamethasone combined with diode laser is promising, additional large-scale prospective studies with prolonged follow-up periods should be conducted to confirm our findings.

Conflict of Interest

None of the authors has conflict of interest with the submission.

Financial Support

No financial support was received for this submission.

Informed Consent

The study was performed with informed consent and approved by the Ethics Committee.

References

1. Smolkin T, Steinberg M, Sujov P, Mezer E, Tamir A, et al. (2008) Late postnatal systemic steroids predispose to retinopathy of prematurity in very-low-birth-weight infants: a comparative study. Acta Paediatr 97: 322-326.

2. Sood BG, Madan A, Saha S, Schendel D, Thorsen P, et al. (2010) Perinatal systemic inflammatory response syndrome and retinopathy of prematurity. Pediatr Res 67: 394-400.

3. Paananen R, Husa AK, Vuolteenaho R, Herva R, Kaukola T, et al. (2009) Blood cytokines during the perinatal period in very preterm infants: relationship of inflammatory response and bronchopulmonary dysplasia. J Pediatr 154: 39-43.

4. Stewart MW (2012) The expanding role of vascular endothelial growth factor inhibitors in ophthalmology. Mayo Clin Proc 87: 77-88.

5. Dammann O, Leviton A (2006) Inflammation, brain damage and visual dysfunction in preterm infants. Semin Fetal Neonatal Med 11: 363-368.

6. Kim TI, Sohn J, PI SY Yoon YH (2003) Postnatal risk factors of retinopathy of prematurity. Semin Neonatol 8:469-73.

7. Genzel-Boroviczény O, MacWilliams S, Von Poblotzki M, Zoppelli L (2006) Mortality and major morbidity in premature infants less than 31 weeks gestational age in the decade after introduction of surfactant. Acta Obstet Gynecol Scand 85: 68-73.

8. Halliday HL, Ehrenkranz RA, Doyle LW (2009) Early (<8days) postnatal corticosteroids for preventing chronic lung disease in preterm infants. Arch Pediatr 17: 999-1004.

9. Rotshild T, Nandgaonkar BN, Yu K, Higgins RD (1999) Dexamethason reduces oxygen-induced retinopathy in the mouse model. Pediatr Res 46: 94-100.

10. Behar-Cohen FF, Parel JM, Pouliquen Y, Thillaye-Goldenberg B, Goureau O, et al. (1997) Iontophoresis of dexamethasone in the treatment of endotoxin-induced-uveitis in rats. Exp Eye Res 65: 533-545.

11. Brenner T, Yamin A, Abramsky O, Gallily R (1993) Stimulation of tumor necrosis

factor-alpha production by mycoplasmas and inhibition by dexamethasone in cultured astrocytes. rain Res 608: 273-279.

12. Yossuck P, Yan Y, Tadesse M, Higgins RD (2000) Dexamethasone and critical effect of timing on retinopathy. Invest Ophthalmol Vis Sci 41: 3095-3099.

13. Wagge A, Bakke O (1998) Glucocorticosteroids suppress the production of tumor necrosis factor by lipopolysaccharide-stimulated human monocyte. Immunology 63: 303-311.

14. Palexas GN, Sussman G, Welsh NH (1992) Ocular and systemic determination of IL-1 beta and tumour necrosis factor in a patient with ocular inflammation. Scand J Immunol Suppl 11: 173-175.

15. International Committee for the Classification of Retinopathy of Prematurity (2005) The International Classification of Retinopathy of Prematurity revisited. Arch Ophthalmol 123: 991-999.

16. Jang SY1, Choi KS, Lee SJ (2010) Delayed-onset retinal detachment after an intravitreal injection of ranibizumab for zone 1 plus retinopathy of prematurity. J AAPOS 14: 457-459.

17. Orozoco- Gómez LP, Hernández-Salazar L, Moguel-Ancheita S, et al. (2011) Laser-ranibizumab treatment for retinopathy of prematurity in umbral-preumbral disease. Three years of experience. Cir Cir 79: 225-32.

18. Andreoli CM, Miller JW (2007) Anti-vascular endothelial growth factor therapy for ocular neovascular disease. Curr Opin Ophthalmol 18: 502-508.

19. Bonsante F, Latorre G, Iacobelli S, Forziati V, Laforgia N, et al. (2007) Early low-dose hydrocortisone in very preterm infants: a randomized, placebo-controlled trial. Neonatology 91: 217-221.

20. Park YJ, Kim YH, Choi WS, Chung IY, Yoo JM (2010) Treatment with triamcinolone acetonide prevents decreased retinal levels of decorin in a rat model of oxygen-induced retinopathy. Curr Eye Res 35: 657-663.

21. Goissen C, Fontaine C, Braun K, Bony H, Al-Hosri J, et al. (2011) [Prospective study at 1 week of life of thyroid function in 97 consecutive pre-term newborns under 32 weeks of gestation]. Arch Pediatr 18: 253-260.

22. Osborn DA, Hunt RW (2007) Postnatal thyroid hormones for preterm infants with transient hypothyroxinaemia. Cochrane Database Syst Rev (1): CD005945.

23. Fujitaka M, Jinno K, Sakura N, Takata K, Yamasaki T, et al. (1997) Serum concentrations of cortisone and cortisol in premature infants. Metabolism 46: 518-521.

24. Ares S, Quero J, Diez J, Morreale de Escobar G (2011) Neurodevelopment of preterm infants born at 28 to 36 weeks of gestational age: the role of hypothyroxinemia and long-term outcome at 4 years. J Pediatr Endocrinol Metab 24: 897-902.

25. Field T, Hernandez-Reif M, Diego M, Figueiredo B, Schanberg S, et al. (2006) Prenatal cortisol, prematurity and low birthweight. Infant Behav Dev 29: 268-275.

26. Rastogi A, Akintorin SM, Bez ML, Morales P, Pildes RS (1996) A controlled trial of dexamethasone to prevent bronchopulmonary dysplasia in surfactant-treated infants. Pediatrics 98: 204-210.

27. Anttila E, Peltonemi O, Haumont D, et al. (2005) Early neonatal dexamethasone treatment for prevention of bronchopulmonary dysplasia. Randomised trial and meta-analysis evaluating the duration of dexamathsone teraphy. European Journal of Pediatrics 164: 472-481.

28. Hafezi-Moghadam A, Simoncini T, Yang E, et al. (2002) Acute cardiovascular protective effects of corticosteroids are mediated by non-transcriptional activation of endothelial nitric oxide synthase. Nat Med 8: 473-479.

29. Charles R, Neal Jr, Brian L. et al. (2003) Dexamethasone exposure during the neonatal period alters ORL1 mRNA expression in the hypothalamic paraventricular nucleus and hippocampus of the adult rat. Developmental Brain Research 146: 15-31.

30. Eriksson L, Haglund B, Ewald U, Odlind V, Kieler H (2009) Short and long-term effects of antenatal corticosteroids assessed in a cohort of 7,827 children born preterm. Acta Obstet Gynecol Scand 88: 933-938.

31. Henderson-Smart DJ, Cools F, Bhuta T, et al. (2007) Elective high frequency oscillatory ventilation versus conventional ventilation for acute pulmonary dysfunction in preterm infants. Cochrane Database Syst Rev (3): CD000104.

32. Msall ME (2006) The panorama of cerebral palsy after very and extremely preterm birth: evidence and challenges. Clin Perinatol 33: 269-284.

33. Modrzejewska M, Grzesiak W, Karczewicz D, Zaborski D (2010) Refractive status and ocular axial length in preterm infants without retinopathy of prematurity with regard to birth weight and gestational age. J Perinat Med 38: 327-331.

34. Dhawan A, Dogra M, Vinekar A, et al. (2008) Structural sequelae and refractive outcome after successful laser treatment for threshold retinopathy of prematurity. J Pediatr Ophthalmol Strabismus 45: 356-361.

35. Chen YZ, Qiu J (2001) Possible genomic consequence of nongenomic action of glucocorticoids in neural cells. News Physiol Sci 16: 292-296.

36. Baud O, Foix-L'Helias L, Kaminski M, Audibert F, Jarreau PH, et al. (1999) Antenatal glucocorticoid treatment and cystic periventricular leukomalacia in very premature infants. N Engl J Med 341: 1190-1196.

37. Baud O, Laudenbach V, Evrard P, Gressens P (2001) Neurotoxic effects of fluorinated glucocorticoid preparations on the developing mouse brain: role of preservatives. Pediatr Res 50: 706-711.

38. Thurau SR, Frosch M, Zierhut M, Gümbel H, Heiligenhaus A (2007) [Topical and systemic corticosteroid therapy for uveitis in childhood]. Klin Monbl Augenheilkd 224: 516-519.

39. Fishman JM, Burgess C, Waddell A (2011) Corticosteroids for the treatment of idiopathic acute vestibular dysfunction (vestibular neuritis). Cochrane Database Syst Rev : CD008607.

40. Bonhomme GR, Mitchell EB (2012) Treatment of pediatric optic neuritis. Curr Treat Options Neurol 14: 93-102.

41. Habot-Wilner Z, Sallam A, Roufas A, Kabasele PM, Grigg JR, et al. (2010) Periocular corticosteroid injection in the management of uveitis in children. Acta Ophthalmol 88: e299-304.

42. Figueroa MS, Noval S, Contreras I, Arruabarrena C, García-Pérez JL, et al. (2010) [Pars plana vitrectomy as anti-inflammatory therapy for intermediate uveitis in children]. Arch Soc Esp Oftalmol 85: 390-394.

43. Leder HA, Jabs DA, Galor A, Dunn JP, Thorne JE (2011) Periocular triamcinolone acetonide injections for cystoid macular edema complicating noninfectious uveitis. Am J Ophthalmol 152: 441-448.

44. Yossuck P, Yan Y, Tadesse M, Higgins RD (2001) Dexamethasone alters TNF-alpha expression in retinopathy. Mol Genet Metab 72: 164-167.

45. Wallace DK, Wu KY (2013) Current and future trends in treatment of severe retinopathy of prematurity. Clin Perinatol 40: 297-310.

14

Multiple Sampling from the Central Veins with their Tributaries can Detect Bilateral Hyperaldosteronism with a Cortisol-Producing Adenoma in a Hypertensive Patient

Ikki Sakuma[1], Jun Saito[1], Yoko Matsuzawa[1], Masao Omura[1], Seiji Matsui[2], Koshiro Nishimoto[3,4], Kuniaki Mukai[5] and Tetsuo Nishikawa[1*]

[1]Endocrinology and Diabetes Center, Yokohama Rosai Hospital, Yokohama, Japan
[2]Department of Radiology, Yokohama Rosai Hospital, Yokohama, Japan
[3]Departments of Urology, School of Medicine, Keio University, Tokyo, Japan
[4]Department of Urology, Tachikawa Hospital, Tokyo, Japan
[5]Department of Biochemistry, School of Medicine, Keio University, Tokyo, Japan

Abstract

A 52-year old woman was admitted to our hospital for evaluation of left adrenal incidenataloma. Endocrinological examination showed Cushing's syndrome (CS) complicated with masked primary aldosteronism (PA). On the other hand, multiple sampling from the central veins and one or two tributaries of the adrenal veins before and after ACTH-stimulation (multiple AVS) clearly revealed bilateral hyperaldosteronism with excess cortisol secretion from the left adrenal. Thus, we diagnosed this case as CS due to left adrenal tumor with bilateral hyperaldosteronism, and left adrenalectomy was done. Immunohistochemical analysis of the removed left adrenal showed cortisol-producing adenoma and multiple aldosterone-producing cell clusters (APCCs) expressing CYP11B2 within the attached adrenal. Bilateral PA is mostly diagnosed as idiopathic hyperaldosteronism (IHA). IHA has not been examined enough pathologically. We first describe here a possible involvement of APCCs inducing hyperaldosteronism in a case of bilateral PA with a cortisol-producing-adenoma.

Keywords: Idiopathic hyperaldosteronism; Aldosterone-producing cell clusters; Adrenal vein sampling; Cushing's syndrome

Introduction

Here, we describe a case of left adrenal incidentaloma in a patient with Cushing's syndrome (CS) simultaneously complicating hyperaldosteronism. In US and Japan, a screening program for primary aldosteronism (PA), which is a major cause of endocrine hypertension, was recently introduced [1,2]. Aldosterone producing adenoma (APA) and idiopathic hyperaldosteronism (IHA) are the main causes of PA. APA usually responds to unilateral adrenalectomy, which corrects hyperaldosteronism and can attenuate hypertension. The medical management of IHA is generally recommended. Therefore IHA has not been examined enough pathologically. On the other hands, Nishimoto et al. have recently established an immunohistochemical technique for detecting CYP11B1 and CYP11B2 and suggested that it would allow the confirmatory pathological diagnosis of APA [3]. They detected areas of variegated zonation, in which the abnormal zones consisted of CYP11B2- expressing subcapsular cell clusters, which are termed as aldosterone- producing cell clusters (APCCs). They proposed that in the human adrenal cortex aldosterone production is constitutive in APCC and inducible in the zona glomerulosa of the conventional tissue [3]. In this case, results of multiple sampling from the central veins and one or two tributaries of the adrenal veins before and after ACTH- stimulation (multiple AVS) and immunohistochemistry of steroidogenic enzymes suggested multiple APCCs, possibly inducing bilateral hyperaldosteronism. We first describe a possible involvement of APCCs-induced hyperaldosteronism in bilateral PA with a cortisol- producing adenoma.

Case Report

A 52-year-old woman was admitted to Yokohama Rosai Hospital in order to have her left adrenal incidentaloma and hypertension eval-

uated. A few months before her referral to our hospital, abdominal CT, which was performed due to abdominal pain, detected a left adrenal tumor. Abdominal pain gradually disappeared and was thought to be caused by gastroenteritis. She had previously been diagnosed with hypertension and had started taking anti-hypertensive medication (nifedipine) at the age of 50. A physical examination revealed that she measured 153 cm in height and weighed 39 kg, indicating emaciation. Her blood pressure was 183/104 mmHg even under taking a antihypertensive drug. She displayed some cushingoid features such as thin skin and hirsutism. Laboratory examination showed dyslipidemia and impaired glucose tolerance. 75g oral glucose tolerance test showed diabetic pattern (0 min, 74 mg/dl; 120 min, 214 mg/dl). A bone X-ray and dual-energy X-ray absorptiometry (DEXA) of lumbar spine revealed osteoporosis (T-score: -3.6).

An endocrinological examination (Table 1) revealed that the circadian rhythm of the patient's hypothalamic-pituitary-adrenal axis had been disturbed by persistently suppressed ACTH levels. Her urine free cortisol level was elevated to 252 (normal range: 11.2~80.3) μg/ day. However, her cortisol level was not suppressed (14.9 μg/dL) by the administration of 1mg dexamethasone. Abdominal CT with contrast medium demonstrated a left adrenal tumor (30 mm in a diameter), while the right adrenal gland was found to be atrophic (Figure 1A and 1B). Plain CT also showed the left adrenal tumor of 33 Hounsfield units. In 131I-adosterol scintigraphy, the radioisotope was taken up by the left adrenal tumor but not by the contralateral adrenal gland (Figure 1C). On the basis of these results, she was diagnosed as CS [4].

*Corresponding author: Tetsuo Nishikawa, Endocrinology and Diabetes Center, Yokohama Rosai Hospital, 3211 Kozukue-cho, Kohoku-ku, Yokohama City, Kanagawa 222-0036, Japan, E-mail: tetsuon@yokohamah.rofuku.go.jp

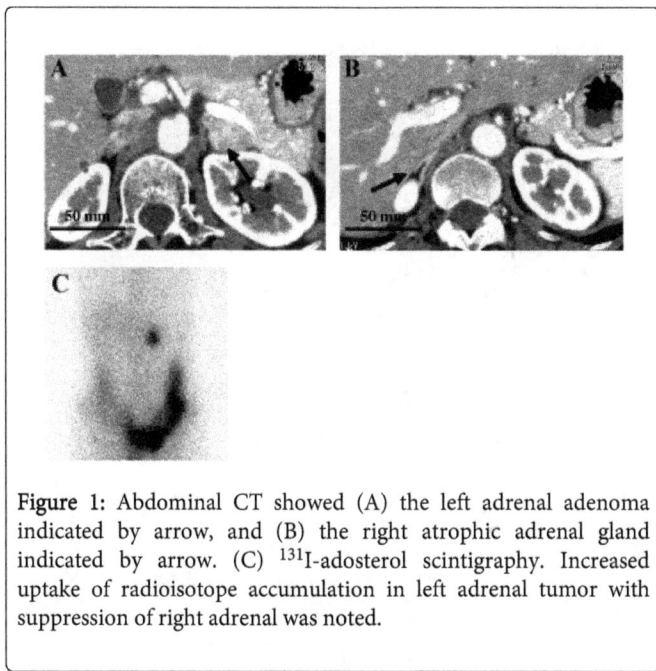

Figure 1: Abdominal CT showed (A) the left adrenal adenoma indicated by arrow, and (B) the right atrophic adrenal gland indicated by arrow. (C) ^{131}I-adosterol scintigraphy. Increased uptake of radioisotope accumulation in left adrenal tumor with suppression of right adrenal was noted.

Serum				
Na	144	mEq/L		
K	3.8	mEq/L		
ACTH	<1.0	pg/mL		
CS	12.4	µg/dL		
PRA	0.5	ng/mL/hr		
PAC	133	pg/mL		
DHEA-S	20	µg/dL		
Urine				
CCr	107.8	mL/min		
Na	140.6	mEq/day		
K	52.3	mEq/day		
free cortisol	252	µg/day		
aldosterone	5.4	µg/day		
Diural rhythm and dexamethasone suppression test				
	8:00	23:00	Dex 1mg	
ACTH (pg/mL)	<1.0	<1.0	<1.0	
CS (µg/dL)	12.4	11.8	14.9	
PRA (ng/mL/hr)	0.1	<0.1		
PAC (pg/mL)	70	74	65	
CRH stimulation test, 100 µg iv				

	0 min	30 min	60 min	120 min
ACTH (pg/mL)	<1.0	1.6	<1.0	1.6
CS (µg/dL)	13.3	16.5	15.4	13.6
ACTH stimulation test, 250 µg iv				
	0 min	30 min	60 min	
CS (µg/dL)	14.6	29.4	35.1	
PAC (pg/mL)	128	384	408	
PRA (ng/mL/hr)	0.4			
Captopril test, 50 mg po				
	0 min	90 min		
PRA (ng/mL/hr)	0.2	0.6		
PAC (pg/mL)	43	56		
ARR	215	93.3		
Saline infusion test, 2L div				
	240 min			
PRA (ng/mL/hr)	0.3			
PAC (pg/mL)	71			
Frosemide upright test, 20 mg iv				
	240 min			
PRA (ng/mL/hr)	2.1			
PAC (pg/mL)	358			
Multiple AVS				

	RAV		LAV	
	PAC (pg/mL)	CS (µg/dL)	PAC (pg/mL)	CS (µg/dL)
Central	36200	200	23400	1100
Inferior	29500	172	21800	853
Lateral	33000	197	4490	1390

Table 1: Results of endocrine function tests before surgical treatment

ARR: Aldosterone Renin Ratio; AVS: Adrenal Vein Sampling; CS: Cortisol; Dex: Dexamethasone; LAV: Left Adrenal Vein; PAC: Plasma Aldosterone Concentration; PRA: Plasma Renin Activity; RAV: Right Adrenal Vein.

Interestingly, in addition to hyper production of cortisol, this case showed slightly elevated PAC of 128 pg/mL, suppressed PRA of 0.4 ng/mL/hr, and elevated aldosterone renin ratio (ARR) of 320, suggesting the possibility of primary aldosteronism (PA) according to the guidelines [2]. Therefore we investigated whether or not PA was also associated. Captopril challenge test showed suppression of ARR from 215 to 93.3, while PAC was not suppressed to less than 60 pg/mL by saline infusion test (71 pg/mL). ACTH stimulation test with 0.25 mg cosyntropin also demonstrated a marked increase in PAC to 408 pg/mL in the present case. These results indicated a high possibility of the autonomous secretion of aldosterone.

Left adrenal tumor was expected to cause CS. However, subtype of PA in this case was considered a variety of adrenal pathologies, such as IHA, left adrenal tumor co-producing aldosterone and cortisol, or double adenomas which consist of left cortisol producing adenoma and micro APA at ipsilateral bilateral or contralateral side. Multiple AVS was performed to determine precisely the subtype of PA because therapeutic approach may differ depending on the disease subtype (Table 1). The central, inferior tributary, and lateral tributary veins of the right adrenal displayed aldosterone levels of 36200, 29500, and 33000 pg/mL, and cortisol levels of 200, 172, 197 μg/dL respectively. On the other hands, the central, superior tributary, and lateral tributary veins of the left adrenal exhibited aldosterone levels of 23400, 21800, and 4490 pg/mL, and cortisol levels of 1100, 853, and 1390 μg/dL respectively. Venography of the left lateral tributary detected tumor staining. CT revealed an adrenal tumor attached to the left lateral adrenal gland. Therefore, we assumed that the left lateral tributary was connected to the tumor. Cortisol level in the left superior tributary was not sufficiently suppressed compared to that in the lateral tributary, indicating hormone secretion from the tumor partially flowed into the superior tributary. Evaluation criteria of hyperaldosteronism based on the aldosterone/cortisol ratio was not used because of autonomous cortisol secretion. We could simply detect the presence of hyperaldosteronism by analysing absolute values of aldosterone in each central and tributary vein. We reported that the cut-off value of hyperaldosteronism was 14,000 pg/mL (adrenal vein PAC after ACTH stimulation) [2]. The left lateral tributary displayed cortisol hypersecretion but not hyperaldosteronism. On the basis of these results, we judged that the left adrenal tumor secreted cortisol without hyperaldosteronism and that bilateral PA due to IHA was responsible for the patient's hyperaldosteronism. In order to control excessive secretion of cortisol (but not that of aldosterone), we performed laparoscopic left adrenalectomy. Left adrenal tumor 28×23×10 mm, and was yellowish in color with lipofuscin granules. A histopathological examination showed that it was composed of compact cells with eosinophilic cytoplasm. An immunohistochemical examination of the tumor detected immunoreactivity to CYP17, 3βHSD and CYP11B1, but not to CYP11B2 (Figure 2A-2C). The adjacent adrenal cortex was grossly atrophic, which was consistent with CS. Multiple CYP11B2-expressing sub capsular cell clusters, which were indicative of APCC, were detected diffusely in the adjacent adrenal cortex (Figure 2D and 2G). 3βHSD was also expressed in the APCCs (Figure 2E). CYP17 was not expressed in the APCCs (Figure 2F). After left adrenalectomy, a second endocrinological examination was performed (Table 2). As a result, it was found that her cortisol levels had markedly decreased, indicating cure of Cushing's syndrome. And her aldosterone levels had halved. An ACTH stimulation test produced an increase in her PAC to 241 pg/mL. Her blood pressure returned to within the normal range soon after surgery without the administration of any medication. The patient was discharged uneventfully at 16th postoperative day under supplementation of 10 mg of hydrocortisone. Hydrocortisone was gradually tapered. And 1-year after surgery, a third endocrinological examination was performed (Table 3). As a result, ACTH and cortisol levels improved, compared to just after surgery. On the other hands, aldosterone response to ACTH stimulation fell within normal range, indicating remission of IHA.

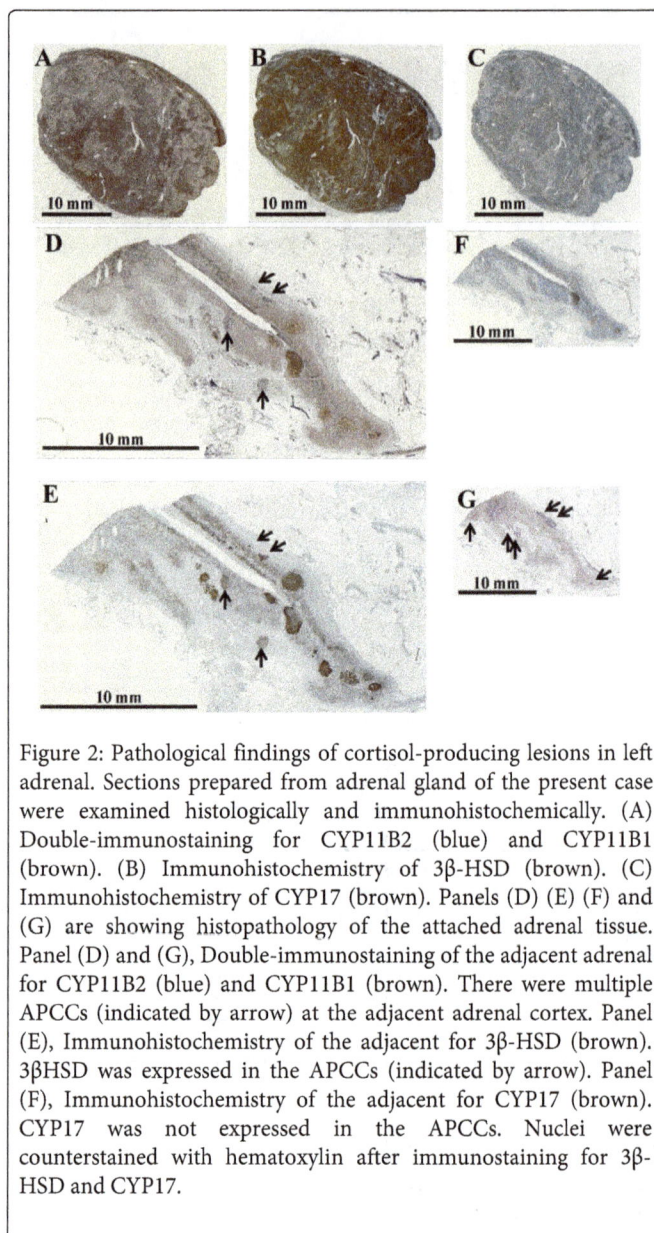

Figure 2: Pathological findings of cortisol-producing lesions in left adrenal. Sections prepared from adrenal gland of the present case were examined histologically and immunohistochemically. (A) Double-immunostaining for CYP11B2 (blue) and CYP11B1 (brown). (B) Immunohistochemistry of 3β-HSD (brown). (C) Immunohistochemistry of CYP17 (brown). Panels (D) (E) (F) and (G) are showing histopathology of the attached adrenal tissue. Panel (D) and (G), Double-immunostaining of the adjacent adrenal for CYP11B2 (blue) and CYP11B1 (brown). There were multiple APCCs (indicated by arrow) at the adjacent adrenal cortex. Panel (E), Immunohistochemistry of the adjacent for 3β-HSD (brown). 3βHSD was expressed in the APCCs (indicated by arrow). Panel (F), Immunohistochemistry of the adjacent for CYP17 (brown). CYP17 was not expressed in the APCCs. Nuclei were counterstained with hematoxylin after immunostaining for 3β-HSD and CYP17.

Discussion

We described a case with CS due to left cortisol producing adenoma and bilateral hyperaldosteronism. We preoperatively diagnosed the patient with bilateral hyperaldosteronism based on the results of multiple AVS and confirmed multiple APCCs as the cause of her excess aldosterone levels via immunohistochemical examinations of her steroidogenic enzyme expression.

Patients with concurrent CS and PA have been reported in several studies [5-8]. Pediatis et al. reported that PA associated with hypercortisolism occured 12.1% in 83 adrenal incidentalomas [7]. Hiraishi et al. detected PA complicated with subclinical CS in 8 of 38 PA patients (21%) [9]. A recent study suggested that the ACTH test can be useful in PA subtype diagnosis [10]. In PA with CS, hyperaldosteronism could be masked because ACTH suppressed by CS may decrease aldosterone production. ACTH stimulation test was reported to be useful for detecting masked hyperaldosteronism with CS [8]. In our case, clinical signs and endocrinological data suggested CS possibly associated with masked PA before performing AVS. PA manifests as several subtypes with different biochemical and pathological characteristics, with APA and IHA accounting for most cases [11]. Concurrent CS and PA cases also could be classified into several subtypes of PA [9]. It is well known that conventional AVS could detect the laterality of hyperaldosteronism. Moreover, multiple AVS could easily detect the portions of localized (APA) or diffuse adrenal lesions (IHA) compared to conventional AVS [12]. By multiple AVS, we preoperatively diagnosed the present case as CS due to a left cortisol-producing adenoma associated with bilateral hyperaldosteronism (IHA). Immunohistochemistry of the tumor detected immunoreactivity to CYP17, 3βHSD and CYP11B1, but not to CYP11B2. These findings suggested that the tumor secreted cortisol and did not be involved in hyperaldosteronism. On the other hands, immunohistochemistry of the adjacent atrophic adrenal cortex detected multiple APCCs. Immunohistochemistry of APCCs detected immunoreactivity to 3βHSD and CYP11B2, but not to CYP17 and CYP11B1, indicating that those APCCs could mainly produce aldosterone. Some APCCs were relatively large (about 2mm), which was estimated to be etiology of hyperaldosteronism. Furthermore, bilateral hyperaldosteronism detected by multiple AVS was possibly caused by APCCs in bilateral adrenals even though right adrenalectomy was not performed yet. On the other hands, Nishimoto et al. suggested that APCCs were found in some cases of normal adrenals and nontumor portions of cortisol producing adenoma [3]. Number of APCCs in our case was not especially higher than that in the previous paper. It has not been elucidated sufficiently that how many and large APCCs cause hyperaldosteronism. Further study should be done to investigate this issue.

Screening for PA is spreading in Japan, and hence, the number of cases of IHA has been on the increase. According to our findings, the incidence of IHA among PA patients was 26~60% [13,14]. Pathologically, adrenal glands in IHA are characterized by diffuse hyperplasia involving cells that resemble those found in the normal zona glomerulosa without nodules [15]. However, most IHA cases are treated with non-surgical methods because unilateral adrenalectomy has been considered ineffective [16]. Therefore, there is insufficient pathological information about IHA. The findings we obtained with multiple AVS and immunohistochemistry suggest that multiple APCCs can cause bilateral hyperaldosteronism. One-year after left adrenalectomy, PA interestingly remitted. We do not fully explain the reason why unilateral adrenalectomy could improve hyperaldosteronism in this case. It is possible to consider that excess cortisol production might affect intra-adrenal renin-angiotensin system, resulting in high aldosterone synthesis induced by locally produced angiotensin II. Thus, it is speculated that APCC existed in adrenal tissues of IHA could produce excess amounts of aldosterone stimulated by cortisol-induced intra-adrenal renin-angiotensin system in this case. On the other hand, unilateral adrenalectomy was reported to be effective on reducing blood pressure and PAC in some case with IHA, not associating with Cushing syndrome [17,18]. Therefore, we need to clarify the effectiveness of unilateral adrenalectomy for the patients with IHA. In conclusion, we first describe here a possible involvement of APCCs-induced hyperaldosteronism in a case of bilateral PA with a cortisol-producing adenoma. It has not been elucidated sufficiently that how many and large APCCs cause hyperaldosteronism. Furthermore we should perform pathophysiological investigations for this issue by multiple AVS and immunohistochemistry.

Acknowledgements

This work was partly supported by the Grant for Research on Intractable Diseases provided from the Japanese Ministry of Health, Labour and Welfare.

We thank Mr. Shinya Sasai, Ms. Yuka Yokomichi, and Ms Hitomi Shimizu in the Department of Pathology, Tachikawa Hospiatal for excellent technical assistance with immunohistochemistry.

References

1. Funder JW, Carey RM, Fardella C, Gomez-Sanchez CE, Mantero F, et al. (2008) Case detection, diagnosis, and treatment of patients with primary aldosteronism: an endocrine society clinical practice guideline. J Clin Endocrinol Metab. 93: 3266-3281.

2. Nishikawa T, Omura M, Satoh F, Shibata H, Takahashi K, et al. (2011) Guidelines for the diagnosis and treatment of primary aldosteronism-- the Japan Endocrine Society 2009. Endocr J 58: 711-721.

3. Nishimoto K, Nakagawa K, Li D, Kosaka T, Oya M, et al. (2010) Adrenocortical zonation in humans under normal and pathological conditions. J Clin Endocrinol Metab 95: 2296-2305.

4. Nieman LK, Biller BM, Findling JW, Newell-Price J, Savage MO, et al. (2008) The diagnosis of Cushing's syndrome: an Endocrine Society Clinical Practice Guideline. J Clin Endocrinol Metab 93: 1526-1540.

5. Morimoto R, Kudo M, Murakami O, Takase K, Ishidoya S, et al. (2011) Difficult-to-control hypertension due to bilateral aldosterone-producing adrenocortical microadenomas associated with a cortisol-producing adrenal macroadenoma. J Hum Hypertens. 25: 114-121.

6. Onoda N, Ishikawa T, Nishio K, Tahara H, Inaba M, et al. (2009) Cushing's syndrome by left adrenocortical adenoma synchronously associated with primary aldosteronism by right adrenocortical adenoma: report of a case. Endocr J. 56: 495-502.

7. Piaditis GP, Kaltsas GA, Androulakis II, Gouli A, Makras P, et al. (2009) High prevalence of autonomous cortisol and aldosterone secretion from adrenal adenomas. Clin Endocrinol (Oxf) 71: 772-778.

8. Kukidome D, Miyamura N, Sakakida K, Shimoda S, Shigematu Y, et al. (2012) A Case of Cortisol Producing Adrenal Adenoma Associated with a Latent Aldosteronoma: Usefulness of the ACTH Loading Test for the Detection of Covert Aldosteronism in Overt Cushing Syndrome. Internal Medicine 51: 395-400.

9. Hiraishi K, Yoshimoto T, Tsuchiya K, Minami I, Doi M, et al. (2011) Clinicopathological features of primary aldosteronism associated with subclinical Cushing's syndrome. Endocr J 58: 543-551.

10. Sonoyama T, Sone M, Miyashita K, Tamura N, Yamahara K, et al. (2011) Significance of adrenocorticotropin stimulation test in the diagnosis of an aldosterone-producing adenoma. J Clin Endocrinol Metab 96: 2771-2778.

11. Somlóová Z, Widimský J Jr, Rosa J, Wichterle D, Strauch B, et al. (2010) The prevalence of metabolic syndrome and its components in two main types of primary aldosteronism. J Hum Hypertens 24: 625-630.

12. Omura M, Saito J, Matsuzawa Y, Nishikawa T (2011) Supper-selective ACTH-stimulated adrenal vein sampling is necessary for detecting precisely functional state of various lesions in unilateral and bilateral adrenal disorders, inducing primary aldosteronism with subclinical Cushing's syndrome. Endocr J. 58: 919-920.

13. Omura M, Sasano H, Saito J, Yamaguchi K, Kakuta Y, et al. (2006) Clinical characteristics of aldosterone-producing microadenoma, macroadenoma, and idiopathic hyperaldosteronism in 93 patients with primary aldosteronism. Hypertens Res. 29: 883-889.

14. Young WF (2007) Primary aldosteronism: renaissance of a syndrome. Clin Endocrinol (Oxf) 66: 607-618.

15. Novitsky YW, Kercher KW, Rosen MJ, Cobb WS, Jyothinagaram S, et al. (2005) Clinical outcomes of laparoscopic adrenalectomy for lateralizing nodular hyperplasia. Surgery 138: 1009-1016.

16. Jeck T, Weisser B, Mengden T, Erdmenger L, Grune S, et al. (1994) Primary aldosteronism: difference in clinical presentation and long-term

follow-up between adenoma and bilateral hyperplasia of the adrenal glands. The Clinical investigator 72: 979-984.

17. Inuzuka M, Tamura N, Sone M, Taura D, Sonoyama T, et al. (2012) A case of myelolipoma with bilateral adrenal hyperaldosteronism cured after unilateral adrenalectomy. Intern Med 51: 479-485.

18. Sukor N, Gordon RD, Ku YK, Jones M, Stowasser M (2009) Role of unilateral adrenalectomy in bilateral primary aldosteronism: a 22-year single center experience. J Clin Endocrinol Metab 94: 2437-2445.

15

Neurosteroid Synthesis in Adult Female Rat Hippocampus, Including Androgens and Allopregnanolone

Yasushi Hojo[1,2], Masahiro Okamoto[1,3], Asami Kato[1], Shimpei Higo[1], Fusako Sakai[1], Hideaki Soya[4], Takeshi Yamazaki[5] and Suguru Kawato[1,2]*

[1]Department of Biophysics and Life Sciences, Graduate School of Arts and Sciences, The University of Tokyo, 3-8-1 Komaba, Meguro, Tokyo 153-8902, Japan, 9 The University of Tokyo, Japan
[2]Bioinformatics Project of Japan Science and Technology Agency, The University of Tokyo, Japan
[3]Research Fellow of the Japan Society for the Promotion of Science, Japan
[4]Laboratory of Exercise Biochemistry and Neuroendocrinology, Institute for Health & Sports Sciences, University of Tsukuba, Tsukuba, Ibaraki, Japan
[5]Laboratory of Molecular Brain Science, Graduate School of Integrated Arts and Sciences, Hiroshima University, Higashi-Hiroshima, Japan

Abstract

Female rat hippocampus synthesizes significant amount of estrogens, including progesterone (PROG), estrone and estradiol (E2). Hippocampal level of PROG and E2 are considerably higher than those in plasma. Female hippocampal estrogens play a significant role in the fluctuation of dendritic spine density across the estrous cycle. Here we extend the study to the investigation of female androgens, including testosterone (T) and Dihydrotestosterone (DHT), in the female rat hippocampus, since female androgens had been largely unknown. By combination of mass-spectrometric analysis with HPLC-purification and picolinoyl-derivatization of sex steroids, we determined the accurate concentration of T and DHT in the hippocampus. The levels of T and DHT in female hippocampus at Proestrus were approximately 1.1 nM and 0.6 nM, respectively, suggesting a significant synthesis of T and DHT. The level of plasma T was approx. 0.1 nM, implying almost no contribution of plasma T to hippocampal T. The concentration of hippocampal DHT had a good correlation with that of hippocampal T, suggesting a significant activity of 5α-reductase (DHT synthase) in the female. Allopregnanolone level was also determined as a useful indicator of 5α-reductase activity. Interestingly mRNA expression level of 5α-reductase and androgen receptor (AR) was not significantly different between the different estrous cycle stages, or between female and male. Nevertheless, sex difference existed with respect to the levels of T, DHT and Allo in hippocampus. Although physiological significance of female hippocampal androgens waits further investigations, the female hippocampus produces T or DHT which may be useful to suppress anxiety, for example.

Keywords: Dihydrotestosterone; Female hippocampus; Androgens; Testosterone; Allopregnanolone

Abbreviations: Allo: Allopregnanolone; AR: Androgen Receptor; D1: Diestrus 1; D2: Diestrus 2; DHT: Di Hydro Testosterone; E2: Estradiol; ER: Estrogen Receptor; Est: Estrus; LC-MS/MS: Liquid Chromatography with Tandem-Mass-Spectrometry; Pro: Proestrus; PROG: Progesterone; PFBz: Pentafluorobenzoxy; StAR: Steroidogenic Acute Regulatory Protein; T: Testosteron

Introduction

In female hippocampus, synthesis and function of androgens have not been well investigated, although estrogens have been extensively studied about synthesis and function. We recently demonstrated that female rat hippocampus synthesizes 17β-estradiol (E2), progesterone (PROG) and estrone [1], which is similar to hippocampus-synthesized steroids in male [2-5]. The estrous cycle-dependent fluctuation of the spine density in female rat hippocampus had a good correlation with the cyclic fluctuation of hippocampal E2 or PROG level [1]. Hippocampal testosterone (T) level in female rats was almost as high as hippocampal E2 level (~1 nM) [1]. The level of Dihydrotestosterone (DHT), the most potent androgen, in female hippocampus, however, remains to be undetermined, although one study reported the presence of very low level DHT (the numerical concentrations were not written) with radioimmunoassay (RIA) [6]. We should determine the accurate concentration of DHT by improvement of the sensitivity of measurements in female hippocampus, since androgen application to the aged female hippocampus decrease a depression-like behavior of aged mice [7]. Concerning the steroid synthesis systems in female

rat hippocampus, mRNA for T synthesis including P450 (17α) and 17β-HSD (type 1 and 3) are expressed [1]. It remains unclear whether 5α-reductase (DHT synthase) and androgen receptor (AR) are expressed in female hippocampus, although one report showed 5α-reductase (type 2) expression with in situ hybridization in female mice brain [8]. In male rat hippocampus, steroidogenic enzymes and steroid receptors are mainly localized in pyramidal neurons in CA1 and CA3, and granule neurons in dentate gyrus [2,4,9-12]. Their neuronal localization of female should be clarified.

5α-reductase produces not only DHT from T, but also allopregnanolone [13] from PROG. Concentration of Allo has been demonstrated using RIA [6,14], GC-MS [15,16] and liquid chromatography with tandem-mass-spectrometry (LC-MS/MS) [17]. Although Allo had been extensively investigated with regard to its anxiolytic and anti-depressive effects [18,19] via modulation of gamma-aminobutyric acid A (GABAA) receptors [20], the physiological significance of DHT in female hippocampus is still unknown and should be investigated. We here examine whether DHT synthase or AR expresses in female rat hippocampus. Localization of P450 (17α), steroidogenic acute regulatory protein (StAR) and AR in female hippocampus is also examined with Immunohistochemical

*Corresponding author: Suguru Kawato, Department of Biophysics and Life Sciences, Graduate School of Arts and Sciences, The University of Tokyo, 3-8-1 Komaba, Meguro, Tokyo 153-8902, Japan, E-mail: kawato@bio.c.u-tokyo.ac.jp

staining. By combination of mass-spectrometric analysis with HPLC-purification and picolinoyl-derivatization of steroids [1,10,21], the accurate concentration of hippocampal DHT and T is determined. Allo in female hippocampus is determined to compare with male Allo [6,14-17]. By comparison of hippocampal androgens and Allo between in male and female, we clarified the profile of steroid synthesis in female rat hippocampus, which is different from male.

Materials and Methods

Animals

Wistar rats (10 weeks old) were purchased from Saitama Experimental Animals Supply (Japan). The estrous cycle of female rats was monitored with morning vaginal smears. Only those rats showing three consecutive 4-day cycles of Pro, Est, D1 and D2 were used at the age of 12 weeks old. Ovariectomy (OVX) and sham operations were performed two-weeks before (at 10w old) the experiments. Male rats were also used at the age of 12 weeks old. All animals were maintained under a 12 h light/12 h dark exposure and free access to food and water. The experimental procedure of this research was approved by the Committee for Animal Research of the University of Tokyo.

Chemicals

T and DHT were purchased from Sigma [22]. Picolinic acid was from Tokyo Chemical Industry (Japan) and, $^{13}C_3$-T, $^{13}C_3$-DHT and Allo-d$_4$ were from CDN Isotope Inc. (Canada). [^{3}H] labeled steroids ([1,2,6,7-^{3}H]-T, [1,2,6,7-^{3}H]-DHT and [1,2,6,7-^{3}H]-Allo) were purchased from Perkin Elmer [22].

RT-PCR

The detailed procedures of mRNA analyses are described in elsewhere [2,4,23]. Total RNAs were isolated from the hippocampus adrenal gland, liver, prostate and testis of adult rats, using a SV total RNA Isolation System (Promega, USA). The purified RNAs were treated with RNase-free DNase to eliminate the possibility of genomic DNA contamination, and quantified on the basis of the absorbance at 260/280 nm. The purified RNAs (100 ng) were reverse-transcribed to obtain cDNAs, using a M-MLV Reverse Transcriptase (Promega, USA). PCR was performed by using these cDNAs. The oligonucleotides for PCR amplification were designed as illustrated in Table S1. The PCR protocols comprised application of a 30 s denaturation period at 95°C, a 20 s annealing period at individual temperature for each enzyme, and a 30 s extension at 72°C, for individual number of cycles for each enzyme (Table S1). For semi-quantitative analysis, the RT-PCR products were separated on 2% agarose gels, stained with ethidium bromide, and analyzed with a fluorescence gel scanner (Atto, Japan) and Image J software. In all the cases we first plotted amplification curves in order to choose the linear phase of PCR cycles. The comparison between different estrous cycle stages can be performed after normalization by glyceraldehyde-3-phosphate dehydrogenase (GAPDH, a house keeping gene) as internal standard. It should be noted that GAPDH expression was not changed across the estrous cycle. The optimal cycle number of GAPDH mRNA was determined as 17 from the amplification curve. The comparison of relative abundance between different estrous stages or between female and male was performed by using the normalized expression. As positive control, we used the reference organ (adrenal gland, liver, prostate and testis)

Mass-spectrometric assay of steroids (T, DHT and Allo)

Detailed procedures are described elsewhere [21].

Step 1: Purification of steroids from hippocampi with normal phase HPLC.

A rat was deeply anesthetized and decapitated at 10-10:30 a.m., since at this time window estradiol (E2) surge at Pro occurs in plasma [24]. The whole hippocampi was removed and homogenized. To calculate the recovery of steroids, radioactive steroids (20,000 cpm) were added as internal standards to hippocampal homogenate. To extract steroid metabolites, ethyl acetate/hexane (3:2 vol/vol) was applied to the homogenates which were then mixed. The mixture was centrifuged at 2,500×g and the organic layer was collected. After evaporation, the extracts were dissolved in 1ml of 40% methanol/H_2O and applied to a C_{18} Amprep solid phase column (Amersham Biosciences, USA) to remove contaminating fats. The extracts were dried, dissolved in an elution solvent of HPLC. The steroid metabolites were separated into T and DHT using a normal phase HPLC system (Jasco, Japan) with an elution solvent of hexane: isopropyl alcohol: acetic acid=98:2:1. A silica gel column (0.46×15 cm, Cosmosil 5SL, Nacalai Tesque, Japan) was used. By monitoring 3H-steroids, the recoveries of T, DHT and Allo were 41 ± 7%, 29 ± 5% and 50 ± 8% respectively, after extraction, C_{18} column treatment and normal phase HPLC separation. As internal standards, 100 pg of isotope labeled steroids ($^{13}C_3$-T, $^{13}C_3$-DHT and Allo-d$_4$) were added to steroid extracts.

Step 2: Derivatization of HPLC-purified steroids before application to LC (reverse 185 phase)-MS/MS.

Preparation and purification of T-17-picolinoyl-ester, DHT-17-picolinoyl-ester and Allo-3-picolinoyl-ester were performed with slight modification of previous methods [1,21]. For preparation of T-17-picolinoyl-ester, DHT-17-picolinoyl-ester and Allo-3-picolinoyl-ester, evaporated steroid extracts from the hippocampus or plasma were reacted with 50 μL of picolinoic acid suspension (4% 191 picolinoic acid, 4% of 4-dimethylaminopyridine, 2% 2-methyl-6-nitrobenzoic anhydride in tetrahydrofuran anhydrous) (i.e., 80 mg of picolinoic acid, 80 mg of 4-dimethylaminopyridine, 40 mg of 2-methyl-6-nitrobenzoic acid in 2 mL of tetrahydrofuran) and 20 μL of triethylamine, for 0.5 h at room temperature. The reaction products dissolved in 1% acetic acid were purified using a Bond Elute C_{18} column (Varian, USA). The dried sample was dissolved in elution solvent of LC. The reaction products were purified with the C_{18} column by using 80% acetonitrile. The purified steroid-derivative was dissolved in elution solvent of LC.

Step 3: Determination of the concentration for T, DHT and Allo using LC-MS/MS.

For determination of the concentration of T and DHT, the LC-MS/MS system, which consists of a Shimadzu HPLC system and an API-5000 triple stage quadrupole mass spectrometer (Applied Biosystems, USA) were employed. LC chromatographic separation was performed on a Kinetex C_{18} column (2.1×150 mm, 1.7 μm, Phenomenex, USA) for T-picolinoyl ester and DHT-picolinoyl ester. For determination of the concentration of Allo, LC chromatographic separation was performed on a preparation column (Unison UK- Phenyl HT (3 μm, 2.0×50 mm, Imtact, Japan)) and an analytical column (Cap cell core C_{18} (2.7 μm, 2.1×100 mm, Shiseido Japan)). After elution of Allo-picolinoyl-ester from the preparation column, Allo-picolinoyl-ester was subsequently loaded to the analytical column. The preparation column enables us to separate Allo (3α-hydroxy-5α-pregnan-20-one) from isomers with equivalent molecular weight (3α-hydroxy-5β-pregnan-20-one, 3b-hydroxy-5α-pregnan-20-one and 3b-hydroxy-5β-pregnan-20-one). MS analysis was operated with electro spray ionization [25] in the positive-ion mode. The isotope-labeled steroid derivatives were used for calibration of retention time by monitoring the m/z transition, from 397 to 256 for $^{13}C_3$-T-picolinoyl-ester, from 399 to 206 for $^{13}C_3$-DHT-picolinoyl-ester, and from 428.4 to 287.3 for Allo-d4-picolinoyl-ester, respectively. Isotope-labeled steroid derivatives were used for internal standards in order to measure recovery of steroids as well as to calibrate the retention time. By monitoring isotope steroids, the recoveries of T, DHT and Allo were determined as 73 ± 3%, 70 ± 2% and 82 ± 6%, respectively, after derivatization, purification and MS/MS detection. In the multiple reaction monitoring mode, the instrument monitored the m/z transition, from 394 to 253 for T-picolinoyl, from 396 to 203 for DHT-picolinoyl, and from 424.4 to 283.3 for Allo-picolinoyl, respectively (Figure S1 and Table S2). Here, m and z represent the mass and charge of a steroid derivative, respectively. The limits of quantification for steroids were measured with blank samples, prepared alongside hippocampal samples through the whole extraction, fractionation and purification procedures. The limits of quantification were 1 pg for T and DHT, and 0.5 pg for Allo per 0.1 g of hippocampal tissue, respectively (Table S2). From the calibration curve using standard T or DHT dissolved in blank samples, the linearity was observed between 1.0 pg and 2000 pg for T and DHT, between 5 pg and 1000 pg for Allo, respectively (Figure S2).

Immunohistochemical staining of hippocampal slices

Detailed procedures are described elsewhere [2,4,10,11]. Hippocampal slices were prepared from 12 week-old female rats at Proestrus stage. Animals were deeply anesthetized and perfused transcardially with PBS (0.1 M phosphate buffer and 0.14 M NaCl, pH 7.3), followed by fixative solution (4% paraformaldehyde/PBS). The hippocampi were post fixed, cryo protected, and frozen-sliced coronally

with a cryostat (CM1510, Leica). Staining for steroidogenic enzymes (P450 (17α), P450arom and StAR) and receptors (AR and ERa) was performed with the avidin-biotin-peroxidase complex technique. Dilution of primary antibody was 1:1000 each for purified anti-guinea pig cytochrome P450(17α) IgG [26], purified anti-human P450arom IgG [27], anti-mouse StAR IgG [28], anti-AR IgG (PG-21, Millipore, USA), or purified anti-rat C terminal of ERa antibody (RC-19) [12]. After application of primary antibody, the slices were incubated for 18 h at 4°C, in the presence of 0.5% Triton X-100. Biotinylated anti-rabbit IgG (1:1000) and streptavidin-horseradish peroxidase complex (Vector Laboratories) was applied. Immuno-reactive cells were detected with a solution of diaminobenzidine with ammonium nickel sulfate. After embedding in Entellan Neu (Merck, Germany), the immuno-reactive cells were observed under microscope.

Statistical analysis

Data are expressed as mean ± SEM. For comparison of the mRNA level of steroidogenic enzymes and receptors, we used a 1-way ANOVA followed by Tukey-Kramer posthoc multiple comparisons. For comparison of the concentration of T or DHT in the hippocampus between male and female, we used Student's t-test. A difference was considered significant at a value of *p<0.05, **p<0.01 or ***p<0.001.

Results

Molecular biological analysis of steroidogenic enzymes and steroid receptors in the female hippocampus

The hippocampal expression of steroidogenic enzymes (StAR, 5α-reductase (Types 1 and 2)) and AR were examined across the estrous

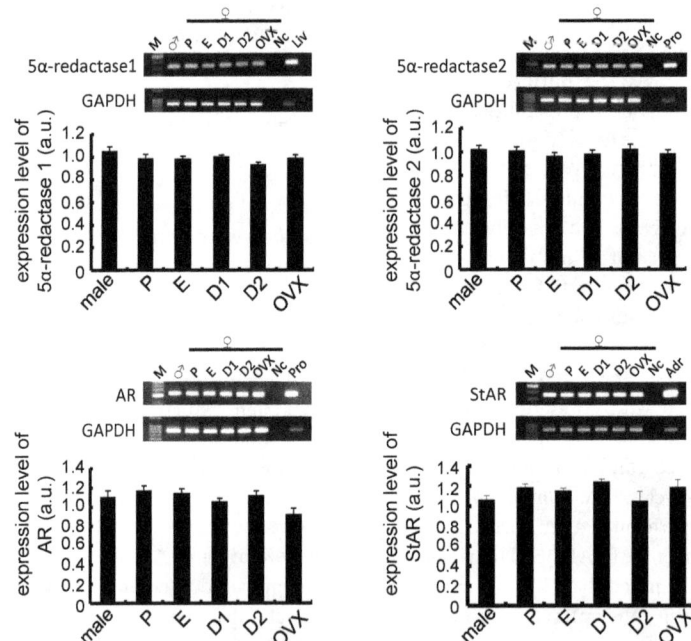

Figure 1: No significant change in expression levels of mRNAs for sex steroidogenic enzymes and receptor (A: 5a-reductase type1, B: 5a-reductase type2, C: AR and D: StAR) in the female hippocampus across the estrous cycle. Upper panels show representative PCR images and lower panels show statistical comparisons. In each images, from left to right, size marker (100 bp ladder) (M), male hippocampus (male), female hippocampus at Pro (P), Est (E), D1 (D1), D2 (D2), and OVX female rats (OVX), the sample without template DNA as negative control (Nc). For each enzyme, the RT-PCR products for mRNAs are visualized with ethidium bromide staining on the top of each panel. As an internal control, the ethidium bromide staining of GAPDH is shown on the bottom of each panel. PCR was performed by using cDNA made by reverse transcription from 100 ng of hippocampal total RNA. Statistical comparisons show no estrous cycle-dependent changes of mRNA expression for sex-steroidogenic enzymes. The vertical axis indicates the expression level for each enzyme calculated from the intensity of EB bands. Each value is mean ± S.E.M. Data are taken from duplicate determinations for each rat of total 4 rats.

cycle. Expression levels of mRNA transcripts normalized by GAPDH are shown as bar graphs in Figure 1. Surprisingly, no significant cyclic fluctuations across the estrous cycle were observed for their expression levels. OVX did not change the expression level of any steroidogenic enzyme and AR. Relative number of transcripts, expressed in the hippocampus of adult female rats, was approx. 1/3 of that in the liver for 5α-reductase type 1, approx. 1/300 of that in the male prostate for 5α-reductase type 2, approx. 1/10 of that in the male prostate for AR, and approx. 1/100 of that in the adrenal for StAR (Table 1).

Mass-spectrometric determination of androgen and allopregnanolone levels in the female hippocampus

The concentration of T, DHT and Allo was determined for adult female and male rat hippocampus using a chromatogram analysis of the fragmented ions of steroid-derivatives. We chose the hippocampus at Proestrus stage for steroid determination since RT-PCR analysis revealed no estrous cycle-related fluctuation of the expression for 5α-reductase (types 1 and 2) which is required for synthesis of DHT

and Allo. Results are summarized in Figures 2 and 3. T, DHT and Allo were derivatized with picolinoyl before application to LC-MS/MS to increase the accuracy of determination by improving the limit of quantification (LOQ) (Table S2).

In the chromatographic profiles of the fragmented ion of T-17-picolinoyl-ester, DHT-17-picolinoyl-ester and Allo-3-picolinoyl-ester, a single clear peak was observed at 4.12, 4.37 and 8.43 min, respectively (Figurea 2A1, 2B1 and 2C1). For these steroids, the retention time of the observed steroid peak was the same as that of standard steroid. To confirm the assay accuracy, the hippocampal homogenate spiked with known amounts of the steroids was prepared and its concentration of steroid was determined 296 (Table S3). The LOQs were defined in Table S2 as the lowest value with an acceptable accuracy (90-110%) and precision (i.e. RSD<10%). The results of intra- and inter-assay were shown in Table S2. The RSD for intra- and inter-assay was less than 5.1% and 7.2%, respectively.

Hippocampal level of androgens in female were 1.1 nM for T and

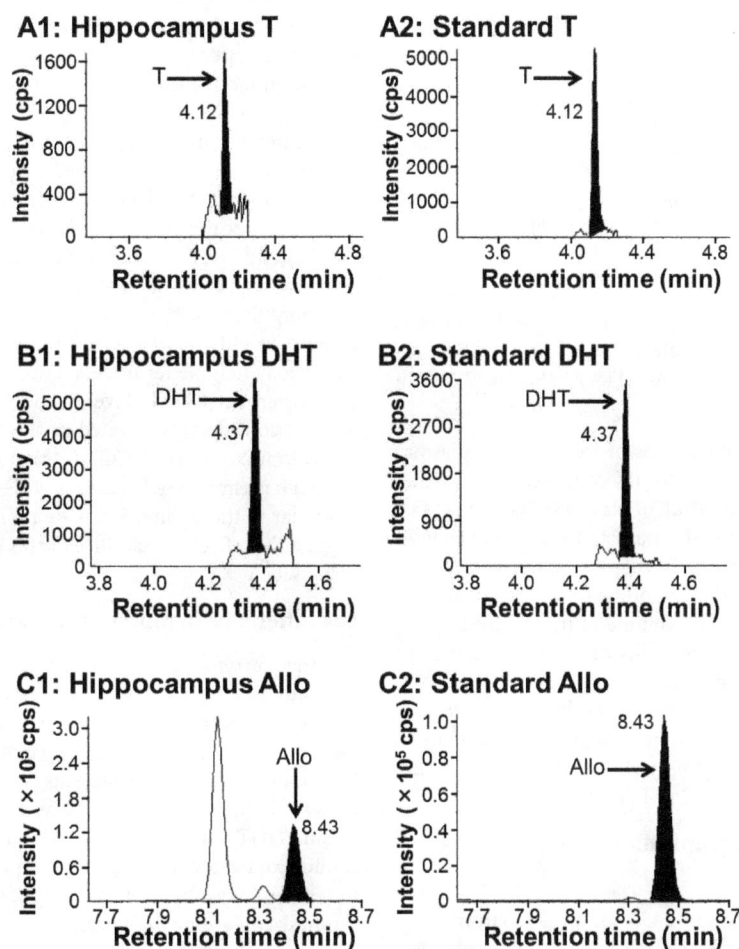

Figure 2: Mass-spectrometric analysis of hippocampal sex-steroids (12-week-old female rats), LC-MS/MS ion chromatograms of T (A), DHT(B) and Allo(C). (A1), (B1) and (C1) represent the chromatograms of the fragmented ions of each steroid from the hippocampus. Shaded portions indicate the intensity of fragmented ions of T (m/z=253), DHT (m/z=203) and Allo (m/z=283.3), respectively. (A2), (B2) and (C2) represent the chromatograms of the fragmented ions of the standard steroids. The vertical axis indicates the intensity of the fragmented ion. The horizontal axis indicates the retention time of the fragmented ion, t=4.12 min for T, 4.37 min for DHT, and 8.43 min for Allo, respectively. The time of sample injection to LC system was defined as t=0 min. Note that pre-purification step using normal phase HPLC before injection to LC system is very important to achieve high precision and good reproducibility of LC-MS/MS determination in order to avoid contamination of other steroids and fats. Steroid-derivatives or steroids were further separated with reversed phase LC-column before MS/MS. In the multiple reaction monitoring modes, the instrument monitored the m/z transition (Table S2).

Enzyme or receptor	Relative expression level in female hippocampus[a]	Reference organ
5a-reductase 1	1 : 3	Liver
5a-reductase 2	1 : 300	Prostate[c]
AR	1 : 10	Prostate
StAR		
	1 : 100	adrenal

[a]Value of Proestrus sample was used because no fluctuation of mRNA level was observed between any stage of estrous cycle

[b]Relative expression level in female hippocampus (Proestrus) is indicated with the ratio to that in reference organ

[c]Prostate was prepared from 12 week-old male rats

Table 1: Comparison of mRNA levels of steroidogenic enzymes or receptors between in hippocampus and in reference organ.

Testosterone (T)		Dihydrotestosterone (DHT)	
(nM)[b]	(ng/g wet weight)	(nM)	(ng/g wet weight)
1.10 ± 0.28[c] (n[d]=12)	0.32 ± 0.08	0.62 ± 0.16 (n=7)	0.18 ± 0.05

(A) Hippocampal androgens (T and DHT) in female[a]

Female (n=3)		Male (n=3)	
(nM)	(ng/g wet weight)	(nM)	(ng/g wet weight)
16.4 ± 2.3	5.2 ± 0.7	1.00 ± 0.71	0.32 ± 0.23

(B) Hippocampal Allo in female and male

[a]All female samples were prepared at Proestrus stage

[b]Concentration in nM is calculated using the average volume of 0.124 mL for one whole hippocampus that has 0.124 ± 0.002 g wet weight (n=44). We assumed that tissue having 1 g of wet weight has an approximate volume of

Table 2: Mass spectrometric analysis of the concentration of androgens (T and DHT) or Allopregnanolone (Kerr JE et al.) in the hippocampus and plasma of adult female rats.

0.62 nM for DHT, respectively (Figure 3a). The level of hippocampal T was much higher than that of plasma T (~0.1 nM) in female. In contrast to androgens, the levels of Allo in the female hippocampus was 16.4 nM which was 16 times higher than that in male (Figure 3B; t=6.52, df=4, p=0.0029).

In order to compare hippocampal levels of steroids with plasma steroids, we converted ng/g wet weight to nM concentration *via* the following estimation (Table 2). First, 1 mL of plasma (93% is water) is assumed to have 1 g weight, as 1 mL of water has 1 g weight. Second, we assume that the hippocampal tissue having 1 g of wet weight has an approx. volume of 1 mL, as nearly 78% of the brain tissue consists of water [29]. Consideration of specific volume of protein and lipids (0.7-1.0 mL/g) in the brain further support this assumption [11,30,31]. After dividing by the individual hippocampal volume (0.124 ± 0.002 wet weight for one whole hippocampus of 12 weeks old female rat, n=44), the levels of T, DHT, Allo in the hippocampus were calculated. Based on these considerations, 0.18 ng/g wet weight of DHT in the hippocampus at Pro corresponds to 0.62 nM (Table 2).

Localization of steroidogenic enzymes and receptors in female hippocampus

The localization and presence of P450 (17α), P450arom and StAR in the hippocampus of adult female rats were demonstrated by Immunohistochemical staining. P450 (17α), P450arom and StAR were mainly localized in pyramidal neurons in CA1-CA3 region as well as granule cells in dentate gyrus [9] (Figure 4A-4C). Immuno staining of glial cells for these enzymes was much weaker than that of principal neurons. In addition to steroidogenic enzymes, we also demonstrated the localization for AR and ERa in hippocampal slices of female. AR and ERa also localized in pyramidal and granule neurons (Figures 4D and 4E). It should be noted that AR immuno reactivity was the

most prominent at CA1pyramidal neurons, whereas region difference in staining pattern of ERa was not observed. The staining pattern of steroidogenic enzymes and receptors in female hippocampus was almost the same as that of male hippocampus [2,4,11,12,32].

Discussion

No significant sex difference in hippocampal steroidogenic systems (mRNA and protein)

Surprisingly, the expression levels of sex steroidogenic enzymes including 5α-reductase (types 1 and 2) and StAR were not significantly different between female and male hippocampus (Figure 1). Furthermore, no cyclic fluctuation of expression levels of these enzymes was observed across the estrous cycle. Other steroidogenic enzymes which are required for androgen or estrogen synthesis including P450 (17α), P450 arom and 17β-HSD (T synthase) also exhibited neither sex difference nor estrous cycle-dependent fluctuation [1], suggesting the constant catalytic activity for steroids in the hippocampus. It may be possible that the localization of enzymes or receptors is sex different even with the equal level of mRNA expression. Therefore, we investigated the localization of enzymes including P450 (17α) and P450arom or receptors including AR and ERa in female hippocampus with immunohistochemistry in current study, resulting in the same pattern as male (Figure 4) [2,4,11,12]. These results suggest that hippocampal synthesis activity of androgen or Allo is independent of sex. In fact, 5α-reductase activity was almost equal between in male and female from the data with high correlation between hippocampal T and hippocampal DHT (Figure 3C). All data of hippocampal T (x-axis) and DHT (y-axis) from both sexes were aligned in a straight line with high correlation (Figure 3C), implying that DHT production was only dependent on substrate T concentration. Here we present analysis at only Proestrus stage, and further analysis at other estrus stages may help better understanding. In addition, we also measured corticosterone (CORT) level in the female hippocampus, and CORT was not considerably elevated upon sacrifice or anesthetics treatment. Only approx. 200 nM CORT was penetrated to the hippocampus, although plasma CORT transiently elevated to approx. 1500 nM, which is similar to the situation in male rat hippocampus [33]. These results suggest that effects by sacrifice -stress on the hippocampus may not be serious.

Sex difference in hippocampal androgen and allo levels

The current study revealed that female hippocampus is able to synthesize androgens (T and DHT) in addition to estrogens. In female, hippocampal T (~1 nM) is much higher (nearly 10 fold) than plasma T (~0.1 nM) [1], implying that the contribution of plasma T to hippocampal T is very weak. This is very different from male in which 70-80% of hippocampal T is derived from plasma T [21]. Since female plasma DHT would be lower than plasma T (~0.1nM), plasma DHT cannot contribute to the production of hippocampal DHT (~0.6 nM) in female. Majority of female hippocampal DHT should be therefore synthesized from hippocampal-synthesized T. Although male hippocampus synthesizes androgens and estrogens [2,11,21,33,34], sex difference exists in the level of hippocampal steroids. The hippocampal level of androgens (T and DHT) is significantly high in male than in the female. The levels of T and DHT in the female hippocampus were 15 times lower than those in male (Figure 3A). In contrast to androgens, hippocampal Allo level was 16 times higher in female than in male. What generates such a sex difference in hippocampal steroid level? It may be due to the difference in precursor steroids supplied via blood circulation between female and male. Most abundant precursor

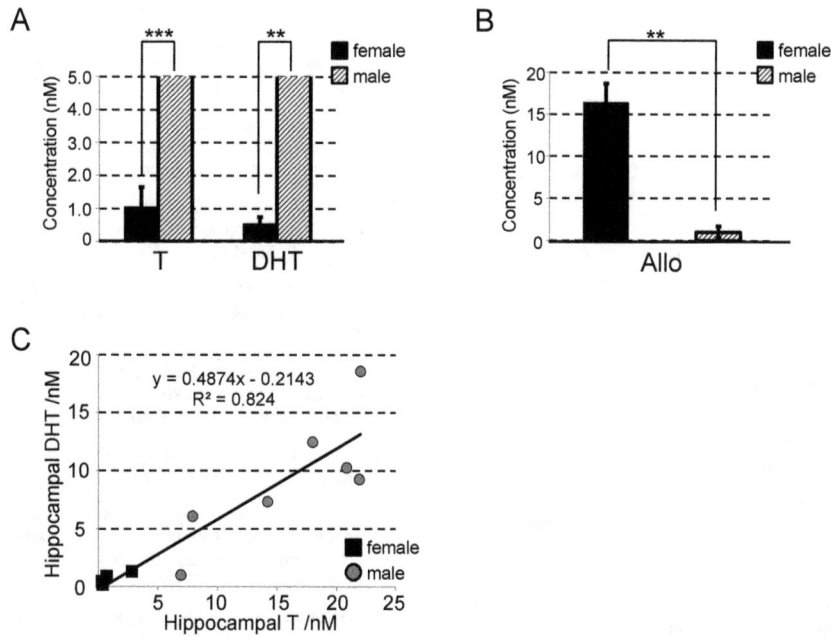

Figure 3: (A) Comparison of hippocampal androgens (T and DHT) level between male and female. Data are expressed as Mean ± SEM. Hippocampal level of androgens was significantly different between female and male (t=5.94, df=7, p=0.00057 for T, and t=4.12, df=6, p=0.0062 for DHT, respectively). (B) Comparison of hippocampal Allo level between male and female. Data are expressed as Mean ± SEM. Hippocampal level of Allo was significantly different between female and male (t=6.52, df=4, p=0.0029). (C) Relationship between hippocampal T and DHT for individual rats. Male data are taken from (Hojo Y et al., 2009). Number of animals is 7 for male and 4 for female, respectively. Statistical significance, **p<0.01, ***p<0.001.

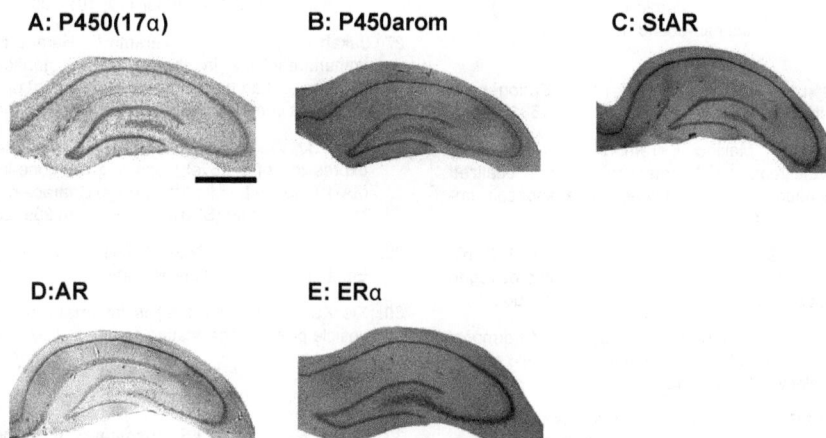

Figure 4: Immunohistochemical staining for P450(17a) (A), P450arom (B) StAR (C), AR (D) and ERa (E) in the hippocampus of 12 week-old female rat at Proestrus stage. The coronal section of whole hippocampus (20 mm thickness) was used. Scale bar, 800 mm.

steroids for synthesis of sex steroids in the hippocampus may be PROG (precursor of Allo) originally produced by ovary or adrenal gland (20-50 nM in plasma) in female, and T (precursor of DHT) from testis (~15 nM) in male, respectively [21,1]. Almost all hippocampal androgens (T and DHT) in female were hippocampus-synthesized from PROG, because the level of plasma T (~0.1 nM) in female was much lower than that of hippocampal T [1].

Earlier studies on female androgens in the brain

The concentration of T and DHT in adult female hippocampus had not yet been accurately determined in previous studies. Although one study reported the presence of androgens with RIA method [6],

the numerical concentrations were not written due to very low levels. On the other hand, a significant concentration of Allo has been demonstrated using RIA [6,14], GC-MS [15,16] and LC-MS/MS [17]. The concentration of Allo was approximately 6 ng/g (~20 nM) in female hippocampus at Proestrus [6,14]. On the other hand Allo was very low approximately 0.4 ng/g (~1 nM) in male adult whole brain [15,16] or undetectable in male cultured hippocampus. These concentrations are qualitatively similar to those observed in the current study. Compared to male, physiological role of androgens in female hippocampus is not clear. One of the possible physiological roles might be suppression of depression, since supplementation of androgens in female decreased a depression-like behavior of aged mice [7]. Extensive studies on physiological roles of female androgen should be needed.

Acknowledgements

Dr. S. Homma (Aska Pharmamedical) is acknowledged for steroid analysis.

References

1. Kato A, Hojo Y, Higo S, Komatsuzaki Y, Murakami G, et al. (2013) Female hippocampal estrogens have a significant correlation with cyclic fluctuation of hippocampal spines. Front Neural Circuits 7: 149.

2. Hojo Y, Hattori TA, Enami T, Furukawa A, Suzuki K, et al. (2004) Adult male rat hippocampus synthesizes estradiol from pregnenolone by cytochromes P45017alpha and P450 aromatase localized in neurons. Proc Natl Acad Sci U S A 101: 865-870.

3. Hojo Y, Murakami G, Mukai H, Higo S, Hatanaka Y, et al. (2008) Estrogen synthesis in the brain--role in synaptic plasticity and memory. Mol Cell Endocrinol 290: 31-43.

4. Kawato S, Hojo Y, Kimoto T (2002) Histological and metabolism analysis of P450 expression in the brain. Methods Enzymol 357: 241-249.

5. Okamoto M, Hojo Y, Inoue K, Matsui T, Kawato S, et al. (2012) Mild exercise increases dihydrotestosterone in hippocampus providing evidence for androgenic mediation of neurogenesis. Proc Natl Acad Sci U S A 109: 13100-13105.

6. Frye CA, Bayon LE (1999) Mating stimuli influence endogenous variations in the neurosteroids 3alpha,5alpha-THP and 3alpha-Diol. J Neuroendocrinol 11: 839-847.

7. Frye CA, Walf AA (2009) Depression-like behavior of aged male and female mice is ameliorated with administration of testosterone or its metabolites. Physiol Behav 97: 266-269.

8. Matsui D, Sakari M, Sato T, Murayama A, Takada I, et al. (2002) Transcriptional regulation of the mouse steroid 5alpha-reductase type II gene by progesterone in brain. Nucleic Acids Res 30: 1387-1393.

9. Pardridge WM, Mietus LJ (1979) Transport of steroid hormones through the rat blood-brain barrier. Primary role of albumin-bound hormone. J Clin Invest 64: 145-154.

10. Higo S, Hojo Y, Ishii H, Komatsuzaki Y, Ooishi Y, et al. (2011) Endogenous synthesis of corticosteroids in the hippocampus. PLoS One 6: e21631.

11. Kimoto T, Tsurugizawa T, Ohta Y, Makino J, Tamura H, et al. (2001) Neurosteroid synthesis by cytochrome p450-containing systems localized in the rat brain hippocampal neurons: N-methyl-D-aspartate and calcium-dependent synthesis. Endocrinology 142: 3578-3589.

12. Mukai H, Tsurugizawa T, Murakami G, Kominami S, Ishii H, et al. (2007) Rapid modulation of long-term depression and spinogenesis via synaptic estrogen receptors in hippocampal principal neurons. J Neurochem 100: 950-967.

13. Kerr JE, Allore RJ, Beck SG, Handa RJ (1995) Distribution and hormonal regulation of androgen receptor (AR) and AR messenger ribonucleic acid in the rat hippocampus. Endocrinology 136: 3213-3221.

14. Frye CA, Petralia SM, Rhodes ME (2000) Estrous cycle and sex differences in performance on anxiety tasks coincide with increases in hippocampal progesterone and 3alpha,5alpha-THP. Pharmacol Biochem Behav 67: 587-596.

15. Ebner MJ, Corol DI, Havlíková H, Honour JW, Fry JP (2006) Identification of neuroactive steroids and their precursors and metabolites in adult male rat brain. Endocrinology 147: 179-190.

16. Meffre D, Pianos A, Liere P, Eychenne B, Cambourg A, et al. (2007) Steroid profiling in brain and plasma of male and pseudopregnant female rats after traumatic brain injury: analysis by gas chromatography/mass spectrometry. Endocrinology 148: 2505-2517.

17. Ishihara Y, Kawami T, Ishida A, Yamazaki T (2013) Allopregnanolone-mediated protective effects of progesterone on tributyltin-induced neuronal injury in rat hippocampal slices. J Steroid Biochem Mol Biol 135: 1-6.

18. Frye CA, Walf AA (2002) Changes in progesterone metabolites in the hippocampus can modulate open field and forced swim test behavior of proestrous rats. Horm Behav 41: 306-315.

19. Frye CA, Walf AA (2004) Hippocampal 3alpha,5alpha-THP may alter depressive behavior of pregnant and lactating rats. Pharmacol Biochem Behav 78: 531-540.

20. Smith SS, Shen H, Gong QH, Zhou X (2007) Neurosteroid regulation of GABA(A) receptors: Focus on the alpha4 and delta subunits. Pharmacol Ther 116: 58-76.

21. Hojo Y, Higo S, Ishii H, Ooishi Y, Mukai H, et al. (2009) Comparison between hippocampus-synthesized and circulation-derived sex steroids in the hippocampus. Endocrinology 150: 5106-5112.

22. Fusani L, Gahr M (2006) Hormonal influence on song structure and organization: the role of estrogen. Neuroscience 138: 939-946.

23. Kimoto T, Ishii H, Higo S, Hojo Y, Kawato S (2010) Semicomprehensive analysis of the postnatal age-related changes in the mRNA expression of sex steroidogenic enzymes and sex steroid receptors in the male rat hippocampus. Endocrinology 151: 5795-5806.

24. Gorski RA, Mennin SP, Kubo K (1975) The neural and hormonal bases of the reproductive cycle of the rat. Adv Exp Med Biol 54: 115-153.

25. Caruso D, Pesaresi M, Maschi O, Giatti S, Garcia-Segura LM, et al. (2010) Effect of short-and long-term gonadectomy on neuroactive steroid levels in the central and peripheral nervous system of male and female rats. J Neuroendocrinol 22: 1137-1147.

26. Shinzawa K, Ishibashi S, Murakoshi M, Watanabe K, Kominami S, et al. (1988) Relationship between zonal distribution of microsomal cytochrome P-450s (P-450(17) alpha,lyase and P-450C21) and steroidogenic activities in guinea-pig adrenal cortex. J Endocrinol 119: 191-200.

27. Jakab RL, Horvath TL, Leranth C, Harada N, Naftolin F (1993) Aromatase immunoreactivity in the rat brain: gonadectomy-sensitive hypothalamic neurons and an unresponsive "limbic ring" of the lateral septum-bed nucleus-amygdala complex. J Steroid Biochem Mol Biol 44: 481-498.

28. Clark BJ, Wells J, King SR, Stocco DM (1994) The purification, cloning, and expression of a novel luteinizing hormone-induced mitochondrial protein in MA-10 mouse Leydig tumor cells. Characterization of the steroidogenic acute regulatory protein (StAR). J Biol Chem 269: 28314-28322.

29. McIlwain H BH (1985) Biochemistry and the Central Nervous System. Edinburgh: Churchill Livingstone.

30. Xie XS, Stone DK (1986) Isolation and reconstitution of the clathrin-coated vesicle proton translocating complex. J Biol Chem 261: 2492-2495.

31. Tanford C, Nozaki Y, Reynolds JA, Makino S (1974) Molecular characterization of proteins in detergent solutions. Biochemistry 13: 2369-2376.

32. Tabori NE, Stewart LS, Znamensky V, Romeo RD, Alves SE, et al. (2005) Ultrastructural evidence that androgen receptors are located at extranuclear sites in the rat hippocampal formation. Neuroscience 130: 151-163.

33. Hojo Y, Higo S, Kawato S, Hatanaka Y, Ooishi Y, et al. (2011) Hippocampal synthesis of sex steroids and corticosteroids: essential for modulation of synaptic plasticity. Front Endocrinol (Lausanne) 2: 43.

34. Kawato S (2004) Endocrine disrupters as disrupters of brain function: a neurosteroid viewpoint. Environ Sci 11: 1-14.

16

Progesterone-induced Maturation and Down Regulation of Membrane Bound Na+, K+-ATPase

Mohanty BK*

School of MVM, 1417 Baramunda Colony, Bhubaneswar-751003, Orissa, India

Abstract

Progesterone induces maturation by releasing oocyte from G2 of MI cell cycle arrest. This process is rate limiting as it produces fertilizable eggs. Therefore, it draws a lot of attention. Na+, K+-ATPase is a membrane bound enzyme molecule that has known to have various functions. One of these functions is to act as receptor for Progesterone. In oocyte maturation to egg entirely depends on progesterone, a hormone that is known to reduce risk of cancer. Using EM Histo-cytochemical novel technique, we have shown that membrane bound Na+, K+-ATPase are gradually down-regulated following Progesterone-induced maturation. By Germinal Vesicle Break down, Na+, K+-ATPase is completely down-regulated from oolemma and only present in the narrow region of Germinal Vesicle Break Down. This is an important phenonmena as this down-regulation coincides with cell entering M-phase. Here, I also briefly introduce you to a technique that only localizes phosphate cleaving membrane bound Na+, K+-ATPase.

Keywords: Na+; K+-ATPase; Down regulation; Progesterone

Introduction

Progesterone induces fully grown Stage VI oocytes to mature that leads to Nuclear Envelope Break Down and the appearance of white spot in the animal hemisphere [1-3]. Na+, K+-ATPase is a P-type ATPase that undergoes E1-E2 transition to translocate 3Na+ outside cell against electrochemical gradient. In all living animal cells it regulates cell pH. It is also involved in firing electrical current in neuronal cells. It has specialized functions in muscles and cardiac cells. The molecular structure and genetic expression of this protein has been extensively studied [4,5]. It is a multigene protein. It is heterodimer of a catalytic α-subunit of approximately 100-110 kD peptide and a β-sununit of 40 kD. Four isoforms of α-subunit have been reported [4,6,7]. Three isoforms of β-subunit have also been identified [6]. The third subunit of Na+, K+-ATPase is γ-subunit of 7-10 kD [8,9]. Experimental evidences suggest that the Na+, K+- ATPase activity is modulated by protein kinase A and protein kinase C by phosphorylation [10,11].

Na+, K+-ATPase is a key instigator of cell polarity [12]. We have shown that Na+, K+-ATPase activity is asymmetrically localized over the animal hemisphere of fully differentiated Stage VI Xenopus oocytes [12]. The Vegetal pole that holds the vegetal cortices comprising VegT, TGF-β and Cyclin-B lacks Na+, K+-ATPase activity completely. These Phosphate-cleaving membrane bound Na+, K+- ATPase sets up an internal gradient of Na+ that is critical in establishing polarity [13]. One important aspect of Progesterone- induced down-regulation of membrane bound Na+, K+-ATPase from animal hemisphere is down-regulation fattens the internal Na+ gradient. Therefore, it releases vegetal cortices from its position and moves upward following Progesterone-induced maturation [14] due to complete down-regulation of Na+, K+-ATPase from the animal hemisphere [12]. This down-regulation causes complete flattening of internal Na+ that is set due to asymmetric localization of Na+, K+- ATPase activity. This asymmetry sets up three internal Na+ gradients [12]. The vegetal hemisphere that lacks

Na+, K+-ATPase activity has a sink for Na+. The animal hemisphere that has Na+, K+-ATPase activity has medium level of Na+. While the equatorial region has negligible to low Na+. We believe, the acidic proteins such as Tgf-β [15], Cyclin-B [16,17] and VegT [14] are localized in the vegetal cortices while the basic proteins such as AP-2 [18], Sox2 and Sox3 [19] are localized in the animal hemisphere and the neutral proteins such as Brachy [20] is localized in the equatorial region. Exceptions are there. As we know myoD is a basic protein and it is localized in the equatorial region possibly due to its binding partner. My estimation is Na+ is the key instigator of cell polarity. Therefore, this asymmetry is critical [12].

Following Progesterone-induced maturation, Na+, K+-ATPase is localized in the animal pole region. It appears that the Dorsal-ventral axis is already set up in the matured eggs with presence of ATPase activity towards the dorsal side (Figure 1) [12]. Na+, K+-ATPase is key receptor molecule [1,2]. We believe, apart from Progesterone and Estradiole it also possibly act as receptor for sperm and we expect an up-regulation of ATPase activity at the sperm entry point. We think Na+, K+-ATPase may be the key receptor for hormones [1,2] and sperm. We are making greater stride to resolve the issue. As we know Na+ is the binding factor between sperm and egg therefore such asymmetric localization is critical. Surely this will be a turning point. Another important point about the down-regulation of Na+, K+- ATPase following Progesterone-induced maturation is arrest of cell cycle at M-phase. Does that means Na+, K+-ATPase activity may have a role in metastasis? It would be interesting to observe Na+, K+- ATPase activity in uterine and cervical cancer by EM Histo- Cytochemical method, the technique that localizes phosphate cleaving Na+, K+-ATPase activity at the resolution of electron microscope. It may resolve what effect progesterone and estrogen have on uterine and cervical cancer (we are open to collaboration).

---

*Corresponding author: Mohanty BK, School of MVM, 1417 Baramunda Colony, Bhubaneswar-751003, Orissa, India, E-mail: bkmohanty_colorado_edu@yahoo.com

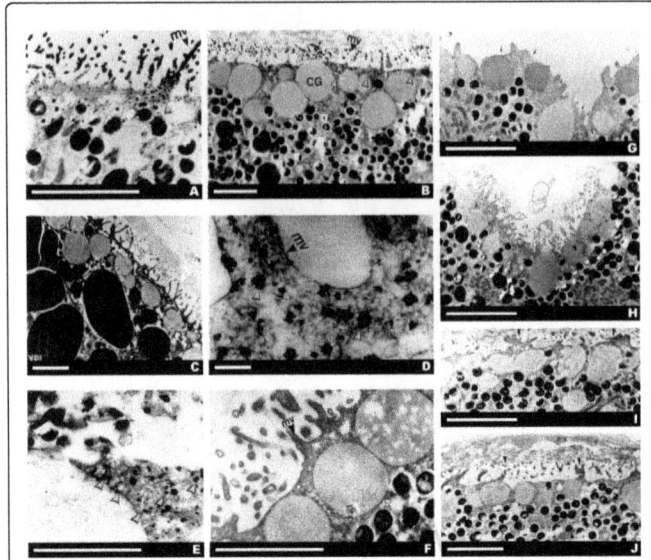

Figure 1: Localization of Na$^+$, K$^+$-ATPase activity following progesterone-induced maturation of stage-VI Xenopus oocytes. We see slight up-regulation (A) and then immediate complete down-regulation of Na$^+$, K$^+$-ATPase activity (B-H). A: An up-regulation of Na$^+$, K$^+$-ATPase activity within 1 hr after progesterone-induction. B: A substantial and near complete down-regulation of Na$^+$, K$^+$-ATPase activity following 3 hr of progesterone induction. C: Complete absence of Na$^+$, K$^+$-ATPase activity over the vegetal hemisphere. (D, E) Presence of vesicle associated reaction deposits in the sub cortical region of the oocyte following 3 hr of progesterone induction, suggesting endocytotic removal of the membrane Na$^+$, K$^+$-ATPase molecules from the plasma membrane. G: Presence of countable number of Na$^+$, K$^+$-ATPase molecules over the animal pole region of polar body extrusion following GVBD. Na$^+$, K$^+$-ATPase activity is completely down-regulated by GVBD, and vesicle-associated reaction deposits are absent from the cytoplasm of subcortical region. We believe the side that has maximum ATPase activity forms the dorsal side of the fertilized egg. This observation was only made possible by EM enzyme Histo-cytochemical technique: (I) Complete absence of reaction deposits, when K$^+$ is completely removed. (F, J) Complete absence and near complete absence of Na$^+$, K$^+$-ATPase activity over two different regions over the animal hemisphere in the presence of 10 μM Ouabain. (H) The presence of countable number of Ca^{2+}, Mg^{2+}-ATPase activity at the region of polar body extrusion over animal pole region following GVBD. Magnifications/bar sizes: (A) 15,000/1 mm; (B) 6,000/1 mm; (C) 5,000/1 mm; (D) 5,000/100 nm; (E) 30,000/1 mm; (F) 15,000/1 mm; (G-I) 10,000/1 mm; (J) 8,000/1 mm. (Adopted from Mohanty and Gupta, 2012).

Progestrone is a steroid hormone involved in female menstrual cycle, pregnancy (supports gestation) and embryogenesis of human and other species [20-22]. In clinical term, reduced progesterone adversely affects endometrium maturation and results in subfertility and pregnancy miscarriage [23,24]. On the contrary Estrogen exposure induces breast and endometrial cancer [25]. It also proliferated epithelial cells to develop into cancer [26]. Progesterone, on the other-hand, inhibits this estrogen-induced cell proliferation and stimulates epithelial differentiation [27]. Consequently, progesterone is used

therapeutically to inhibit the proliferation of estrogen- dependent endometrial cancers [28-30].

It is also important to know why a down-regulation is necessary before fertilization. The reason could be very rewarding. I believe the vegetal cortices released from vegetal hemisphes eggs following Progesterone-induced maturation has a significant role. Cyclin B moves upward and enters into the nucleus to complete division. Similarly, down-regulation makes eggs quiescent and prepares eggs to hostile environment and any damage to DNA. In Xenopus, eggs are laid in wetland that remains hostile. We were the first to show a detailed analysis of Na+, K+-ATPase activity in any vertebrate oocytes and in maturing eggs [12] and the experiment using EM Histo- cytochemical technique was repeated 7 times with constistant results. In the process we realized Na+, K+-ATPase activity can be different if localize by EM Histo-cytochemical technique and immune- cytochemical localization as later can localize epitope both from active and inactive Na+, K+-ATPase [31]. This protection allows organogenesis and patterning to proceed normally following fertilization to production of normal embryos.

EM Histo-cytochemical localization is the best technique to localize Na+, K+-ATPase activity. It gives most consistent results compare to immunocytochemical localization. The biochemical localization only shows presence of Na+, K+-ATPase activity but not their spatial distribution. For present study, we have used Mayahara et al. 1980 technique. It's a direct one-step method. In this technique we fixed the progesterone-induced and uninduced stage stage VI oocytes in 2% paraformaldehyde and 0.005% glutaraldehyde for 30 mins and then both group of oocytes were processed as method completely described in Mohanty and Gupta [12]. The technique is so versetile that one can count individual phosphate cleaving ATPase molecules. We estimated upto 20 times higher ATPase activity over the animal hemisphere than the vegetal hemisphere.

Acknowledgements

I thank my colleagues for input and my mother for her blessings.

References

1. Morrill GA, Erlichman J, Gutierrez-Jurez R, Kostellow AB (2005) The steroid-binding subunit of the Na+,K+-ATPase as a progesterone receptor on the amphibian oocyte plasma membrane. Steroids 70: 933-945.

2. Morrill GA, Kostellow AB, Askari A (2008) Progesterone binding to the Î±1-subunit of the Na+,K+-ATPase on the cell surface: insights from computational modeling. Steroids 73: 27-40.

3. Ferrell Jr JE (1999) Xenopus oocyte maturation: new lessons from a good egg. Bioessays 21:833-842.

4. Lingrel JB, Orlowski J, Shull MM, Price EM (1990) Molecular genetics of Na,K-ATPase. Prog Nucleic Acid Res Mol Biol 38: 37-89.

5. Sachs G, Munson K (1991) Mammalian phosphorylating ion-motive ATPase. Curr.Opin. Cell Biol 3:685-694.

6. Blanco G, Mercer RW (1998) Isozymes of the Na-K-ATPase: heterogeneity in structure, diversity in function. Am J Physiol 275: F633-650.

7. Jorgensen PL, Andersen JP (1988) Structural basis for E1-E2 conformational transition in Na+,K+-pump and Ca2+-pump proteins. J Memb Biol. 103: 95-120.

8. Mercer RW, Biemesderfer D, Bliss DP, Collins LH, Forbrus B (1993) Molecular cloning and immunological characterization of the gamma- polypeptide, a small protein associated with Na,K-ATPase. J Cell Biol 121: 579-586.

9. Geering K (2008) Functional roles of Na,K-ATPase subunits. Curr Opin Nephrol Hypertens 17: 526-532.

10. Vasilets LA, Schamalzing G, Madefessel WH, Hasse W, Schwarz W (1990) Activation of protein kinase C by phobol ester induces down- regulation of Na+,K+-ATPase in the oocytes of Xenopus laevis. J Mem. Biol 118: 131-142.

11. Chibalin AV, Vasilets LA, Hennekes H, Pralong D, Geering K (1992) Phosphorylation of Na,KATPase Î±1-subunits in microsomes and in homogenates of Xenopus oocytes resulting from the stimulation of Protein Kinase A and Protein Kinase C. J BiolChem 267: 22378-22384.

12. Mohanty BK, Gupta BL (2012) A marked animal-vegetal polarity in the localization of Na+, K+-ATPase in Xenopus oocytes and their progesterone-induced down-regulation. Molecular Reproduction and Development 79: 138-160.

13. De Loof A (1986) The electrical dimensions of cells: the cell as a miniature electrophoresis chamber. Int Rev Cytol 104: 251-352.

14. Horb ME, Thomsen GH (1997) A vegetally localized T-box transcription factor in Xenopus eggs specifies mesoderm and endoderm and is essential for embryonic mesoderm formation. Development 24: 1689-1698.

15. Melton DA (1987) Translocation of a localized maternal mRNA to the vegetal pole of Xenopus oocytes. Nature 328: 80-82.

16. Dalby B, Glover DM (1993) Discrete sequence elements control posterior pole accumulation and translational repression of maternal cyclin B RNA in Drosophila. EMBO J 12: 1219-1227.

17. Ford HLH, Pardee AB (1999) Cancer and the cell cycle. J Cell Biochem Suppl 32-33: 166-172.

18. Luo T, Matsuo-Takasaki M, Thomas ML, Weeks DL, Sargent TD (2002) Transcription factor AP-2 is an essential and direct regulator of epidermal development in Xenopus. Dev Biol 245: 136-144.

19. Mohanty BK, Akpan I, Klymkowsky MW (2001) Sox3 is an essential factor in early Xenopus development. Mol Biol of Cell 12: 237a.

20. Cunncliffe V, Smith JC (1992) Ectopic mesoderm formation in Xenopus embryos caused by widespread expression of Brachyury homologue. Nature 358: 427-430.

21. Ace CI, Okuliecz WC (1995) Differential gene regulation by estrogen and progesterone in the primate endometrium. Mol Cell Endocrin 115: 95-105.

22. Whitehead MI, King RJB, McQueen J, Campbell S (1979) Endometrial histology and biochemistry in chimeric women during oestrogen and oestrogen/progesterone therapy. J R Soc Med 72: 322-327.

23. Jones GS (1991) Luetal phase defect: a review of pathophysiology. Curr Opin Obstet Gynecol 3: 641-648.

24. Wentz AC (1980) Endometrial biopsy in evaluation of infertility. Fertil Steril 33: 121-124.

25. Key TJA, Pike MC (1977) The role of oestrogen and progesterone in the epidermiology and prevention of breast cancer. Eur J Cancer Clin Onco 24: 29-43.

26. Finn CA, Martin L (1970) The role of oestrogen secreted before oestrus in the preparation of the uterus for implantation in the mouse. J Endocrinol 47: 431-438.

27. Finn CA, Porter DG (1975). Handbook in reproductive biology. 1. The Uterus. Elek Science. London.

28. Cohen CJ, Bruckner HW, Deppe G (1984) Multidrug treatment of advanced and recurrent endometrial carcinoma: a gynecologic oncology group study. Obstet Gynecol 63: 719-726.

29. Henderson BE, Ross RK, Pike MC (1993) Hormonal chemoprevention of cancer in women. Science 259: 633-638.

30. Mayahara H, Fujimoto K, Saito T, Ogawa K (1980) A new one-step method for the cytochemical localization of ouabain-sensitive, potassium-dependent p-nitrophenyl phosphatase activity. Histochemistry 67: 125-138.

31. Mohanty BK (2014). Biochemical vs. Immuno, Histo-cytochemical estimation of Na+,K+-ATPase. Sky J of Biochem Res 3: 65-71.

17

Regulation of Expression of Secretory Leukocyte Protease Inhibitor by Progesterone in BeWo Choriocarcinoma Cells

Neelima P. Sidharthan and Addicam Jagannadha Rao*

Department of Biochemistry, Indian Institute of Science, Bangalore, India

Abstract

Secretory leukocyte protease inhibitor is a multifunctional protein with a variety of activities attributed to it. A significant increase in the expression of Secretory leukocyte protease inhibitor was noticed in syncytiotrophoblasts following differentiation of cytotrophoblasts in to syncytiotrophoblasts by addition of Forskolin. Using the BeWo cells which are derived from choriocarcinoma, the effect of addition of progesterone and estradiol on the expression of Secretory leukocyte protease inhibitor by Reverse Transcription Polymerase Chain Reaction was assessed. It was found that while addition of low concentration of progesterone resulted in a significant increase in expression of Secretory leukocyte protease inhibitor, addition of estradiol even at high concentration had no effect. The specificity of effect of progesterone was established by the observation that addition of Progesterone along with progesterone receptor antagonist (RU484) resulted in decrease in the level of expression of Secretory leukocyte protease inhibitor. These results suggest that Secretory protease leukocyte protease inhibitor is a progesterone regulated gene.

Keywords: Progesterone; Estrogen; Regulation; SLPI; BeWo cells.

Introduction

Secretory Leukocyte Protease Inhibitor (SLPI) is a nonglycosylated hydrophobic cationic 12 kDa protein with a variety of activities attributed to it. During our studies on the profiling of genes during differentiation of uni-nucleated cytotrophoblasts (CT) into multinucleated syncytiotrophoblasts (ST) by DDRT-PCR and micro array analysis of RNA from CT and ST we found several fold increase in the expression of SLPI in the ST [1]. It is also known that it exhibits a variety of activities, which includes anti-protease, anti-inflammatory, anti-bacterial activities [2]. SLPI is a highly conserved protein and murine SLPI appears to be structurally highly similar to human SLPI [3]. However, it is reported that while the human SLPI is regulated by progesterone (P4) [4], in the case of rat, it is regulated by estrogen [5]. In view of the apparent differential regulation of SLPI in rodents and human and considering the fact that SLPI structure is highly conserved, it was of interest to investigate the regulation of SLPI by P4 in BeWo cells which is derived from human choriocarcinoma.

Materials and Methods

Cell culture and induction of differentiation in human trophoblastic BeWo cells

BeWo cells (a human choriocarcinoma cell line, generously gifted by Dr. Susan Fisher, University of California, San Francisco, California) were cultured in DMEM/Ham's F-12 medium (Sigma Chemical Co., St. Louis, MO) containing 10 % FCS (Hyclone laboratories Inc., UT) and antibiotics (100 U/ml Penicillin, 50μg/ml Gentamycin and 5 U/ml Nystatin), at 37°C, in an atmosphere of 5% CO_2. For experiments involving induction of differentiation, cells were maintained in serum-free medium as described by Taylor et al. [6], with minor modifications prepared with DMEM/Ham's F-12 medium supplemented with insulin (1μg/ml), transferrin (5 μg/ml), Bovine Serum Albumin (500 μg/ml) and antibiotics (100U/ml penicillin, 50 μg/ml Gentamycin and 5U/ml Nystatin)

The following chemicals Insulin, Transferrin, MEM, Ham's F12 medium; Bovine serum; Albumin were obtained from Sigma chemicals Co., St. Louis, MO, USA. P4 and Estradiol 17β (E2) were obtained from Steraloids Inc, Wilton, NH, USA, ICI 182780 (a pure antiestrogen is a gift from Dr. A.E. Wakeling of Zeneca Pharmaceuticals, UK). RU486 (17α-hydroxy-11β-(4-dimethylamino-phenyl)-17β-(1-propynyl) estra-4, 9-dien-3-one) was obtained from Roussel-Uclaf, Paris, France. Fadrazole (aromatase inhibitor) CGS 16949A was a gift from CIBA Geigy Ltd. Basel, Switzerland.

Hormonal regulation of SLPI expression in BeWo cells

0.5×10^5 cells/ml/well were plated in 6 well multi-dishes and after overnight culture, the cells were incubated in the presence of 1μM of P4 or 2. 5μM of E2 or 1μM RU486 or 1μM of Fadrazole (Aromatse inhibitor) in serum free medium supplemented with insulin, transferrin and BSA. After different duration of incubation i.e, 0, 6, 12, 24h, cells were harvested for RNA isolation using Trizol reagent (Sigma Chemical Co., St. Louis, MO, USA), according to manufacture's instructions. Parallel control experiments were performed with cells incubated with vehicle control (ethanol). MTT assay was carried out to check the viability of the cells before and after the treatment (Data not provided). The integrity of the isolated RNA was checked on a 1% MOPS-HCHO agarose gel and the quantity of RNA estimated spectrophotometrically. RT-PCR was performed as described earlier [7]. The PCR reaction mix contained 0.4 μM of the forward and reverse primers, 200 μM of the dNTP mix, in 10 mM Tris-1 mM MgCl2 buffer and 1 unit of Taq Polymerase [Bangalore Genie, India]. cDNA amplifications used highly specific forward and reverse primers (for SLPI or GAPDH) with an initial heating at 94°C for 3 min, followed by the required number of cycles of 94°C for 1 min, annealing temperature for 1 min and 72°C for 2 min, on a PCR Thermal Cycler (MJ Research Inc., USA). PCR reactions were performed within the linear range of amplificatio

***Corresponding author:** Prof. A. J Rao , Department of Biochemistry, Indian Institute of Science, Bangalore, India,
E-mail: ajrao@biochem.iisc.ernet.in, ajrao2000@yahoo.com

for each amplicon (which ranged from 25-35 cycles) to facilitate quantitation. To ensure accurate quantification, PCR products were assessed by melt curves and also electrophoresed on 2% agarose gels to ensure a single product of the correct size was being amplified. A 12 µl aliquot of the PCR products was electrophoresed on a 1.5% agarose gel and visualized upon staining with ethidium bromide (EtBr). Each figure is representative of three independent experiments. Signal intensities of various bands were determined using the Kodak Electrophoresis and Gel Documentation Analysis System (EDAS-120). The expression levels of specific transcripts were inferred upon normalizing their signal intensities to that of glyceraldehyde 3-phosphate-dehydrogenase (GAPDH), which served as an internal control in this semi-quantitative analysis. Values so obtained were used to determine mean ± S.E. for a graphical representation. 'Significance or *P*-value' was determined using standard statistical test. The authenticity of the RT-PCR products was confirmed by sequencing, following their purification from low-melting agarose gels using the commercially available GFXTM PCR DNA/Gel Band Purification kit (Amersham Pharmacia Biotech., UK). Sequencing was performed at the DNA Sequencing Facility, IISc, using the ABI Prism 377 automated DNA sequencer.

The effect of addition of P4 was also tested at a concentration ranging from 0.01µM to 1µM and a time course study was also carried out. The effect of addition of P4 receptor antagonist RU486 on the expression of SLPI was also monitored. A dose dependent study was carried out using different concentrations of E2 at a concentration of 5, 7.5, and 10µM.

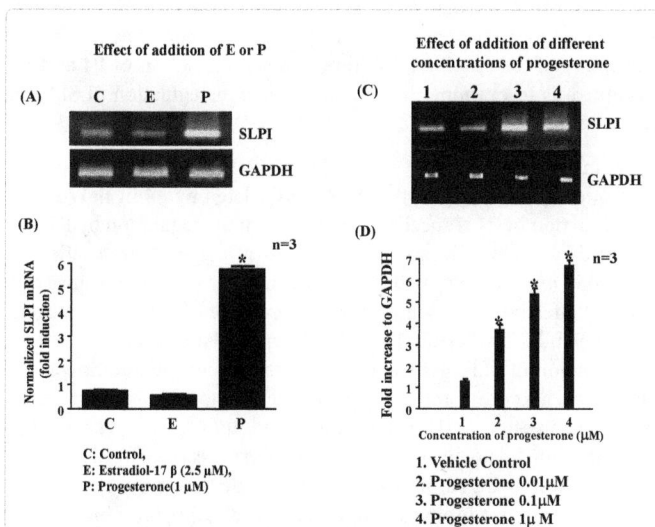

Figure 2: Effect of addition of Progesterone on SLPI expression in BeWo cells. A & B: Time course and C&D: Specificity of progesterone action. A) Cells incubated with or without P4 (1 µM) for 0–24 h. RNA isolated reverse transcribed cDNA was subjected to semi-quantitative PCR in the linear range of amplification with GAPDH as an internal control. B) Graphical representation of results presented in A, (values expressed as fold increase over control mean ± S.E. from three independent experiments). C) RT-PCR analysis for expression of SLPI 1) control, (2) P4 (1µM), (3) RU486 (1µM), (4) P4 + RU486 (both at 1µM) and incubations were carried out for 24 h. RNA was reverse transcribed and cDNA was subjected to semi-quantitative PCR in the linear range of amplification with GAPDH as an internal control. D) Graphical representation of results presented in C (values expressed as fold increase over control; mean ± S.E. from three independent experiments). * Significantly different from group 2 p<0.001.

Results

Regulation of SLPI expression by P4 and E2

Initially the effect of addition of P4 or E2 to BeWo cells on the expression of SLPI after 24h of addition was examined. It can be seen from the results presented in Figure 1 (A&B) that addition of 1µM P4 resulted in a very significant increase in the level of expression of SLPI gene while E2 at 2.5 µM had no effect.

The effect of P4 was also tested at concentrations ranging from 0.01µM to 1µM. It can be seen from the results presented in the Figure 1 (C&D). P4 was effective in stimulating the expression of SLPI gene at all the concentrations tested and even 0.01µM was quite effective in stimulating the expression of SLPI.

A time course study on the effect of incubation of BeWo cells with and without P4 (1 µM) for 0, 6, 12 and 24h on the expression of SLPI was carried out to assess the expression of SLPI by RT-PCR. It can be seen from the results presented in the Figure 2 (A&B) that by as early as 6 h there was a distinct increase in expression of SLPI gene.

The specificity of P4 effect was established by incubating the BeWo cells along with a specific P4 receptor antagonist RU486. It can be seen from the results presented in the Figure 2 (C&D) that incubation of P4 along with RU486 decreased the stimulatory effect of P4 on SLPI gene expression.

Regulation of SLPI gene expression by E2 in BeWo cells

As placenta has high expression of aromatase enzyme, it was essential to rule out the possibility that increase in SLPI expression is not due to conversion of P4 into E2. This was established by addition of Fadrazole (Aromatase inhibitor AI) along with P4 and it can seen from the results presented in Figure 3 (A&B) that incubation of BeWo cells with P4 along with AI also had no effect on the increase in SLPI gene expression as assessed by RT-PCR analysis.

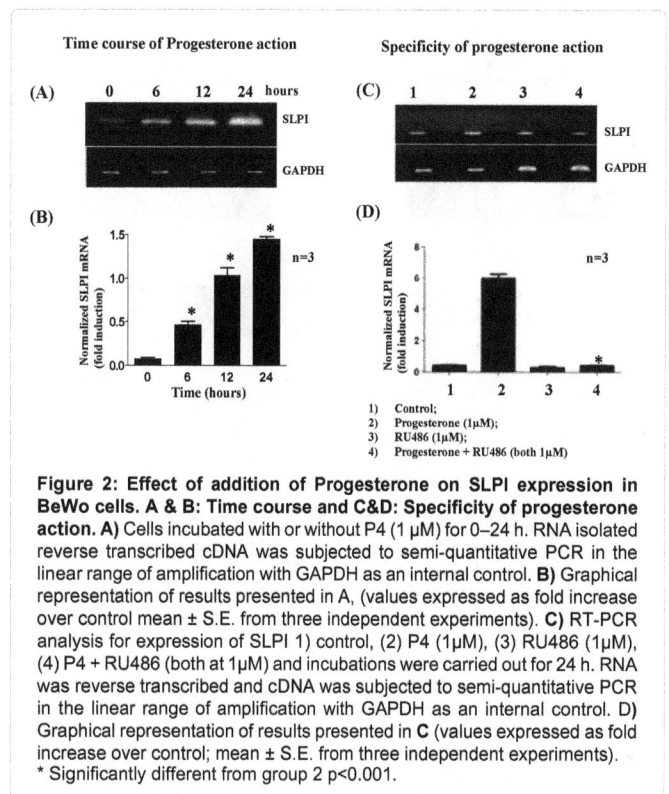

Figure 1: Regulation of expression of SLPI by steroid hormone in BeWo cells. A & B: Effect of addition of E2 or Progesterone and C&D: Different concentrations of progesterone. (A) Cells were incubated with 1 µM P4 or 2.5µM E2 for a period of 12h. RNA isolated was reverse transcribed and cDNA was subjected to semi-quantitative PCR in the linear range of amplification with GAPDH as an internal control. B) Graphical representation of results presented in A, after normalizing to GAPDH used as an internal control (values expressed as fold increase over control mean ± S.E. from three independent experiments). C) Cells were incubated with different concentrations of P4 ranging from 0.01µM to 1µM for 12h. RNA was reverse transcribed and cDNA subjected to semi-quantitative PCR in the linear range of amplification. D) Graphical representation of results presented in C, (values expressed as fold increase over control mean ± S.E. from three independent experiments).
* Significantly different from Control p<0.001.

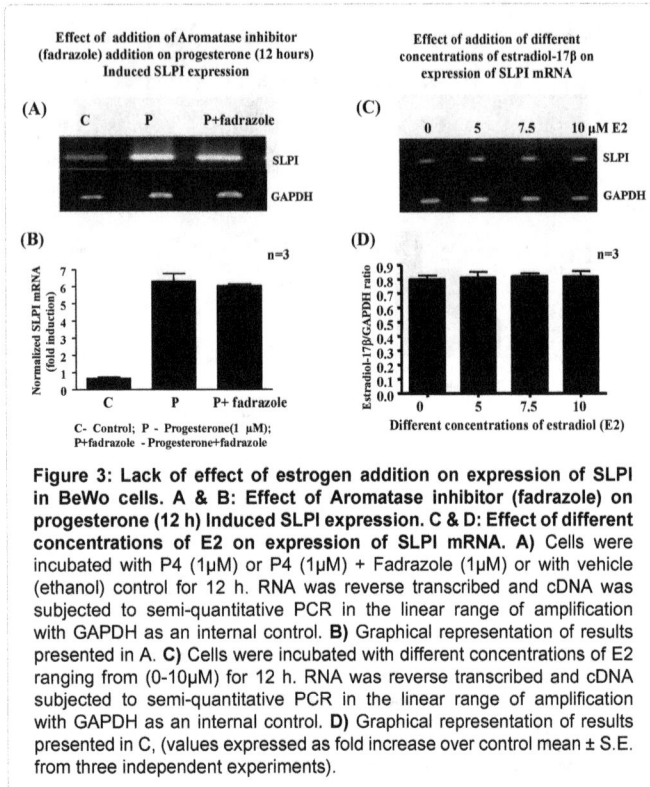

Figure 3: Lack of effect of estrogen addition on expression of SLPI in BeWo cells. A & B: Effect of Aromatase inhibitor (fadrazole) on progesterone (12 h) Induced SLPI expression. C & D: Effect of different concentrations of E2 on expression of SLPI mRNA. A) Cells were incubated with P4 (1µM) or P4 (1µM) + Fadrazole (1µM) or with vehicle (ethanol) control for 12 h. RNA was reverse transcribed and cDNA was subjected to semi-quantitative PCR in the linear range of amplification with GAPDH as an internal control. B) Graphical representation of results presented in A. C) Cells were incubated with different concentrations of E2 ranging from (0-10µM) for 12 h. RNA was reverse transcribed and cDNA subjected to semi-quantitative PCR in the linear range of amplification with GAPDH as an internal control. D) Graphical representation of results presented in C, (values expressed as fold increase over control mean ± S.E. from three independent experiments).

The results of study in which the effect of addition of different concentration of E2 also revealed that even at a very high concentration of 10 µM, E2 had no effect on the expression of SLPI in BeWo cells as assessed by RT-PCR (Figure 3 C&D).

Discussion

Over the years the differentiation of proliferating mononuclear cytotrophoblasts into non-proliferative multi nucleated but highly functional syncytiotrophoblasts has been employed to address several questions related to regulation of growth, stage specific expression of genes as well as cytoskeletal changes that occur during the differentiation process. We have successfully employed both primary cell culture of cells isolated from first trimester and term placenta as well as the BeWo choriocarcinoma cell line to address several questions regarding regulation of telomerase as well as role of E2 in differentiation of CT into ST [1,7,8].

In our attempts to understand the molecular players of trophoblastic differentiation using two approaches of DD-RT-PCR and microarray analysis we found that SLPI is one of the transcripts is highly expressed following differentiation of CT into ST. Before proceeding with DD-RTPCR analysis we have validated the system both at morphological as well as at the functional level. By 72 h, following addition of Forskolin, clear multinucleated syncytia were observed in the treated groups. We have also observed that by 48 h there is a decrease in proliferation markers like PCNA and Cyclins and the appearance of ST specific markers like β hCG and endoglin as assessed by RT-PCR thus validating the system employed [1].

SLPI expression increased during differentiation in a time dependent manner and as the cells differentiated, there was an increase in SLPI starting from 24 h of incubation with Forskolin. It is well known that pregnancy hormones like P4 and E2 control gene expression in

placental cells [8]. It is likely that the anti-protease and anti-microbial actions of SLPI will be involved in key reproductive events such as fertilization, implantation and pregnancy.

P4 is also required for maintenance of the pregnancy by stimulating and maintaining uterine functions, necessary for early embryonic development, implantation, placentation and fetal development. After the luteo-placental shift in steroidogenesis (at around the 7th or 8th week of human gestation), the placenta becomes the principal source for production of P4 and the synthesis in P4 increases rapidly throughout the course of pregnancy.

Cyclical expression of SLPI and elafin, particularly in endometrium, suggests that their expression may also be influenced by steroid hormones such as P4 [9]. There are relatively few studies examining this aspect, although it has been reported that SLPI expression is upregulated by P4 treatment of cervical explants [10]. There is new evidence showing that SLPI is a P4-regulated gene and that the hormone is likely to regulate its expression in female reproductive tract tissues [11]. Serum P4 concentrations are in the nanomolar range during the secretory phase of the menstrual cycle and are in the micromolar range in the feto-placental unit during pregnancy. Considering this it was felt important to check the effect of addition of different concentrations of P4. Furthermore, it has been reported that 90% of P4 is metabolized within 24 h in cell culture experiments [11-13]

SLPI gene is shown to be P4 regulated in Ishikawa endometrial epithelial cells and its presence has been demonstrated in this cell type in humans and non-human primates [11,14]. Velarde et al. [15] have demonstrated that BTEB1 (basic transcription element binding protein-1) as a functional P4 receptor-A and P4 receptor -B interacting partner in the P4 mediated transcriptional activation of SLPI gene in Ishikawa endometrial epithelial cells [15]. These reports as well as the availability of the specific inhibitors to block the action of P4 and E2 prompted us to examine the role of steroids in regulation of SLPI in BeWo cells.

Results of our studies which involved the quantitation of the mRNA, clearly established that SLPI is regulated by P4 in BeWo cells and the action of P4 is specific, as the effect of up-regulation by P4 was inhibited by RU486. The above studies clearly suggest that the effect of P4 on SLPI expression is mediated via the nuclear P4 receptor since this action is effectively antagonized in the presence of the anti-gestogen, RU486. Similar studies on T47D breast epithelial cell line showed an up-regulation of SLPI gene and protein expression on addition of P4 and RU486 and other anti-gestogens were able to inhibit this increase in SLPI expression [11]. In our studies, addition of E2 even at high concentration did not have any effect on the expression of SLPI in BeWo cells. This was again emphasized by the fact that aromatase inhibitors fadrazole could not inhibit the upregulation of expression induced by P4. These studies with BeWo cells as well as studies on non-human primates [14] and the present study using human choriocarcinoma cells clearly demonstrate SLPI is a P4 regulated gene.

Acknowledgement

AJR is thankful to the Department of Science and Technology for the award of Rajarammanna Fellowship. The authors also thank the Indian Institute of Science; the Department of Science and Technology; the Department of Biotechnology, Indian Council of Medical Research, Government of India, and the Mellon Foundation USA, Conrad, USA, Rockefeller Foundation for the financial assistance provided during the course of the work.

References

1. Neelima PS, Rao AJ (2008) Gene expression profiling during Forskolin induced

differentiation of BeWo cells by differential display RT-PCR. Mol Cell Endocrinol 281: 37-46.

2. Zhang Q, Shimoya K, Moriyama A, Yamanaka K, Nakajima A, et al. (2001) Production of secretory leukocyte protease inhibitor by human amniotic membranes and regulation of its concentration in amniotic fluid. Mol Hum Reprod 7: 573–579.

3. Kikuchi T, Abe T, Yaekashiwa M, Tominaga Y, Mitsuhashi H, et al. (2000) Secretory leukoprotease inhibitor augments hepatocyte growth factor production in human lung fibroblasts. Am J Respir Cell Mol Biol 23: 364–370.

4. King AE, Morgan K, Sallenave JM, Kelly RW (2003) Differential regulation of secretory leukocyte protease inhibitor and elafin by progesterone. Biochem Biophys Res Commun 23: 594-599.

5. Chen D, Xu X, Cheon YP, Bagchi MK, Bagchi IC (2004) Estrogen induces expression of secretory leukocyte protease inhibitor in rat uterus. Biol Reprod 71: 508-514.

6. Taylor RN, Newman ED, Chen SA (1991) Forskolin and methotrexate induce an intermediate trophoblast phenotype in cultured human choriocarcinoma cells. Am J Obstet Gynecol 164: 204-210.

7. Rama S, Petrusz P, Rao AJ (2004) Hormonal regulation of human trophoblast differentiation: A possible role for 17-β-estradiol and GnRH. Mol Cell Endocrinol 218: 79-94.

8. Soundararajan R,   Rao AJ (2004) Trophoblast 'pseudo-tumorigenesis': significance and the contributory factors. Reprod Biol Endocrinol 2: 15.

9. King AE, Critchley HO, Kelly RW (2000) Presence of secretory leukocyte protease inhibitor in human endometrium and first trimester decidua suggests an antibacterial protective role. Mol Hum Reprod 6: 191-196.

10. Denison FC, Calder AA, Kelly RW (1999) The action of prostaglandin E2 on the human cervix: stimulation of interleukin 8 and inhibition of secretory leukocyte protease inhibitor. Am J Obstet Gynecol 180: 614-620.

11. King AE, Morgan K, Sallenave JM, Kelly RW (2003) Differential regulation of secretory leukocyte protease inhibitor and elafin by progesterone. Biochem Biophys Res Commun 310: 594-599.

12. Nelson DM, Johnson RD, Smith SD, Anteby EY, Sadovsky Y (1999) Hypoxia limits differentiation and up-regulates expression and activity of prostaglandin H synthase 2 in cultured trophoblast from term human placenta. Am J Obstet Gynecol 180: 896-902.

13. Arici A, Marshburn PB, MacDonald PC, Dombrowski RA (1999) Progesterone metabolism in human endometrial stromal and gland cells in culture. Steroids 64: 530-534.

14. Ace CI, Okulicz WC (2004) Microarray profiling of progesterone-regulated endometrial genes during the rhesus monkey secretory phase. Reprod Biol Endocrinol 2: 54.

15. Velarde MC, Iruthayanathan M, Eason RR, Zhang D, Simmen FA, et al. (2006) Progesterone receptor transactivation of the secretory leukocyte protease inhibitor gene in Ishikawa endometrial epithelial cells involves recruitment of Kruppel-like factor 9/basic transcription element binding protein-1. Endocrinol 147: 1969-1978.

18

The Role of Fulvestrant in the Treatment of Metastatic Breast Cancer

Bánhegyi RJ[1], Laczó I[1*], Fülöp F[2], Mellár E[2] and Pikó B[1]

[1]Oncology Centre, Pandy Kalman Bekes County Hospital, Hungary
[2]Department of Radiology, Pandy Kalman Bekes County Hospital, Hungary

Abstract

Nowadays we cannot find a cancer, in which the targeted therapy based on targeted diagnostics (immunohisto-chemistry, FISH, etc.) would not stand in the centre of the investigations. Breast cancer is not an exception either. Although the optimally performed surgery and the adequately planned radiotherapy are still important elements in the treatment of breast cancer and the achievement of effective local tumor control but their role has essentially changed in the last few years. In the treatment of patient who has been suffering from breast cancer for years either with or without his/her knowledge, the surgery should not be performed as soon as possible but when the patient "benefits" the most from this procedure. If distant metastases are present the removal of the tumor from the breast which means only the tip of the iceberg is absolutely unnecessary or it is required only in special cases. Systemic tumor control can be reached only by medicinal treatment. Regarding these treatments the importance of endocrine therapies (antiestrogens, aromatase inhibitors, LH-RH analogues etc.) traditional and modern chemotherapies (antracyclines, taxanes, platinum and pyrimidine derivatives, eribulin etc.) and the targeted biological therapies (trastuzumab, lapatinib, bevacizumab, olaparib etc.) can be emphasized. The targets of these biological therapies are either extracellular or intracellular molecular targets, such as estrogen receptor (tamoxifen, anastrazole, letrozole, exemestane, fulvestrant etc.) HER2 (trastuzumab, lapatinib, etc.), VEGF (bevacizumab, etc.) PARP (olaparib). It is well-known that due to frequent hormone sensitivity of breast cancer drugs influencing the hormonal effect are very effective. From these the importance of fulvestrant is discussed in our article. Based on literature data fulvestrant proved to be efficient both in locally advanced and metastatic breast cancers even if it was administered not as first (or second) line therapy.

Keywords: Hormone resistance; Fulvestrant; Long-term survival

Introduction

The hormone sensitivity of breast cancer and the idea of hormonal treatment have been known since the end of 19th century. Probably Schnizinger was the first, who suggested in 1889 the surgical removal of ovaries as a treatment in women suffering from breast cancer [1]. Following this in 1895 Beatson performed the first therapeutic bilateral oophorectomy and one year after this procedure reported about regression in locally advanced and metastatic breast cancer [2]. In the years of 1930 Taylor observed that the time to developing metastasis after mastectomy followed by bilateral ovarian irradiation prolonged [3]. These realizations created finally the basis of the hormone therapy of breast cancer. In the years of 1950 the surgical intervention and bilateral ovarian irradiation were routinely used as a part of adjuvant therapy and also in the treatment of metastatic breast cancer [4]. After these artificial castrations which were otherwise irreversible, the next big step in the hormonal therapy of breast cancer was the appearance of the drugs with reversible effects (anti-estrogens, GNRH analogs) in the second half of the 20th century. The anti-estrogen Tamoxifen, which was originally developed as a contraceptive and has residual estrogen effect as well, has been used successfully since 1973 for the treatment of breast cancer and even nowadays this is one of the most frequently ordered anticancer drugs [5]. It is suitable for the treatment of localized as well as metastatic breast cancer, even for chemoprevention [6].

There were great expectations to the efficacy of novel hormonal drugs, so-called "pure" anti-estrogens with no residual estrogen effect at all, appearing in the years of 1990, these expectations proved true to a certain extent. Administration of fulvestrant is indicated if breast cancer was proved to be sensitive for endocrine therapy, i.e. in hormone receptor positive breast cancer (ER: estrogen receptor, PR: progesterone receptor). It can be indicated both in clinically tumor- free status (for adjuvant therapy) and for the treatment of locally – locoregionally advanced and metastatic breast cancer (for palliative therapy considering the summary of product characteristics and the financial regulations). Nowadays there are a lot of drugs available, called slightly inaccurately- hormone medications which are in fact chemically hormone related drugs, but regarding their mechanism of action they can be called as hormone receptor blocking drugs [7]. The adequate individual selection and the optimal administration sequence of these treatments raise a lot of questions among oncologists. However, there is now a broad professional consensus that a significant survival benefit can be observed with the administration of the modern, third generation aromatase inhibitors compared to the former drugs (progestagens and tamoxifen) [8]. Clinical studies supporting these findings were conducted around the turn of the millennium, when there were no data available about such hormone receptor blocking drugs like fulvestrant [9,10].

*Corresponding author: Ibolya Laczó Adress: Oncology Centre, Pandy Kalman Bekes County Hospital, Hungary, E-mail: laczoibolya@freemail.hu

Fulvestrant decreases the effect of the body's own estrogen in several ways. Chemically it is a synthetic 17-beta estradiol analogue which binds to the estrogen receptor with similar affinity as the endogenous estradiol and this binding leads to an increased receptor degradation which results in a decrease of cell division normally induced by the own estradiol in the originally hormone sensitive- cancer cells. Additionally, it inhibits the intracellular signal pathway responsible for the receptor associated cell proliferation which results in anti-tumorigenic effect as well [11]. Fulvestrant is a steroidal anti- estrogen with a selective ER down-regulating (SERD) effect. In fact, it is a targeted drug, the target of which is the estrogen receptor. It is a competitive antagonist of the ER receptor binding to the estrogen receptor with high affinity and completely blocking its functions. Fulvestrant has a „pure anti-estrogen" effect which means it has no agonist, i.e. estrogen like effect on estrogen-receptor [12]. These chemical characteristics explain its high endocrine therapeutic efficacy. Patients responding well for the treatment show typically a long-term remission, probably the above mentioned estrogen receptor degradation effect stand in the background of postponing the resistance development. Its efficacy after tamoxifen resistance was proved by several investigations [11,12]. Administering fulvestrant in second or third line after anti-estrogen therapy proved to be more effective than the other hormone combinations (especially the progestagens), while in clinical studies administered as first line therapy it had equivalent effect than the other drugs (aromatase inhibitors, tamoxifen). The initial positive expectations were not supported by randomized early clinical studies (comparative studies with tamoxifen, anastrozole and exemestane which served as a basis in the registration procedure to certain extent), they confirmed only its equivalence with the above mentioned drugs [13-16]. Searching for its cause finally the (evidently negative) role of under-dosage was proved as a slightly significant survival benefit were observed in certain new clinical trials in which fulvestrant was administered in a monthly dose of 500-1000 mg instead of the previous 250 mg [9,17,18]. Several data refer to that the use of fulvestrant -similarly to other oncotherapies- may offer more benefit for the patients regarding both the progression free and the overall survival, if it was administered differently from current financial Hungarian regulations, i.e. not only in palliative circumstances as salvage therapy but considering the adequate predictive factors - it could be an option in the early treatment which is otherwise permitted by the summary of the product characteristics [19,20].

In Hungary the trade license of the drug was given first on 10. March 2004 and was renewed after 5 years. The active agent fulvestrant can be found only in one hormonal product in Hungary which is indicated according to the currently valid summary of product characteristics for the treatment of postmenopausal women with estrogen receptor positive, locally advanced or metastatic breast cancer for disease relapse during or after adjuvant anti-estrogen therapy, or disease progression on therapy with an anti-estrogen. In contrary to this the prescription availability is much more limited by the Hungarian National Health Insurance Fund: it can be prescribed in locally, locoregionally advanced or metastatic hormone receptor positive breast cancer in case of disease progression (defined as 25% increase in the size of the detected lesions or the development of new lesions) after treatment with tamoxifen and aromatase inhibitor – or aromatase inhibitor if the patient did not receive tamoxifen previously. After the first two week loading dose the drug is administered as 2x250 mg intramuscular injection monthly. The contraindications of its administration are limited to known hypersensitivity to its active agents or components, pregnancy, lactation

and severe hepatic impairment. The most frequent side effects include: increase of liver enzyme levels (ALT, AST, ALP, sometimes GGT), elevation of serum bilirubin, nausea, vomiting, diarrhea, fatigue, headache, backache, hot flashes, skin rashes, allergic reactions, urogenital infections, thrombosis, and pulmonary embolism. The tightened lumen of the needle of pre-filled syringe in which the drug is distributed can provide the prescribed slow administration rate.

When administering fulvestrant arthralgia is reported less frequently compared to the use of aromatase inhibitors, hot flashes occur more often compared to tamoxifen and almost every side effects are less fess frequent than with use of progestagens.

Methods

After reviewing the literature data we searched for a patient in our practice in the treatment of whom the fulvestrant proved to be efficient after a second or third line treatment.

Case Report

In the Oncology Centre of Pandy Kalman Békés County Hospital numerous patients suffering from advanced breast cancer were treated successfully with fulvestrant during the last 8-9 years. In this report the case of an old menopausal woman (J.K.) treated with metastatic breast cancer and also suffering from hypertension will be presented.

The patient is now 66 years old, and she was screened by mammography in March 2010 because of suspicious right breast mass. After the mammography an ultrasound scan of breast and axilla was performed and a core needle breast biopsy was taken from the suspicious mass. Histology found an invasive ductal carcinoma with strong hormone receptor positivity (ER: 90%, PR: 80%), a HER2 immunhistochemistry 1+ (that is negative) status. On the basis of the radiological examinations, in accordance with the physical examination, there was a 4-5 cm large irregular mass in the upper outer quadrant of the right breast and also enlarged nodes were detected in the right axilla. There was no metastasis detected by baseline staging examinations (chest X-ray, abdominal ultrasound scan, whole-body bone scintigraphy) and tumor markers (CEA, CA 15-3) were in normal range.

The patient at that moment was in good performance status (ECOG PS:0) with an appropriate cardiac status (LVEF: 66%) therefore an epirubicine-paclitaxel (EPI-TAX) combination was started as neoadjuvant chemotherapy. After 2 cycles a significant regression was observed both in the primary tumor and the regional metastatic lymph nodes, therefore following a negative PET-CT scan mastectomy with axillary block dissection was performed in May 2010. The histological finding were accordant with the result of the core biopsy: an invasive ductal carcinoma was proved with a diameter of 2.2 cm, strong ER and PR positivity, HER2 negativity, KI-67 was about 20%. 3 out of 8 removed axillary lymph nodes found to be metastatic and in 1 an extension through the capsule could be detected. According to these findings the pathological TNM status was pT2pN1aMx, so regarding the clinically M0 status the breast cancer was classified to IIB (early) stage.

Following this, based on the decision of our multidisciplinary team 3 cycles of epirubicine-cyclophosphamide (EC) and 3 cycles of paclitaxel (TAX) polychemotherapy were administered. Following the chemotherapy adjuvant hormonal therapy (anastrozole) was started and in November and December 2010 postoperative irradiation was performed. After completing the radiotherapy the patient was on continuous anastrozole therapy and came for follow up visits in every 3 months and underwent staging examinations required according to the protocol.

In October 2011, after one year treatment with of anastrozole - hydrothorax was detected on the right side, causing dyspnoea, so following immediate puncture of pleural effusion a chest CT scan was performed which revealed a solitary pulmonary metastasis on the left side (Figure 1). The cytological examination of the pleural fluid supported our suspicion, it referred to pleural involvement. Meanwhile a whole-body bone scintigraphy proved multiple osseous metastases. Considering these findings parenteral ibandronic acid therapy and chemotherapy were started together with administration of low-molecular-weight heparin (LMWH). Between November 2011 and May 2012 the patient received altogether 8 cycles docetaxel and carboplatin (TXT-CBPL) combination as palliative chemotherapy and after a temporary stable disease a progression in the size of the lung metastasis was detected. At the same time the general status of the patient significantly worsened (ECOG PS: 2), anemia developed, due to which red blood cell transfusion was necessary several times. A Jamshidi bone marrow biopsy was already scheduled; however the patient was referred to the emergency department due to acute chest pain, where acute myocardial infarction was diagnosed. After short cardiology rehabilitation, in the middle of June we tried to administer tamoxifen therapy, but the patient did not tolerate it, she complained of insomnia, and therapy was stopped by herself.

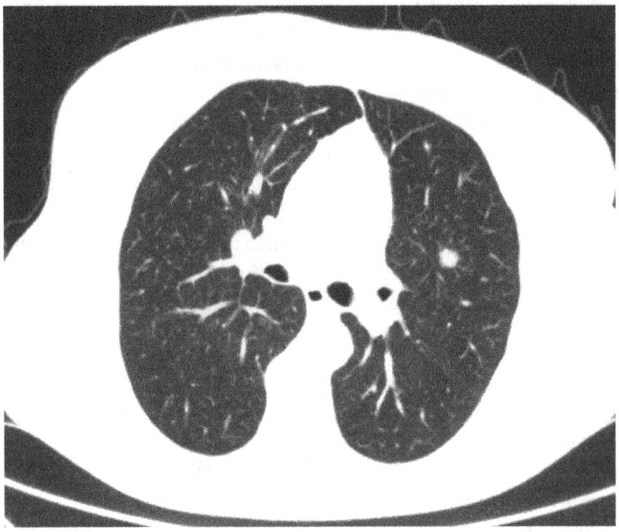

Figure 1: October 2011; solitary left pulmonary metastasis after one-year anastrazole treatment

Based on a new proposal of our multidisciplinary team at the beginning of July 2012 we started fulvestrant therapy. After the first 2- week loading dose the patient has been receiving monthly 2×500 mg fulvestrant injections, the therapy resulted in complete remission regarding the pulmonary metastasis by April 2013 (Figure 2.), bone metastases showed stable status with the previously started bisphosphonate therapy. The patient performance status improved significantly during this period of time (ECOG PS: 1), there is no need for transfusions, and nowadays (February in 2014) she live almost a full-value life, only minimal help is needed for her everyday life.

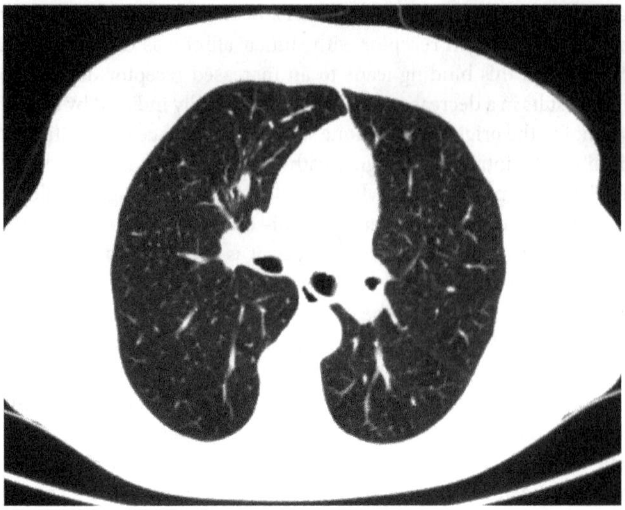

Figure 2: April 2013; Complete remission of the solitary pulmonary metastasis after 10-month fulvestrant treatment

Conclusion

We can conclude that in the complex treatment of strongly hormone dependent (ER positive in at least 50%) and HER2 negative, locally-locoregionally advanced or metastatic breast cancers the endocrine therapy plays a central role in addition to the classic chemotherapies. If the tumor is locally advanced, but there are no distant metastases or there are distant metastases localized mainly to the bones and peripheral lymph nodes, visceral organs or body cavity lymph nodes are not or barely affected, or if the patient performance status is poor and/or the patient has severe co-morbidities or does not agree to receive chemotherapy endocrine therapy can be first choice of treatment. In case of extended visceral involvement with good cardiac and adequate performance status chemotherapy is the preferred first choice; hormonal treatments come into consideration only in second or third line. In our case with the relapse of breast cancer and becoming a metastatic disease we experienced both therapeutic situations. At the beginning, considering the patient's good performance and cardiac status and the pulmonary metastasis, we preferred the chemotherapy then after the patient's status worsened and she suffered a myocardial infarction, the hormonal therapy was preferred. 9 months after the introduction of fulvestrant therapy the staging examinations showed total regression of the pulmonary metastases and a stabile disease of the bone metastases, these results can be regarded as a significant success considering the more and more improving performance status of our patient as well.

References

1. Schinzinger A (1889) Über carcinoma mammae. Verh Dtsch Ges Chir 18: 28-29.

2. Beatson GT (1896) On the treatment of inoperable cases of carcinoma of the mamma: suggestions for a new method of treatment with illustrative cases. Lancet. 11: 104-107.

3. Taylor GW (1934) Artificial menopause in carcinoma of the breast. N Engl. J Med. 211: 1138-1140.

4. Chen WY (2007) Az emlőrák kezelése. In: Chen WY, Wardley A (szerk.): Emlőrák (Dana-Farber Cancer Institute Handbook Series). Lélekben Otthon Kiadó Kft, Budapest: 85-92.

5. Kahán Zs, Bordás P (1996) Emlőrák ma. Springer-Verlag Kiadó, Budapest: 105-131.

6. Bush TL, Helzlsouer KJ (1993) Tamoxifen for the primary prevention of breast cancer: a review and critique of the concept and trial. Epidemiol Rev 15: 233-243.

7. Nagykálnai T (2003) Az emlőrák endokrin kezelése. Springer Tudományos Kiadó, Budapest: 13.

8. Mauri D, Pavlidis N, Polyzos NP, Ioannidis JP (2006) Survival with aromatase inhibitors and inactivators versus standard hormonal therapy in advanced breast cancer: meta-analysis. J Natl Cancer Inst 98: 1285-1291.

9. Di Leo A, Jerusalem G, Petruzelka L, Torres R, Bondarenko IN, et al. (2010) Results of the CONFIRM Phase III trial comparing fulvestrant 250 mg with fulvestrant 500 mg in postmenopausal women with estrogen receptor–positive advanced breast cancer. J Clin Oncol 28: 4594-4600.

10. Howell A, Bergh J (2010) Insights into the place of fulvestrant for the treatment of advanced endocrine responsive breast cancer. J Clin Oncol 28: 4548-4550.

11. Kahán Zs, Horváth Zs (2011) Emlőrák. In: Kásler M (szerk.): Az onkológia alapjai (Egyetemi tankönyv). Medicina Könyvkiadó Zrt, Budapest: 918.

12. Nagykálnai T (2006) Az emlőrák hormonális kezelése. In: Dank M, Demeter J (szerk.): Hatóanyagok, készítmények, terápia. Fókuszban az onkológia és az onkohematológia. Melinda Kiadó, Budapest: 139-158.

13. Howell A, Robertson JF, Quaresma Albano J, Aschermannova A, Mauriac L, et al. (2002) Fulvestrant, formerly ICI 182,780, is as effective as anastrozole in postmenopausal women with advanced breast cancer progressing after prior endocrine treatment. J Clin Oncol 20: 3396-3403.

14. Osborne CK, Pippen J, Jones SE, Parker LM, Ellis M, et al. (2002) Double-blind, randomized trial comparing the efficacy and tolerability of fulvestrant versus anastrozole in postmenopausal women with advanced breast cancer progressing on prior endocrine therapy: Results of a North American trial. J Clin Oncol 20: 3386-3395.

15. Robertson JF, Nicholson RI, Bundred NJ, Anderson E, Rayter Z, et al. (2001) Comparison of the short-term biological effects of 7alpha-[9- (4,4,5,5,5-pentafluoropentylsulfinyl)-nonyl]estra-1,3,5,10)-triene-3,17beta-diol (Faslodex) versus tamoxifen in postmenopausal women with primary breast cancer. Cancer Res 61: 6739-6746.

16. Robertson JF, Osborne CK, Howell A, Jonas SE, Mauriac L, et al. (2003) Fulvestrant versus anastrozole for the treatment of advanced breast carcinoma in postmenopausal women – a prospective combined analysis of two multicenter trials. Cancer 98: 229-238.

17. Kuter I, Hegg R, Singer CF, Badwer R, Lowe E (2008) Fulvestrant 500 mg vs. 250 mg: First results from NEWEST, a randomized, phase II neoadjuvant trial in postmenopausal women with locally advanced, estrogen receptor-positive breast cancer. Breast Cancer Res Treat 109: 585-594.

18. Young OE, Renshaw L, Macaskill EJ, White S, Faratian D, et al. (2008) Effects of fulvestrant 750 mg in premenopausal women with oestrogen- receptor-positive primary breast cancer. Eur J Cancer 44:391-399.

19. Nagy Zs (2010) Emlőrákos betegek kezelése fulvesztranttal – lehetne hatékonyabb? Lege Artis Medicinae 20: 733-736.

20. Pritchard KI, Rolski J, Papai Z, Mauriac L, Cardoso F, et al. (2010) Results of a phase II study comparing three dosing regimens of fulvestrant in postmenopausal women with advanced breast cancer (FINDER2). Breast Cancer Res Treat 123: 453-461.

The Role of Steroids and Hormones in Gynecomastia-Factors and Treatments

Pooja Shree*

Department of Biotechnology, SSIET-Anna University, Chennai, India

Abstract

Gynecomastia is an endocrine disorder where the male breast tissue swells and growth in the size abnormally. All men and women have breast glands; however they're no longer significant in males, because they have a tendency to be small and undeveloped. Drugs which include steroids motive 10%-25% of cases of gynecomastia. They throw off the hormonal stability which increases in estrogen (the female sex hormone) and/or a lower in testosterone (the male sex hormone), which reasons the breast tissue to develop. Almost all reasons of gynecomastia may be in a single manner or different much like excess production of the hormone estrogen inside the male frame because of different factors. In this article, we overview the reasons and treatment of gynecomastia.

Keywords: Estrogen; Gynecomastia; Steroids; Breast tissue

Introduction

Gynecomastia is a benign growth of the male breast tissue. Gynae which means "lady" and mastos means "breast" in Greek. It can be characterized as the nearness of >2 cm of palpable, firm and ductal breast tissue. Before digging profound into the reasons for gynecomastia, let's get straight about what is gynecomastia and what it isn't. Breast enlargement in male caused by inordinate bosom tissue development is authentic gynecomastia. Breast enlargement in men can likewise be caused by fat being developed behind and around the areola and this is to be recognized from pseudogynecomastia or adipomastia or lipomastia. This is to be prominent from pseudogynecomastia, which lacks presence of this sort of disk of tissue, as it is a boom in sub areolar fat without growth of the breast glandular aspect [1-3].

Gynecomastia is found in 60%–90% of newborns and commonly resolves spontaneously within few weeks. Most pubertal young men create gynecomastia, by the age of 14 years 60% of boys have gynecomastia. Beyond the pubertal age, gynecomastia is found in 33%-41% ordinary men matured 25-45 years and in 55%-60% of men over the age of 50 years (Figure 1).

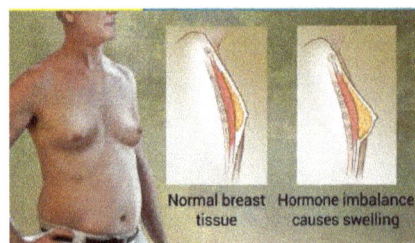

Figure 1: Swollen male breast tissue caused by a hormone imbalance.

Gynecomastia pathophysiology

The imbalance between estrogen actions relative to androgen action at the breast tissue level appears to be the main etiology of gynecomastia.

Depending on the hormonal conditions within the body, any demanding elements, and other issues will determine the rate of progression within the improvement of gynecomastia and the depth and severity of the formation of breast tissue include: The sort of anabolic steroid(s) utilized, measurements of anabolic steroids utilized, span of utilization of the anabolic steroids, and perhaps the most critical persuasive deciding component, personal individual hereditary qualities and responsiveness [4,5].

Steroidal abuse

Steroid clients are one of the sub bunches among men who have gynecomastia. The un-methodical utilization of it is the thing that causes gynecomastia. When a steroid client begins his cycle, the regular hormonal adjust in his body is changed by concealment of the creation of the male hormone testosterone. This triggers a progression of chain response coming full circle in the improvement of gynecomastia.

Not all steroids prompt Gynecomastia, but rather they all have their consequences. Anadrol and Dianabol are large reasons for Gynecomastia, yet there are others. Estrogen goes about as the essential offender in the arrangement and the advancement of gyno where it will append to the Estrogen receptors situated on cells inside breast tissue and signal growth. What comes about is then a continuous improvement of greasy tissue, stringy tissue, and glandular tissue that inevitably after some time will detail full Gynecomastia [6-11].

***Corresponding author:** Pooja Shree, Department of Biotechnology, SSIET-Anna University, Chennai, India, E-mail: Shrithushree@gmail.com

Hormonal imbalance

All individuals regardless own both female sex hormones (estrogens) and male sex hormones (androgens). During pubescence, levels of these hormones may change and ascend at various levels, bringing about a transitory state in which estrogen fixation is tremendously high. Gynecomastia caused by temporary adjustments in hormone tiers with increase usually disappears on its own within six months to 2 years. Occasionally, gynecomastia that develops in pubescence holds on past two years and is called persistent pubertal gynecomastia [12-14].

Low testosterone levels

Illegal testosterone medications utilized for building up can cause breast development in males. Anabolic steroids are manufactured synthetic variants of testosterone. While testosterone treatment can assist enhance your sexual coexistence, muscle mass, vitality, disposition and it could also purpose some transient breast development. This is on account of all men have an enzyme called aromatase that converts testosterone to a shape of estrogen. Taking a medication to hinder the transformation of testosterone to estrogen additionally is certifiably not a smart thought [15-18].

High estrogen levels

The female sex hormone estrogen inside the male may cause the breast development. It may be over abundance estrogen persisted from pubescence, due to a pre-current medical circumstance, as a reaction of medicines or because of drug abuse. Once there is an abundance of estrogen, it sets off a sequence response with the aid of decreasing the generation of testosterone and bringing down digestion. Abundance estrogen will likewise signal the body to hold more fat in the chest and in the belly. When fat is stored in the chest and belly, they emit a catalyst called aromatase that converts testosterone to estrogen. So pectoral fat basically turns into an auxiliary organ that produces estrogen [19-21].

Medical Conditions that Can Cause Gynecomastia

Around 20% of gynecomastia is caused by medications or exogenous chemicals. Drugs and chemicals that cause decreased testosterone levels either by causing direct testicular damage, by blocking testosterone synthesis, or by blocking androgen action can produce gynecomastia. For instance, phenothrin, a chemical component in delousing agents, possessing antiandrogenic activity, has been attributed as the cause of an epidemic of gynaecomastia among Haitian refugees in US detention centers in 1981 and 1982. Chemotherapeutic drugs, such as alkylating agents, cause Leydig cell and germ cell damage, resulting in primary hypogonadism.

One of the traditional examples of a scientific condition that motives gynecomastia is Klinefelter Syndrome. This disorder is described by a chromosomal oddity with men having an extra X chromosome. Studies have demonstrated that men with this medicinal condition have gynecomastia as a typical side effect [22-24].

Hyperthyroidism

The thyroid organ is in charge of the creation of thyroid hormones and hyperthyroidism takes place when this gland turns over-energetic. Hyperthyroidism is sexually unbiased and can happen to the two people yet in men, it is considered as one of the reasons of gynecomastia.

Early recognition of this condition and auspicious intercession has been located to effectively reverse gynecomastia [25,26].

Kidney failure

Kidney failure is one of the medicinal conditions that can cause gynecomastia when our kidneys can't do their ordinary sifting process, it triggers a progression of bodily reactions and hormonal brokenness is one among them. The final product is a concealment of the generation of Testosterone. In this situation, estrogen levels tip the hormonal stability inflicting gynecomastia.

Treatment and Medication

Treatment of Gynecomastia is not constantly important. It relies on its motive, period, and severity and whether it causes agony or uneasiness. Since early stages of gynecomastia happens in puberty stage, normally resolves on its very own without treatment within three years in 90% of cases, no active remedy is needed. But if the breast increases >4 cm in measurement may not be reduced totally. If medicines are the reason for gynecomastia, halting the culpable medication can be effective in decreasing gynecomastia. Treatment of any basic therapeutic conditions is likewise imperative. Both pharmaceuticals and surgical procedures have been effectively used to treat gynecomastia [27-29].

Once gynecomastia is established, testosterone treatment of hypogonadal men with gynecomastia often fails to produce breast regression. Unfortunately, testosterone treatment may actually produce the side effect of gynecomastia by being aromatized to estradiol. Thus, although testosterone is used to treat hypogonadism, its use to specifically counteract gynecomastia is limited. Dihydrotestosterone, a non-aromatizable androgen, has been used in patients with prolonged pubertal gynecomastia with good response rates.

From previous series, the patients with gynecomastia show no significant improvement after the medications. This may be related to the stage of disease at which medical treatment is initiated. It has been suggested that the patient with a long history of gynecomastia, in which the breast tissue becomes fibrotic, tends to be resistant to medical treatment.

Breast surgery

Reduction mammoplasty is taken into consideration for patients with macromastia or long-status gynecomastia or in persons in whom medical therapy has failed. Minimally invasive surgery is available and it may be associated with few complications and prompt recovery.

It is also considered for beauty reasons. The aims of surgery are: (1) to get rid of painful breast tissue. (2) To restore the patient's chest to acceptable beauty form. Complications of surgical procedure consist of removal of tissue because of a compromised blood supply, contour irregularity, hematoma or sarcoma formation, and everlasting numbness inside the nipple-areolar place, doughnut deformity, nipple necrosis, nipple flattening [30].

Liposuction

This surgical procedure removes breast fats, but no longer the breast gland tissue itself. Liposuction/lipoplasty ("fat modeling") is best remedy as it is associated with few sequelae. In this technique, a limited cannula is embedded in breast tissue and used to vacuum fat tissue after that cannula pushed and pulled to break all adipocytes and suctioning them out. This method is known as suction-helped liposuction [31,32].

Mastectomy

The commonly utilized method is subcutaneous mastectomy that includes coordinate resection of the glandular tissue utilizing a peri-areolar or trans-areolar approach, with or without liposuction. Liposuction alone might be adequate if bosom growth is absolutely because of overabundance greasy tissue without considerable glandular hypertrophy. This less invasive sort of surgical operation entails much less recovery time [33].

Selective estrogen receptor modulators (SERMs)

SERMs are tamoxifen and raloxifene can help reduce the amount of breast tissue, even though they are not ready to completely dispense with the issue [34]. Tamoxifen, an estrogen antagonist, is effective for recent-onset and gentle gynecomastia Up to 80% of patients report partial to finish resolution. These medicinal drugs are most often used for excessive or painful gynecomastia With the management of clomiphene, an antiestrogen about 50% of sufferers acquire partial diminishment in breast size, and approximately 20% of patients observe entire resolution. Adverse outcomes are uncommon and consist of visual problems, rashes, and nausea. Other capsules used, albeit less often, includes danazol [35]. Danazol, a synthetic subsidiary of testosterone, inhibits pituitary secretion of LH and follicle- stimulating hormone (FSH), which decreases estrogen synthesis from the testicles [36].

Radiotherapy

Radiation therapy is compelling for counteractive action, and treatment of gynecomastia, caused by androgen ablation in sufferers of prostate tumor. Radiation treatment is more successful if given prophylactically before administration of hormone therapy. However, it has been utilized with some achievement in overseeing painful gynecomastia [37].

Discussion

Gynecomastia associated with medicinal conditions can be counteracted by using appropriate therapeutic interventions or via avoidance of the incriminated agent. When age-associated hormonal fluctuations result in gynecomastia, it isn't avoidable prophylactically [38]. When administering lengthy-time period hormonal remedy to prostate most cancer sufferers, prophylactic irradiation of bilateral breasts can save you subsequent development of gynecomastia [27].

Making intelligent lifestyle choices offers the best option for preventing gynecomastia not associated with an underlying disorder. Various factors have been tied to imbalances in hormones. Body builders should avoid anabolic steroids that disturb hormone production and cause other health problems [39]. Use of marijuana has been connected with increased levels of estrogen. Proper diet and exercise can reduce the risk of pseudogynecomastia, the buildup of fat tissue. Prevention of gynecomastia caused by other therapies or underlying disorders may be possible with medications that reduce the effect those factors have on male and female hormones [40].

Conclusion

Treatments for gynecomastia have now not been drastically studied, No tablets have yet been permitted by using the U.S. Food and Drug Administration for remedy of gynecomastia. Fortunately, in lots of instances, gynecomastia resolves spontaneously without the want for unique remedy. Medical and surgical remedies can be effective for con-tinual gynecomastia. Typically gynecomastia is itself not threatening; however guys with gynecomastia have an improved hazard (approximately five-fold) for growing male breast cancer when as compared with the general population. It is possibly that the hormonal adjustments that produce gynecomastia in male additionally boom their danger of developing breast most cancers. This is a commonly identified entity and consciousness to diagnose and attention to analyze and treat it properly is justified.

References

1. Yordanov YP, Shef A (2017) Acute tissue trauma as a trigger for gynecomastia development and progression. J Trauma Treat 6: 409.

2. Sankaranantham M (2017) Hypogonadism and gynecomastia in 3 adolescent boys on ART- 3. HIV Curr Res 2: 123.

3. Bhattacharya SK (2016) Gynecomastia in a young male. J Mol Imag Dynamic 6: 106.

4. Campos PMR, Rosa BP, Barros AS, Karmali S, Almeida JF, et al. (2017) A rare case of bilateral patellar tendon rupture associated with anabolic androgenic steroids use. Orthop Muscular Syst 6: 238.

5. Nuzzi R, Dallorto L (2017) Efficacy and safety of combined intravitreal bevacizumab and retrobulbar corticosteroids for neovascular age-related macular degeneration. J Clin Exp Ophthalmol 8: 659.

6. Somani S, Meghani S (2016) Substance abuse among youth: a harsh reality. Emerg Med (Los Angel) 6: 330.

7. Giardino PA (2016) Child abuse and neglect: Are cases increasing or decreasing after 50+ years of paediatric attention? Clinics Mother Child Health 13: 235.

8. Linder JM, Silverstone PH (2016) Initial long-term findings from a multimodal treatment program for child sexual abuse victims demonstrate reduction of ptsd frequency and symptoms. J Child Adolesc Behav 4: 297.

9. Ahmadi J (2016) Conduct disorder related to poly substance abuse in adolescence. J Psychiatry 19: 371.

10. Raiker N, Aouthmany M, Ezra N (2016) Dermatologic signs and symptoms of substance abuse. J Clin Exp Dermatol Res 7: 337

11. Carmen M Sarabia-Cobo (2016) Screening and interventions in elderly abuse. Glob J Nurs Forensic Stud 1: e104.

12. Onwubuya EI, Ukibe NR, Kalu OA, Agbo BS, Ukibe SN, et al. (2018) Assessment of the effects of oxidative stress on some reproductive hormones in male hypertensive subjects at nauth, nnewi. J Bioanal Biomed 10: 64-69.

13. Kelleni MT (2017) Diabetogenic drugs and hormones, what every physician should know and be aware of ? Gen Med (Los Angeles) 5: e114.

14. Ginneken VV, Ham L, de Vries E, Verheij E, van der Greef J, et al. (2016) Comparison of hormones, lipoproteins and substrates in blood plasma in a c57bl6 mouse strain after starvation and a high fat diet: A metabolomics approach. Anat Physiol 6: 233.

15. Azad N, Sakla N, Bahn G (2018) The effect of testosterone replacement therapy on glycemic control in hypogonadal men with type 2 diabetes mellitus. J Clin Diabetes 1: 101.

16. Hadlow N, Hamilton K, Joseph J, Millar D, Zentner A, et al. (2017) Relationships between anti-mullerian hormone, testosterone, luteinizing hormone and follicle stimulating hormone in men on testosterone therapy. Clin Med Biochem 3: 128.

17. Ueshiba H (2017) The efficacy of testosterone ointment on insulin resistance in men with metabolic syndrome. J Metabolic Synd 6: 225.

18. Gunnels TA, Bloomer RJ (2014) Increasing circulating testosterone: impact of herbal dietary supplements. J Plant Biochem Physiol 2: 130.

19. Zhang K (2014) Epigenetic reprogramming induced by environmental estrogens. Mol Biol 3: e115.

20. Bazin I, Hassine AIH, Mnif W, Gonzalez C (2013) YES as a tool for detecting estrogenic activity of some food additives compounds: E 104, E 122, E 124, E 132 and E 171. J Ecosys Ecograph 3: 128.

21. Suba Z (2013) Low estrogen exposure and/or defective estrogen signaling induces disturbances in glucose uptake and energy expenditure. J Diabetes Metab 4: 272.

22. https://www.mayoclinic.org/diseases-conditions/gynecomastia/symptoms-causes/syc-20351793

23. https://www.gynecoma.com/gynecomastia-diagnosis-treatment/

24. Väre T, Galassi FM, Niinimäki J, Junno JA (2018) Potential case of gynecomastia in mummified remains of an early modern period northern finnish vicar. Clin Anat 31: 641-644.

25. Arya R, Rathi AK, Singh K, Srivastava A, Panda D, et al. (2016) Gynecomastia: A review of literature. MAMC J Med Sci 2: 69-75.

26. Al Jurayyan NA (2016) Childhood gynecomastia: a mini review. Int J Clin Endocrinol Metab 2: 012-015.

27. Cuhaci N, Burcak Polat S, Evranos B, Ersoy R, Cakir B (2014) Gynecomastia: Clinical evaluation and management. Indian J Endocrinol Metab 18: 150-158.

28. Arvind A, Abbas Khan MA, Srinivasan K, Roberts J (2014) Gynaecomastia correction: A review of our experience. Indian J Plast Surg 47: 56-60.

29. Narula H, Carlson H (2014) Gynaecomastia- pathophysiology, diagnosis and treatment. Nat Rev Endocrinol 10: 684-698.

30. Mangla M, Singla D (2017) Gestational gigantomastia: A systematic review of case reports. J Midlife Health 8: 40-44.

31. Moskovitz MJ, Baxt SA, Jain AK, Hausman RE (2007) Liposuction breast reduction: a prospective trial in african american women. Plast Reconstr Surg 119: 718-726.

32. Bellini E, Grieco MP, Raposio E (2017) A journey through liposuction and liposculture: Review. Ann Med Surg (Lond) 24: 53-60.

33. Lazaraviciute G, Chaturvedi S (2017) Mastectomy-a critical review. J Clin Diagn 7: 58-66.

34. Maximov PY, Lee TM, Jordan VC (2013) The discovery and development of selective estrogen receptor modulators (serms) for clinical practice. Curr Clin Pharmacol 8: 135–155.

35. Goodsell DS (2002) The molecular perspective: tamoxifen and the estrogen receptor. The Oncol 7: 163-164.

36. Dmowski WP (1990) Danazol, a synthetic steroid with diverse biologic

effects. J Reprod Med 35: 69-74.

37. Luh JY, Harmon MW (2010) Radiation therapy for gynecomastia. Mayo Clin Proc 85: 398-399.

38. Johnson RE, Murad HM (2009) Gynecomastia: Pathophysiology, evaluation, and management. Mayo Clin Proc 84: 1010-1015.

39. Sansone A, Romanelli F, Sansone M, Lenzi A, Di Luigi L (2017) Gynecomastia and hormones. Endocrine 55: 37-44

40. Carlson HE (2011)Approach to the patient with gynecomastia. J Clin Endocrinol Metab 96: 15-21.

20

Validation of Reference Genes for qPCR Analysis of Resistance Training and Androgenic Anabolic Steroids on Hypothalamus, Adrenal Gland and Fat Tissue

Renan Pozzi, Leandro Fernandes, Bruno FA Calegare and Vânia D'Almeida*

Department of Psychobiology, Universidade Federal de São Paulo, UNIFESP, São Paulo, Brazil

Abstract

Background: Real-time quantitative Polymerase Chain Reaction (qPCR) is a technique used for quantification of gene expression and the use of reference genes is very important to normalize the quantification results.

Aim: To validate the most suitable reference genes for resistance exercise training (REx) and use of nandrolone decanoate (DECA) in three different rat tissues.

Methods: A total of 40 adult male Wistar rats were distributed into four groups: exposed to vehicle three times per week (wk) (CT); eight wk of REx exposed to vehicle three times per wk (T); exposed to DECA three times per wk (D); eight wk of REx exposed to DECA three times per wk (TD). Stability of the following genes was evaluated: *beta actin (Actb), alpha Tubulin (Tubulin), Glyceraldehyde-3-phosphate dehydrogenase (Gapdh), Hypoxanthine phosphoribosyltransferase-1 (Hprt1)* and *18s Ribossomal RNA (18s)* in hypothalamus, adrenal gland and mesenteric fat tissue using GeNorm, NormFinder and BestKeeper software.

Results: In hypothalamus and adrenal, all genes were suitable and none was rejected by statistical analysis; however, in fat tissue, *Actb, Gapdh* and *Hprt1* genes were rejected by geNorm but not the others two software.

Conclusion: In hypothalamus and adrenal all selected genes analized were stable and can be used for qPCR gene expression analysis. However, in fat tissue we suggest the *Tubulin* gene as most stable gene.

Keywords: qPCR; Endogenous control gene; Resistance training; Androgenic anabolic steroids; Rats

Abbrevations: *18s*: 18s Ribossomal RNA; AAS: Androgenic Anabolic Steroids; *Actb*: Beta Actin; Bp: Base Pair; Cq: Cycle Quantification; CT: Control Group; D: Nandrolone Group; DECA: Nandrolone Decanoate; *Gapdh* Glyceraldehyde-3-phosphate Dehydrogenase Hypoxanthine; *Hprt1*: Phosphoribosyltransferase-1; REx: Exercise Training; qPCR: Real-time Quantitative Polymerase Chain Reaction; T: Training group; TD: Training and Nandrolone Group; *Tubulin*: Alpha Tubulin; Wk: Week

Introduction

Real-time quantitative chain reaction (qPCR) relative or absolute analysis requires appropriated endogenous gene as reference gene for data normalization, which are known by: housekeeping gene, normalization gene, endogenous control gene, internal reference gene and suitable reference genes [1]. The reference gene is used to normalize the target gene expression and, for this reason, the incorrect choice of reference genes can alter final results [1].

Our group has validated reference genes for rat models of sleep deprivation [2] and hypoxia [3]. To our knowledge, there are no studies concerning validation of reference genes to analyze the effects of resistance exercise (REx) and androgenic anabolic steroids (AAS) use on gene expression. A good reference gene must show minimum variation of expression in all experimental groups or, in other words, its expression should not be influenced by experimental conditions. Considering the increasing number of exercise-related and/or anabolic steroids articles, validation of the most stable reference genes for qPCR was considered of interest.

AAS are manipulated compounds derivatives of testosterone, whose main function is to isolate the anabolic effect. They are important for the treatment of growth-related diseases, osteoporosis and anemia; however, when used at supraphysiological doses, they may produce side effects such as water retention, early closing of the bone epiphysis [4], aggressiveness [5,6], irritability, hostility, cognitive symptoms such as distractibility, forgetfulness and confusion, testicular atrophy, changes in the prostate and seminal vesicles, gynecomastia, growth changes [7], development of hepatic cysts [5], cardiovascular events such as myocardial infarction, cerebral infarction and pathological hypertrophy, increasing the likelihood of arrhythmias and stroke [8,9]. Thus, despite the abovementioned risks and being prohibited in many countries, athletes and amateur practitioners use supra physiological dosages of steroids to increase the performance and free fat mass.

Resistance exercise, commonly called weight training, is a type of exercise that has as main objective muscle strength gaining. The authors suggest that REx training is a valid strategy to improve blood pressure, insulin resistance, muscle mass and reduce circulating levels of inflammatory markers [10]. Furthermore, physiological and psychological benefits of REx are considered important in physical rehabilitation and treatment programs [11]. Therefore, a number of gene expression and molecular biological studies has been conducted in Rex training and steroids models, including ladder exercise models [12-15]. There is a methodological gap, in which there is a lack of studies that identify the best reference gene in these areas of knowledge.

Corresponding author: Vânia D'Almeida, Department of Psychobiology, Universidade Federal de São Paulo. Street Botucatu, 862-1st floor-Vila Clementino, São Paulo-SP-CEP: 04023062. Brazil, E-mail: vaniadalmeida@uol.com.br

It is known that there is no universal reference gene although *Actb*, *Gapdh*, *Hprt1* and *β2M*, among others are the most commonly used [16]. There are no studies regarding reference genes in this area; therefore, the aim of this study was to validate reference genes for REx and AAS use in rat hypothalamus, adrenal gland and mesenteric fat tissue.

Materials and Methods

Animals

The study was performed using 40 male Wistar rats (10-wk-old; 300-350 g) from CEDEME (Centro de Desenvolvimento de Modelos Experimentais para Medicina e Biologia). Animals were maintained in the Department of Psychobiology facility (Universidade Federal de São Paulo). Room temperature was 22°C (± 1) with 12:12 h light-dark cycle and access to food and water *ad libitum* was allowed. This study was conducted according to the Ethical of the use of Laboratory Animals Guidelines and its experimental protocol was approved by the Ethical Committee of Universidade Federal de São Paulo (#177700/2013).

Groups

A total of 40 Wistar rats (10 wk old) was distributed into four groups: exposed to vehicle (peanut oil-subcutaneous administration 1 ml/kg) 3 times/wk during 8 wk (CT); resistance exercise during 8wk and exposed to vehicle (peanut oil-subcutaneous administration 1 mL/kg) 3x/wk during 8 wk (T); exposed to DECA (subcutaneous administration 5 mg/kg) 3 times/wk during 8 wk (D); submitted to resistance exercise during 8 wk and exposed to DECA (subcutaneous administration 5 mg/kg) 3 times/wk during 8 wk (TD).

Exercise training and drug treatment

The training protocol consisted of progressive REx, 5 times/wk during 8 wk [adapted from 17-19]. A vertical ladder (110 cm high by 18 cm wide, inclined at 80° with 2 cm spacing between rungs) was used; at the top of the ladder there was a dark box (20 cm × 20 cm ×20 cm), where the animal could rest between sets (1 min). Every week, the maximum carrying loading (MCL) was tested, so that the periodization could be determined (Table 1).

Supraphysiological nandrolone decanoate doses (5 mg/kg) were injected subcutaneously to each animal 3 times/wk for 8 wk (15 mg/kg/wk). This dosage was chosen for being equivalent to that used by athletes in physical exercise [20,21]. The peanut oil was used as vehicle at the same volume of DECA (1 ml/kg).

Gene selection

Exercise training and androgenic anabolic steroids affect several systems at cellular level; thus, candidate reference genes were selected among the most common reference genes from animal models in the literature. Reference genes selected were *beta actin (Actb)*, *alpha Tubulin (Tubulin)*, *glyceraldehyde-3-phosphate dehydrogenase (Gapdh)* *hypoxanthine phosphoribosyltransferase-1 (Hprt1)* and *18s ribossomal RNA (18s)*. Primers (Table 2) were designed and synthesized by IDT (Integrated DNA Technologies - www.idtdna.com) according to published Genbank sequences.

RNA extraction, cDNA and qPCR

After 24 h of experimental issue, the animals were euthanized by decapitation between 07:00 am to 10:00 am. Fasting for at least 2 hours was established.

The hypothalamus and adrenal gland were collected and RNA extraction was performed using TRizol⁺ Plus RNA Puification Kit (CAT#12183-555 Ambion RNA, Life Technologies). Mesenteric fat tissue was also collected and total RNA was extracted using the RNeasy Plus Universal Mini Kit (CAT#73404, QIAGEN), according to manufacturer's specifications. RNA was pretreated with DNAse I (2 U/μl), 10X DNase I Buffer (100 mM Tris- pH 7.5, 25 mM MgCl$_2$, 5 mM CaCl$_2$) and incubated for 37°C for 30 sec (Invitrogen) according to manufacturer's specifications. The 28S and *18s* integrity of RNA was evaluated using agarose gel electrophoresis. RNA quantification was performed using spectrophotometry (NanoDrop) and purity was evaluated using two optimal wavelengths: ratio of 260/280 for nucleic acids (1.8<sample>2.2) and ratio of 260/230 for organics contaminations (1.8<sample>2.2).

cDNAs were synthesized using 1 μg of total RNA were placed in the presence of first mixture containing 0.5 μg/μl of Random Primers (Promega) and 3 mM of MgCl$_2$ (Promega), after that incubated at 70°C for 5 minutes. Then were placed in second mixture using Reaction Buffer 5X (Promega), 25 mM of deoxyribonucleotide triphosphates (dNTP), 40 U/μl of RNase inhibitor (RNAsin) (Promega) and enzyme Improm II (Reverse Transcriptase) (Promega). The final volume was 20 μl. The conditions used for reverse transcription were as follows: 25°C for 5 min, 42°C for 60 min and 70°C for 15 min, according to manufacturer's specifications.

qPCR was performed using SYBR Green PCR Master Mix (AppliedBiosystem, Warrington, UK) and StepOnePlus Real-Time PCR (AppliedBiosystem, Warrington, UK). Each reaction was performed using 2 μl of cDNA, 6 μl of H$_2$O, 2 μl of primers (forward and reverse at 0.5 μM each) and 10 μl SYBR green PCR Master Mix to the final volume of 20 μl. All samples were analyzed in duplicates and the average values were used. Design layout was: Holding stage: 3 min at 50°C and 10 min at 95°C; Cycling stage (no of cycles: 40): 15 sec at 95°C and 30 sec at 60°C. Melt curve stage: 15 sec at 95°C and 60° up 3°C each 15 sec to 95°C.

Data analysis

GeNorm, NormFinder and BestKeeper: Three software were used to assess the stability of selected reference genes by different methods. All software are freely available to download permanently or as a demo for free for 14 days: geNorm (https://www.biogazelle.com/qbaseplus); NormFinder (http://moma.dk/normfinder-software); and

BestKeeper		(http://www.gene-quantification.de/bestkeeper. html#download).

The software geNorm uses the M-value as a stability variable, directly assessing linear scale expression quantities by using the standard curve and absolute quantification. The gene with the lower value of M

Sessions/wk	1 wk	2 wk	3 wk	4 wk*	5 wk*	6 wk*	7 wk*#	8 wk*¥
1st Session	50	50	50	50	50	50	50	75
2nd Session	50	50	50	50	50	50	75	75
3rd Session	50	75	75	75	75	75	75	75
4th Session	75	75	75	75	75	75	75	75
5th Session	75	75	75	75	90	90	90	90
6th Session	75	75	90	90	90	90	90	90
7th Session		90	90	90	100	100	100	100
8th Session				100	100	100	100	100

3rd day of training, all session were done using 50% of MCL. # 4th day, day-off. ¥ 4th day, all session was done using 75% of MCL. MCL (Maximum Carrying Loading).

Table 1: Resistance training periodization in % of MCL.

Gene	ID GeneBank	Forward (5' – 3')	Reverse (5' – 3')	Bp	Efficiency*	T°C	Primer [ ]
Beta Actin	NM_031144.3	GTGTGGATTGGTGGCTCTATC	CAGTCCGCCTAGAAGCATTT	122	Hyphotalamus: 97.8% Adrenal Gland: 100.7% Fat Tissue: 97.4%	60°C	I: 10 µM F: 0.5 µM
Alpha Tubulin	NM_022298.1	GACCTGGAACCCACAGTTATT	ATCTTCCTTGCCTGTGATGAG	90	Hyphotalamus: 97.3% Adrenal Gland: 100.8% Fat Tissue: 98.8%	60°C	I: 10 µM F: 0.5 µM
Gapdh	NM_017008.4	CATGGCCTTCCGTGTTCCTA	GCGGCATGTCAGATCCA	55	Hyphotalamus: 103.6% Adrenal Gland: 102.6% Fat Tissue: 101.6%	60°C	I: 10 µM F: 0.5 µM
Hprt1	NM_012583	GCGAAAGTGGAAAAGCCAAGT	GCCACATCAACAGGACTCTTGTAG	76	Hyphotalamus: 98.7% Adrenal Gland: 98.0% Fat Tissue: 99.0%	60°C*	I: 10 µM F: 0.5 µM
18s	NR_046237	CGGACAGGATTGACAGATTG	CAAATCGCTCCACCAACTAA1	83	Hyphotalamus: 99.5% Adrenal Gland: 94.0% Fat Tissue: 97.8%	60°C	I: 10 µM F: 0.5 µM

Bp: Base pair; T°C: Temperature; Primer [ ]: Primer concentration in initial and final volume; I: Initial; F: Final. *In fat tissue, was the addition of stretch of 30 sec at 72°C for cycle. *r²>99 was established. The amplification efficiency is calculated using the slope of the regression line in the standard curve.

Table 2: Reference genes ID and primers design.

is considered the "most stable". NormFinder also uses the values from absolute quantification to calculate stability, which indicates as Stability value the best candidate by the lower value. BestKeeper uses the HKG index which calculates the geometric average of the „most stable" reference genes by Repeated Pair-wise Correlation Analysis and p-value (p<0.05). GeNorm and Normfinder use $2^{-\Delta Ct}$ and the BestKeeper uses Cq values for analysis.

Results

Cycle quantification (Cq) distribution

The results related to fractional qPCR cycles are represented as follow: 1) Hypothalamus (Figure 1)-*Gapdh* showed the lowest standard deviation (± 0.69), followed by *Actb* (± 1.27), *Hprt1* (± 1.35), *Tubulin* (± 1.69) and *18s* (± 2.05); 2) Adrenal gland (Figure 2)-results showed that *Hprt1* had the lowest standard deviation (± 0.96) followed by *Gapdh* (± 1.25), *Actb* (± 1.33), *Tubulin* (± 1.87) and *18s* (± 1.92); 3) Fat tissue (Figure 3), *Gapdh* showed the lowest variation Cqs (± 1.52), followed by *Hprt1* (± 1.65), *Tubulin* (± 2.26), *18s* (± 2.48) and *Actb* (± 2.83).

BestKeeper analysis

In hypothalamus, when comparing all experiments groups, CT *vs.* D, CT *vs.* D or CT *vs.* TD the most stable gene was *18s* gene followed by *Actb, Tubulin, Hprt1* and *Gapdh* genes.

For adrenal gland, *18s* gene was the most stable when analyzing all groups, CT *vs.* D, and CT *vs.* T *vs.* D groups and the less stable was *Hprt1*. Rank sequence are available in Table 3.

In fat tissue when all groups were compared, as well as CT *vs.* T, the most stable gene was *Tubulin* followed by *Actb, 18s, Hprt1* and *Gapdh*. However, when CT *vs.* D and CT *vs.* TD were compared *Tubulin* remains the most stable gene and *Hprt1* was rejected (Table 3).

Normfinder analysis

Analysis in Normfinder software showed that all genes in all groups were suitable, in other words, all genes showed stability values less than 0.15 [22], value considered by software. Moreover, this software showed best combination and stability value of two genes, e.g. in hypothalamus when compared all groups the best combination stability were *Actb* and *18s* wih 0.02 M-value. The other values are presented in Table 4.

In hypothalamic tissue, the *Actb* gene was the most stable gene when compared all groups and CT *vs.* D groups. Moreover, when comparing

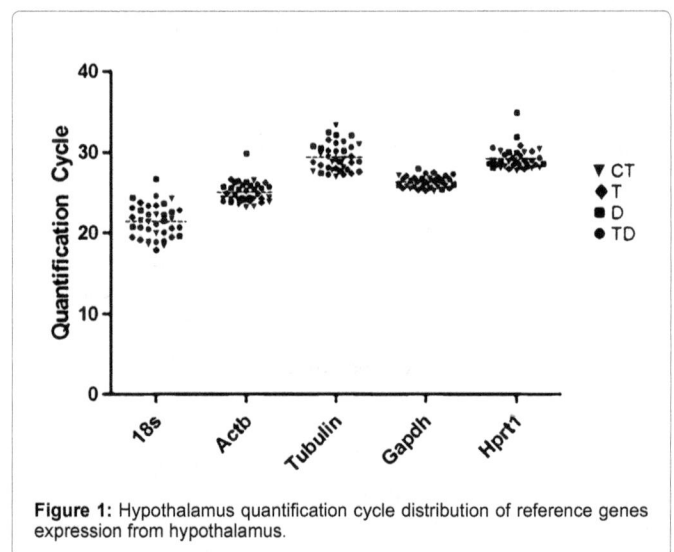

Figure 1: Hypothalamus quantification cycle distribution of reference genes expression from hypothalamus.

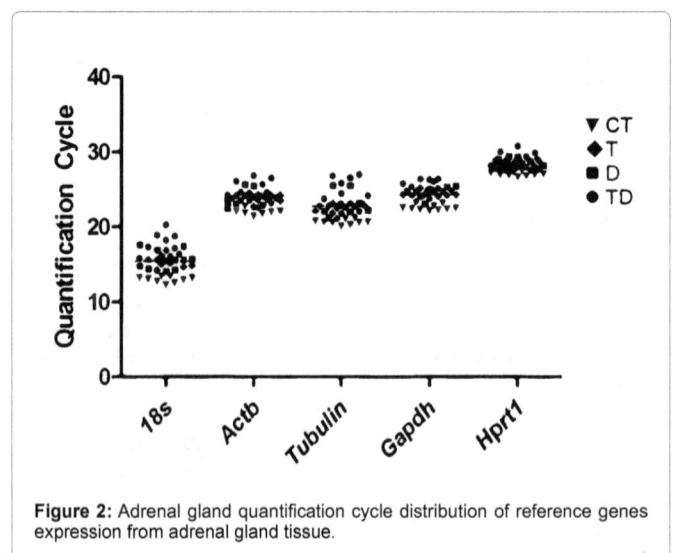

Figure 2: Adrenal gland quantification cycle distribution of reference genes expression from adrenal gland tissue.

CT *vs.* T and CT *vs.* TD groups, the *Hprt1* gene was considered the most stable gene. When all groups were analyzed the following rank was obtained: *Actb, 18s, Hprt1, Tubulin* and *Gapdh* genes. When comparing CT *vs.* D groups, *Actb*, followed by *18s*, *Tubulin*, *Hprt1* and *Gapdh* genes. At CT *vs.* T and CT *vs.* TD groups, *Hprt1*, followed by *18s*, *Tubulin*, *Gapdh* and *Actb* genes.

At adrenal gland, the ranks considering all groups and CT *vs.* TD groups were: *18s*, followed by *Tubulin*, *Gapdh*, *Actb* and *Hprt1* genes; for the CT *vs.* T groups: *Tubulin*, followed by *Actb*, *18s*, *Gapdh* and *Hprt1* genes; and for the CT *vs.* D groups: *Tubulin*, followed by *18s*, *Gapdh*, *Hprt1* and *Actb* genes.

The *Tubulin* gene was considered the most stable gene for fat tissue in all moments and *Gapdh* was the less stable gene, except in CT *vs.* D the *Hprt1* gene was the less suitable gene (Table 4).

GeNorm analysis

Analysis made by software showed that in hypothalamus and adrenal gland all candidates are stable and could be used as reference genes but in mesenteric fat tissue, only *Tubulin* gene was stable in all analysis. The others genes (*Hprt1*, *Actb*, *18s* and *Gapdh* genes) had a 1.5 M-value and it , was not considered good reference genes at least one time.

In hypothalamus the most stable gene was *Actb* when comparing

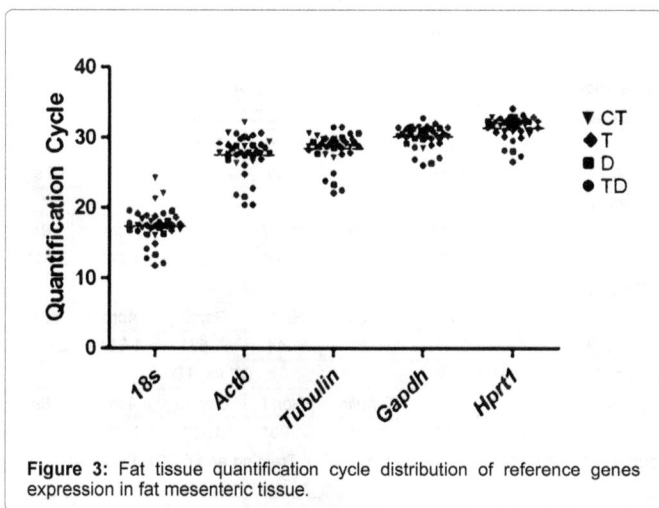

Figure 3: Fat tissue quantification cycle distribution of reference genes expression in fat mesenteric tissue.

all groups, CT *vs.* D and CT *vs.* TD groups, followed by *Hprt1*, *Tubulin*, *Gapdh* and *18s* genes; and for the CT *vs.* T groups: *Actb*, followed by *Hprt1*, *Gapdh*, *Tubulin* and *18s* genes.

In adrenal gland, it was observed that the *Hprt1* gene had the lower rank in all analysis. In all groups and CT *vs.* TD groups the *Actb* gene had the higher rank, following by *Gapdh*, *Tubulin*, *18s* and *Hprt1* genes. For the CT *vs.* T groups, *Gapdh* was the most stable gene, followed by *Actb*, *Tubulin*, *18s* and *Hprt1* genes; and for the CT *vs.* D, *Gapdh* was most suitable gene followed by *Actb*, *18s*, *Tubulin* and *Hprt1* genes.

Considering the mesenteric fat tissue the unique stable gene was the *Tubulin* in all analyzes. *Hprt1* was stable when all groups and CT *vs.* T were compared. The other genes exceeded the M-value allowed by the software (Table 5).

Discussion

To determination of relative expression of target gene in any assay there is a necessity of use a reference gene. Accordingly, the reference gene is usually an endogenous gene in which expression is unchanged regardless of intervention [23]. The use of reference genes is appropriated only if they are tested, normalized and considered stable, some authors believe that it is wrong any gene as reference gene without validating their suitability before running the experiment [24]. In this study, this amount of genes gives us an overview of what can be used in the experiments using AAS and REx.

A simple way to find the most stable reference gene is to analyze the Cq variation and use the one with the lowest variation between experimental groups [25]. However, there are specific software for this type of analysis; the most used in the literature are BestKeeper, Normfinder and geNorm [24]. To our knowledge, there are no studies investigating the most stable genes regarding exercise and anabolic steroids use; therefore, our study will contribute to a more adequate choice of reference genes for those experiments. We separate the analysis group to group to have a more complete analysis, so analyze all groups and then each separate factor, so there is an interpretation according to each intervention.

The analysis of more than one reference gene has been shown to be useful to validate the data, as well as to confirm the results. The authors suggest the use of three reference genes; if the results with the first

Tissue		Hypothalamus					Adrenal gland					Mesenteric fat			
Groups		CT, D, T and TD					CT, D, T and TD					CT, D, T and TD			
Gene	18s	Actb	Tubulin	Hprt1	Gapdh	18s	Tubulin	Actb	Gapdh	Hprt1	Tubulin	Actb	18s	Hprt1	Gapdh
r	0.96	0.93	0.91	0.89	0.77	0.98	0.97	0.96	0.95	0.86	0.98	0.95	0.89	0.86	0.82
p-value	0.001	0.001	0.001	0.001	0.001	0.001	0.001	0.001	0.001	0.001	0.001	0.001	0.001	0.001	0.001
Groups		CT vs. T					CT vs. T					CT vs. T			
Gene	18s	Actb	Tubulin	Hprt1	Gapdh	18s	Gapdh	Tubulin	Actb	Hprt1	Tubulin	Actb	18s	Hprt1	Gapdh
r	0.94	0.91	0.88	0.88	0.68	0.98	0.98	0.96	0.95	0.87	0.96	0.92	0.85	0.78	0.64
p-value	0.001	0.001	0.001	0.001	0.001	0.001	0.001	0.001	0.001	0.001	0.001	0.001	0.001	0.001	0.002
Groups		CT vs. D					CT vs. D					CT vs. D			
Gene	18s	Actb	Tubulin	Hprt1	Gapdh	18s	Tubulin	Gapdh	Actb	Hprt1	Tubulin	Actb	18s	Gapdh	Hprt1
r	0.98	0.96	0.92	0.90	0.85	0.98	0.96	0.95	0.95	0.81	0.92	0.88	0.87	0.57	0.234
p-value	0.001	0.001	0.001	0.001	0.001	0.001	0.001	0.001	0.001	0.001	0.001	0.001	0.001	0.008	0.321
Groups		CT vs. TD					CT vs. TD					CT vs. TD			
Gene	18s	Tubulin	Actb	Hprt1	Gapdh	18s	Tubulin	Actb	Gapdh	Hprt1	Tubulin	Actb	18s	Gapdh	Hprt1*
r	0.96	0.96	0.88	0.87	0.79	0.99	0.98	0.97	0.96	0.94	0.97	0.96	0.92	0.73	0.025
p-value	0.001	0.001	0.001	0.001	0.001	0.001	0.001	0.001	0.001	0.001	0.001	0.001	0.001	0.00	0.922

Data expressed as Pair-Wise Analysis Correlation (r). Higher r correlation indicates the most stable gene. p<0.05 was used in Pearson Correlation. CT: Control Group; D: DECA Group; T: Training Group; TD: Training and DECA Exposed Group. *Result above the limit considered adequate by software analysis.

Table 3: Ranking of reference genes by Bestkeeper software analysis.

Tissue	Hypothalamus					Adrenal gland					Mesenteric fat				
Groups	CT, D, T and TD					CT, D, T and TD					CT, D, T and TD				
Genes	Actb	18s	Hprt1	Tubulin	Gapdh	18s	Tubulin	Gapdh	Actb	Hprt1	Tubulin	18s	Hprt1	Actb	Gapdh
Stability Value	0.04	0.04	0.05	0.05	0.06	0.03	0.03	0.05	0.05	0.06	0.00	0.02	0.02	0.02	0,02
Best Comb.					Actb and 18s					Tubulin and 18s					18s and Tubulin
Stability value for best combination					0.02					0.03					0.01
Groups	CT vs. T					CT vs. T					CT vs. T				
Genes	Hprt1	18s	Tubulin	Gapdh	Actb	Tubulin	Actb	18s	Gapdh	Hprt1	Tubulin	Actb	Hprt1	18s	Gapdh
Stability Value	0.05	0.07	0.07	0.08	0.08	0.04	0.05	0.05	0.06	0.08	0.00	0.00	0.00	0.01	0.01
Best Comb.					Hprt1 and Gapdh					Actb and 18s					Actb and Tubulin
Stability value for best combination					0.05					0.03					0.00
Groups	CT vs. D					CT vs. D					CT vs. D				
Genes	Actb	18s	Tubulin	Hprt1	Gapdh	Tubulin	18s	Gapdh	Hprt1	Actb	Tubulin	Actb	Gapdh	18s	Hprt1
Stability Value	0.01	0.03	0.04	0.05	0.05	0.03	0.03	0.05	0.05	0.06	0.00	0.01	0.01	0.01	0.01
Best Comb.					Actb and 18s					Tubulin and 18s					Actb and Tubulin
Stability value for best combination					0.02					0.03					0.00
Groups	CT vs. TD					CT vs. TD					CT vs. TD				
Genes	Hprt1	18s	Tubulin	Gapdh	Actb	18s	Tubulin	Gapdh	Actb	Hprt1	Hprt1	18s	Tubulin	Actb	Gapdh
Stability Value	0.06	0.06	0.07	0.07	0.07	0.03	0.04	0.06	0.06	0.06	0.00	0.00	0.01	0.01	0.03
Best Comb.					Hprt1 and 18s					Tubulin and 18s					18s and Hprt1
Stability value for best combination					0.04					0.03					0.00

Data expressed as Stability value. Lowest Stability value indicates most stable gene. Best Comb. (Best combination of two genes); CT: Control Group; D: DECA group; T: Training Group; TD: Training and DECA Exposed Group.

Table 4: Ranking of reference genes by the NormFinder software analysis.

Tissue	Hypothalamus					Adrenal gland					Mesenteric fat				
Groups	CT, D, T and TD					CT, D, T and TD					CT, D, T and TD				
Genes	Actb	Hprt1	Tubulin	Gapdh	18s	Actb	Gapdh	Tubulin	18s	Hprt1	Tubulin	Hprt1	Gapdh	Actb	18s
M-Value	0.95	1.02	1.14	1.23	1.26	0.75	0.77	0.87	0.88	0.99	1.21	1.39	1.50*	1.63*	1.79*
Groups	CT vs. T					CT vs. T					CT vs. T				
Genes	Actb	Hprt1	Gapdh	Tubulin	18s	Gapdh	Tubulin	Actb	18s	Hprt1	Tubulin	Hprt1	Gapdh	Actb	18s
M-Value	0.93	0.94	1.14	1.22	1.35	0.43	0.49	0.50	0.63	0.69	1.32	1.50*	1.69*	1.79*	2.01*
Groups	CT vs. D					CT vs. D					CT vs. D				
Genes	Actb	Tubulin	Hprt1	18s	Gapdh	Gapdh	Actb	Tubulin	18s	Hprt1	Tubulin	Hprt1	Gapdh	Actb	18s
M-Value	0.96	1.14	1.14	1.16	1.36	0.66	0.69	0.78	0.79	0.94	1.25	1.44	1.57*	1.63*	2.03*
Groups	CT vs. TD					CT vs. TD					CT vs. TD				
Genes	Actb	Hprt1	Tubulin	Gapdh	18s	Actb	Gapdh	Tubulin	18s	Hprt1	Tubulin	Hprt1	Gapdh	Actb	18s
M-Value	0.92	0.95	1.01	1.04	1.21	0.84	0.89	0.95	1.02	1.10	1.34	1.60*	1.72*	1.77*	2.07*

Data expressed as M-Value. Lowest M-value indicates most stable gene. CT: Control Group; D: DECA Group; T: Training Group; TD: Training and DECA Exposed Group. *Result above the limit considered adequate by software analysis.

Table 5: Ranking of reference genes by GeNorm software analysis.

two are different, a third reference gene must be used, and, if they are similar, it is not necessary to evaluate a third gene [26]. Dheda et al. [27] demonstrated after three experiments with different reference genes that the results can be significantly different from those obtained when an invalidated reference gene is used. This incorrect choice, therefore, results may be erroneous. The same authors also suggest strongly supporting the argument for validation of reference genes prior to their use.

We conducted a search in PubMed and selected 20 articles that investigated the effects of physical exercise and/or androgenic anabolic steroids on gene expression, through qPCR (SYBR Green method), in order to verify if there were common reference genes in these studies. Two groups used only the 18s gene [13,28], five used only Actb gene [29-33]. Other authors used the Cyclophilin gene [15,31] and eight authors used Gapdh as a reference gene in their studies [12,14,34-40]. Only three studies used more than one gene as internal control: Gapdh and large ribosomal protein P0 (RPLP0) genes [41]; Gapdh, Actb, Hprt1 and Cyclophilin gene [42]; the other authors used Ubiquitin C gene as reference gene [43]. Considering the abovementioned articles, the most used reference genes were Gapdh and Actb in different species as human, monkey, rat, and mouse.

The results of the reference gene is controversial, some authors did not find stable results for Actb and Gapdh genes in injured muscle, the results were rejected by geNorm and BestKeeper [44]. In other study, also did not find stable results for Actb gene from hypothalamus of an obesity rat model [45]. Actb and Gapdh genes were rejected in muscle tissue by qBase, software that uses M-Value to analyze reference genes [26]. In our study, Actb and Gapdh genes were shown to be stable in all tissues analyzed by three different software; the only exception was for mesenteric fat analysis through geNorm, which rejected both genes, along with Hprt1.

In hypothalamus and adrenal gland, the three software used in our study showed similar results using different analyses (all groups together or separately, as in CT vs. T, CT vs. D or CT vs. TD). Many types of exercise and/or AAS could alter gene expression in different ways but, in most of our analyses, the values and ranking of genes were similar in all experimental groups. None of the genes were rejected by any of the software; therefore, they are all suitable reference genes for qPCR analysis in rat hypothalamus and adrenal gland.

In mesenteric fat tissue, however, there were some discrepancies between results. All genes were stable and considered suitable as reference genes by Normfinder, but not by BestKeeper and geNorm analysis. GeNorm shows that the only stability gene was *Tubulin* (in all analysis) and when used Bestkepper software, the only exception was *Hprt1* gene, showed above the limit considered adequate.

All software used to check the stability of genes are validated and considered replicated. Most often, results are repeatable despite using different calculations, as M-value and pair-wise correlation. Whereas two of the three software considered all stable candidates and only geNorm considered only *Tubulin* as stable, we suggest that the best gene to be used of adipose tissue is indeed *Tubulin*, however, could be used the other candidates for qPCR analysis if confirm with other reference gene.

It is also valid to emphasize that when we analyze different groups with different interventions, the software will also modify the results. When the NormFinder was used for each analysis groups, the software put genes in a different position and we showed the best combination.

In our study the three software utilized in these analyses produced similar results but the order of the results was not identical and in some cases was considerably different, which corroborate the findings reported by other study [46]. This difference may be attributed to different mathematical models used in each program [24]. On the other hand, there was found similar results for the software geNorm and Normfinder but not for BestKeeper, this can be justified by the fact that this software used the Pearson correlation method to classify the reference genes, a different method compared to the others software [3].

This study is the first to validate reference genes for the evaluation of REx and AAS use effects in different rat tissues. It is important to note that there is no ideal universal reference gene. This work can help you find good candidates, though, for each experiment, species, tissue and other conditions, it is necessary to perform and confirm a specific validation of reference genes, in order to analyze gene expression results more adequately.

Conclusion

In conclusion, our results do not suggest a specific reference gene for hypothalamus and adrenal gland, since all genes analyzed (*Actb*, *18s*, *Hprt1*, *Tubulin* and *Gapdh*) were stable and suitable for gene expression normalization through qPCR. However, in mesenteric fat tissue, the only suitable reference gene accepted by three software was *Tubulin* gene.

Competing Interests

None of the authors has any conflict of interest in submitting this manuscript.

Funding Resource

This project was supported by: FAPESP (Fundação de Amparo à Pesquisa do Estado de São Paulo # 2013/05549-0; # 2013/17587-4), CAPES (Coordenação de Aperfeiçoamento de Pessoal de Nível Superior), CNPq (Conselho Nacional de Desenvolvimento Científico e Tecnológico) and AFIP (Associação Fundo de Incentivo à Pesquisa).

Contribution

Design and experimental procedures: RP, LF, BFAC and VDA. Data analysis: RP, LF and VDA. Contribution with reagents, materials and analysis tools: RP and VDA. Article writer: RP, LF, BFAC and VD.

Acknowledgements

The authors would like to thank Vanessa Gonçalves Pereira for English review writing.

References

1. Bustin SA, Benes V, Garson JA, Hellemans J, Huggett J, et al. (2009) The MIQE guidelines: minimum information for publication of quantitative real-time PCR experiments. Clin Chem 55: 611-622.

2. Lee KS, Alvarenga TA, Guindalini C, Andersen ML, Castro RM, et al. (2009) Validation of commonly used reference genes for sleep-related gene expression studies. BMC Mol Biol 10: 1-45.

3. Julian GS, de Oliveira RW, Perry JC, Tufik S, Chagas JR (2014) Validation of housekeeping genes in the brains of rats submitted to chronic intermittent hypoxia, a sleep apnea model. PLoS One 9: e109902.

4. Alves MJ, Dos Santos MR, Dias RG, Akiho CA, Laterza MC, et al. (2010) Abnormal neurovascular control in anabolic androgenic steroids users.Med Sci Sports Exerc 42: 865-871.

5. Bronson FH (1996) Effects of prolonged exposure to anabolic steroids on the behavior of male and female mice.Pharmacol Biochem Behav 53: 329-334.

6. Farrell SF, McGinnis MY (2003) Effects of pubertal anabolic-androgenic steroid (AAS) administration on reproductive and aggressive behaviors in male rats. Behav Neurosci 117: 904-911.

7. Su TP, Pagliaro M, Schmidt PJ, Pickar D, Wolkowitz O, et al. (1993) Neuropsychiatric effects of anabolic steroids in male normal volunteers. JAMA 269: 2760-2764.

8. Hall RC, Hall RC (2005) Abuse of supraphysiologic doses of anabolic steroids. South Med J 98: 550-555.

9. Scharhag J, Urhausen A, Kindermann W (2003) Anabolic steroid-induced echocardiographic characteristics of professional football players? J Am CollCardiol 42: 588-589.

10. Ogawa K, Sanada K, Machida S, Okutsu M, Suzuki K (2010) Resistance Exercise Training Induced Muscle Hypertrophy Was Associated with Reduction of Inflammatory Markers in Elderly Women. Mediators of Inflammation 2010: 1-7.

11. Teixeira PC, Costa RF, Matsudo SM, Cordas TA (2009) A prática de exercícios físicos em pacientes com transtorno alimentar. Revista de Psiquiatria Clínica 36: 145-152.

12. MacKenzie MG, Hamilton DL, Pepin M, Patton A, Baar K (2013) Inhibition of myostatin signaling through Notch activation following acute resistance exercise. PLoS One 8: e68743.

13. Kim JS, Park YM, Lee SR, Masad IS, Khamoui AV, et al. (2012) β-hydroxy-β-methylbutyrate did not enhance high intensity resistance training-induced improvements in myofiber dimensions and myogenic capacity in aged female rats. Mol Cells 34: 439-448.

14. Domingos MM, Rodrigues MF, Stotzer US, Bertucci DR, Souza MV, et al. (2012) Resistance training restores the gene expression of molecules related to fat oxidation and lipogenesis in the liver of ovariectomized rats. Eur J Appl Physiol 112: 1437-1444.

15. Tanno AP, das Neves VJ, Rosa KT, Cunha TS, Giordano FC, et al. (2011) Nandrolone and resistance training induce heart remodeling: role of fetal genes and implications for cardiac pathophysiology. Life Sci 89: 631-637.

16. Hruz T, Wyss M, Docquier M, Pfaffl MW, Masanetz S, et al. (2011) RefGenes: identification of reliable and condition specific reference genes for RTqPCR data normalization. BMC Genomics 12:156.

17. Cassilhas RC, Lee KS, Fernandes J, Oliveira MG, Tufik S, et al. (2012) Spatial memory is improved by aerobic and resistance exercise through divergent molecular mechanisms. Neuroscience 202: 309-317.

18. Pereira GB, Prestes J, Leite RD, Magosso RF, Peixoto FS, et al. (2010) Effects of ovariectomy and resistance training on MMP-2 activity in rat calcaneal tendon. Connect Tissu e Res 51: 459-466.

19. Hornberger TA, Farrar RP (2004) Physiological hypertrophy of the FHL muscle following 8 weeks of progressive resistance exercise in the rat. Can J Appl Physiol 29: 16-31.

20. Pope JR, Katz DL (1988) Affective and psychotic symptoms associated with anabolic steroids use. Am J Psychiatry 145: 487-490.

21. Pozzi R, Fernandes KR, de Moura CF, Ferrari RA, Fernandes KP, et al. (2013) NandroloneDecanoate Induces Genetic Damage in Multiple Organs of Rats. Arch Environ ContamToxicol 64: 514-518.

22. Vandesompele J, De Preter K, Pattyn F, Poppe B, Van Roy N, et al. (2002) Accurate normalization of real-time quantitative RT-PCR data by geometric averaging of multiple internal control genes. Genome Biol. 3: RESEARCH0034.

23. Svingen T, Jørgensen A, Rajpert-De Meyts E (2014) Validation of endogenous normalizing genes for expression analyses in adult human testis and germ cell neoplasms. Mol Hum Reprod 20: 709-718.

24. Dundas J, Ling M (2012) Reference genes for measuring mRNA expression. Theory Biosci 131: 215-223.

25. Martínez-Beamonte R, Navarro MA, Larraga A, Strunk M, Barranquero C, et al. (2011) Selection of reference genes for gene expression studies in rats. J Biotechnol 151: 325-334.

26. An Y, Reimers K, Allmeling C, Liu J, Lazaridis A, et al. (2012) Validation of differential gene expression in muscle engineered from rat groin adipose tissue by quantitative real-time PCR. Biochem Biophys Res Commun 421: 736-742.

27. Dheda K, Huggett JF, Chang JS, Kim LU, Bustin SA, et al. (2005) The implications of using an inappropriate reference gene for real-time reverse transcription PCR data normalization. Anal Biochem 344: 141-143.

28. 283. Liu XH, Wu Y, Yao S, Levine AC, Kirschenbaum A, et al. (2013) Androgens up-regulate transcription of the Notch inhibitor Numb in C2C12 myoblasts via Wnt/β-catenin signaling to T cell factor elements in the Numb promoter. J Biol Chem 288: 17990-17998.

29. Li R, Ferreira MP, Cooke MB, La Bounty P, Campbell B, et al. (2015) Co-ingestion of carbohydrate with branched-chain amino acids orL leucine does not preferentially increase serum IGF-1 and expression of myogenic related genes in response to a single bout of resistance exercise. AminoAcids 47: 1203-12013.

30. Koga S, Kojima A, Ishikawa C, Kuwabara S, Arai K, et al. (2014) Effects of diet induced obesity and voluntary exercise in a tauopathy mouse model: implications of persistent hyperleptinemia and enhanced astrocytic leptin receptor expression. Neurobiol Dis 71: 180-192.

31. Ebersbach-Silva P, Alves T, Fonseca AT, Oliveira MA, Machado UF, et al. (2013) Cigarette smoke exposure severely reduces peripheral insulin sensitivity without changing GLUT4 expression in oxidative muscle of Wistar rats. Arq Bras Endocrinol Metabol 57: 19-26.

32. Shaker OG, Sadik NA (2013) Vaspin gene in rat adipose tissue: relation to obesity-induced insulin resistance. Mol Cell Biochem 373: 229-239.

33. Brännvall K, Bogdanovic N, Korhonen L, Lindholm D (2005) 19-Nortestosterone influences neural stem cell proliferation and neurogenesis in the rat brain. Eur J Neurosci 21: 871-878.

34. Ellefsen S, Vikmoen O, Zacharoff E, Rauk I, Slettaløkken G, et al. (2014) Reliable determination of training-induced alterations in muscle fiber composition in human skeletal muscle using quantitative polymerase chain reaction. Scand J Med Sci Sports 24: e332-e342.

35. Pekkala S, Wiklund P, Hulmi JJ, Pöllänen E, Marjomäki V, et al. (2015) Cannabinoid receptor 1 and acute resistance exercise - In vivo and in vitro studies in human skeletal muscle. Peptides 67: 55-63.

36. Passos E, Pereira CD, Gonçalves IO, Rocha-Rodrigues S, Silva N, et al. (2015) Role of physical exercise onhepatic insulin, glucocorticoid and inflammatory signaling pathways in an animal model of non-alcoholic steatohepatitis. Life Sci 123: 51-60.

37. Tiss A, Khadir A, Abubaker J, Abu-Farha M, Al-Khairi I, et al. (2014) Immunohistochemical profiling of the heat shock response in obese non-diabetic subjects revealed impaired expression of heat shock proteins in the adipose tissue. Lipids Health Dis 13: 106.

38. Stefanetti RJ, Zacharewicz E, Della GP, Garnham A, Russell AP, et al. (2014) Ageing has no effect on the regulation of the ubiquitin proteasome-related genes and proteins following resistance exercise. Front Physiol 5: 30.

39. Chen R, Feng L, Ruan M, Liu X, Adriouch S, et al. (2013) Mechanical-stretch of C2C12 myoblasts inhibits expression of Toll-like receptor 3 (TLR3) and of autoantigens associated with inflammatory myopathies. PLoS One 8: e79930.

40. Marques-Neto SR, Ferraz EB, Rodrigues DC, Njaine B, Rondinelli E, et al. (2014) AT1 and aldosterone receptors blockade prevents the chronic effect of nandrolone on the exercise-induced cardioprotection in perfused rat heart subjected to ischemia and reperfusion. Cardiovasc Drugs Ther 28: 125-135.

41. Marqueti RC, Heinemeier KM, Durigan JL, de Andrade Perez SE, Schjerling P, et al. (2011) Gene expression in distinct regions of rat tendons in response to jump training combined with anabolic androgenic steroid administration. Eur J Appl Physiol 112: 1505-1515.

42. Ambar G, Chiavegatto S (2009) Anabolic-androgenic steroid treatment induces behavioral disinhibition and downregulation of serotonin receptor messenger RNA in the prefrontal cortex and amygdala of male mice. Genes Brain Behav 8: 161-173.

43. Riedmaier I, Tichopad A, Reiter M, Pfaffl MW, Meyer HH (2009) Influence of testosterone and a novel SARM on gene expression in whole blood of Macaca fascicularis. J Steroid Biochem Mol Biol 114: 167-173.

44. Sun JH, Nan LH, Gao CR, Wang YY (2012) Validation of reference genes for estimating wound age in contused rat skeletal muscle by quantitative real-time PCR. Int J Legal Med 126: 113-120.

45. Li B, Matter EK, Hoppert HT, Grayson BE, Seeley RJ, et al. (2014) Identification of optimal reference genes for qPCR in the rat hypothalamus and intestine for the study of obesity. Int J Obes 38: 192-197.

46. Kim I, Yang D, Tang X, Carroll JL (2011) Reference gene validation for qPCR in rat carotid body during postnatal development. BMC Res Notes 4: 440.

21

A Review of the Estrous Cycle and the Neuroendocrine Mechanisms in the Mare

Satué K[1] and Gardón JC[2]

[1]Department of Animal Medicine and Surgery, Cardenal Herrera University, Spain
[2]Department of Experimental Sciences and Mathematics, Catholic University of Valencia "San Vicente Mártir", Spain

Abstract

With an understanding of basic reproductive science, veterinarians and breeders can be better positioned to achieve their goals. It is important to understand the heat or estrus cycle in order to maximize the chances of success when breeding the mare. Reproductive activity in horses is seasonally dependent, as it is primarily affected by the length of daylight. Therefore the mare has a seasonally polyestrous type of estrous cycle. This means they have breeding season in which they have multiple heat cycles, is receptive to the stallion and ovulates; and a period where they will not go into heat or anestrus. During the anestrus period, most mares show no behavioral signs of sexual receptivity and fail to develop follicles that ovulate. There are exceptions in that a small percentage of mares that do not express a seasonal pattern in that they stay both behaviorally and physiologically receptive to stallions throughout the year. During the ovulatory season, the mare is cycling, thereby exhibiting sexual receptivity to the stallion on a regular basis and is producing follicles that ovulate. The equine estrous cycle is commonly described as a combination of a follicular phase, or estrus, and a luteal phase, or diestrus. The endocrinology of the estrous cycle involves a balance between hormones produced by the pineal gland, hypothalamus, pituitary gland, ovaries, and endometrium. Growth of antral follicles in the ovary occurs in wave-like patterns, and is influenced by several factors such as stage of the estrous cycle, season, pregnancy, age, breed and the individual. In this article will describe the neuroendocrine mechanisms related to breeding seasonality, the hormonal changes that occur during the estrus cycle as well as the variations among mares in regards to the understanding the physiological mechanisms related with the estrous cycle in the mare.

Keywords: Endocrinology; Estrous cycle; Mare

Introduction

The mare is a "seasonally polyestrus" female, meaning that she undergoes regular estrus cycles during a portion of the year and none at others. This is nature's way of preventing the arrival of a foal during bad weather. These cycles are controlled by the mare's hormones, which in turn respond to an increase or decrease in daylight duration with the onset of spring or fall, which affects the pineal gland. The normal estrous cycle in the mare is 21 to 22 days long as defined by the intervals between ovulation. Estrus is the time the mare is "hot", or it is the "follicular phase", as the overt signs of estrus are attributable to the estrogen production by the follicle on the ovary. The duration essentially varies with time of year and is inversely proportional to day length, which means it becomes shorter at the peak of the cycling season. The duration of estrus, however can vary (3 to 9 days), so the most regular period in the estrous cycle is the length of diestrus. Diestrus or the luteal phase is dominated by progesterone produced by the corpus luteum has a duration of 14 day (hormonal) or 15 day (behavioral). It is important to understand that there is a closely linked feedback system between many of the reproductive hormones present in the mare which will alter the level or presence of some hormones as levels of other different hormones increase or decrease. This means that many hormonal changes do occur naturally, but when something becomes unbalanced either naturally or artificially, we can see estrous cycle problems develop in the mare. For this reason the mare is unique compared to the other livestock species because the estrous cycle differs between individuals and between cycles in the same individual. Consequently, to be successful in the breeding of horses is essential that owners of mares and technicians understand the reproductive cycle of the mare.

Reproductive Seasonality in the Mare

From the viewpoint of breeding, the mare is defined as a seasonally polyestrous of long days, or positive phototropic in which breeding activity is regulated directly by the photoperiod. The photoreceptors of the retina capture light stimulus information and transform it into nerve impulses. The nerve impulse is transported through the optic nerve to the suprachiasmatic nucleus and then to the superior cervical ganglion. This last ganglion has adrenergic neuronal endings reaching the pineal gland where the neurotransmitter serotonin is released. Through N-acetyl serotonin, serotonin is transformed into N-acetilserotonina, also called normelatonina. Normelatonina together with the N-acetilserotonina o-methyltransferase (ASMT) involved in the synthesis of melatonin [1].

Melatonin is released during the hours of darkness, following a pattern of secretion inversely proportional to the amount of daylight hours. As a result of increased exposure to photoperiod in the spring and summer, the secretion of melatonin decreases, which in turn stimulates the release of gonadotropin-releasing factor (GnRH) in the hypothalamus. The GnRH enters the hypothalamic-pituitary portal vascular system, and then transported to the adenohypophysis [2], place were follicle stimulating hormones (FSH) and luteinizing hormone (LH) are synthesized. Both gonadotropins are transported through the blood to the ovary place where specifically exert their

*Corresponding author: Katy Satué, Department of Animal Medicine and Surgery, School of Veterinary Medicine, University CEU-Cardenal Herrera, Av. Seminary, s/n, 46113 Moncada, Valencia, Spain,
E-mail: ksatue@uch.ceu.es

functions [3,4]. FSH acts on the granulosa cells of the preovulatory follicle stimulating the growth, follicular maturation and estrogen biosynthesis. On the theca cells, LH is involved in oocyte maturation, ovulation, establishment and maintenance of corpus luteum (CL) as well as development and in the synthesis of P4. Both ovarian steroids control the Hypothalamus-Hypophysis axis (HHA) by feedback mechanisms that determine the estrous cycle in the mare [5-7].

Changes in the length of photoperiod determine reproductive seasonality in the mare, establishing a character circannual reproductive cycle integrated in turn by four periods differing endocrine and physiologically: spring transition period, ovulatory season or breeding season, autumn transition and winter anestrus [8,9].

The spring transition period is occurs after winter anestrus in early spring due to the increased number of hours of daylight or photoperiod, and ends after a period of two months, with the onset of reproductive activity fertile regular feature ovulatory station. Although this period is of great variability both in features and duration, mares show a pattern of erratic sexual activity, characterized by the presence of irregular and long estrous [9].

The increase of FSH at the beginning of this period causes smaller follicular waves, characterized by the development of multiple follicles from 6 to 21 mm of diameter, that regress simultaneously in absence of a dominant follicle [10,11]. Low levels of estradiol-17β (E2) and inhibin, due to the absence of preovulatory follicles, simultaneously inhibit the negative feedback on FSH so that gonadotropin levels remain high. However, the seasonal LH deficiency results in low concentrations of E2, inhibin and other factors present in the follicular fluid as the insulin-like growth factor 1 (IGF-I), causing ovulatory failure. Therefore, when performing rectal palpation or ultrasound examination is often the occurrence of various small antral follicles of similar size (20-30 mm) in the ovary [5]. Due to the influence of photoperiod, the end of spring transition period is represented by larger follicular waves which develop a set of follicles. Most of these follicles undergo atresia but one reaches a larger size than the others. Increasing concentrations of E2 by the preovulatory follicle induced LH surge, leading to first ovulation, indicating the onset of ovulatory season at which fertile cyclical activitybegins [9].

The ovulatory season or breeding season runs from April to September in the northern hemisphere and from October to March in the southern hemisphere. The beginning of the reproductive period occurs when the number of hours of light is adequate to suppress the inhibitory reflex of melatonin on GnRH. GnRH secretion is continuous, pulsed every hour during estrus and every two hours in diestrus. On each estrous cycle may have one or two major follicular waves under uni-or bimodal pattern of FSH secretion. The bimodal pattern occurs specifically at the beginning of the ovulatory season, while the middle or end of this period showed a unimodal pattern [12,13]. In contrast to the transition period, characterized by lower follicular waves, in the breeding season follicular waves develop larger, leading to the formation of a dominant follicle. The influence of these hormonal patterns, determines some variability on the duration of the cycles. In North Hemisphere, estrual cycles become more durable at the beginning (April or May), that the end of the breeding season (June or July). It has been hypothesized that the purpose of reproductive seasonality is to ensure the births in the most favorable time of the year, with better environmental conditions and food availability, for the proper development of the foal [8,9].

The high temperatures and decreased influence of photoperiod

in late summer, promote the onset of autumn transition period, which in the northern hemisphere covers the months from October to December. Both environmental factors involve a series of gradual changes intended to temporarily end with the activation of antral follicles and the ovulatory process. FSH returns to present a bimodal pattern, as the onset of the breeding season, with a discharge rate of one pulse every two days, so that the diameter of the largest follicle decreases gradually as the period progresses and with it the E2 synthesis [14]. This decrease in estrogens inhibits the preovulatory surge of LH culminating in the absence of follicular growth and ovulation arrest in early winter [8,15].

The loss of ability to cycle in mares in anestrus is given by the limited influence of photoperiod on gonadotropin levels and covers the months of December, January and mid-February in the northern hemisphere. The increasing number of hours of darkness during the winter promotes the release of high concentrations of melatonin, while blocking the Hypothalamus-Hypophysis-Gonadal axis (HHGA). Thus, GnRH secretion becomes pulsatile with very low amplitude and frequency, being not enough to stimulate the secretion of gonadotropins FSH and LH [3]. Performing rectal palpation ovaries showed small and hard due to the absence of follicles larger than 15 mm. The uterus loses muscle tone and becomes flaccid. Sometimes, we prefer to call this stage as anovulatory and not as anoestrus, because some mares show signs of heat due the release of estrogen by the adrenal glands [9].

Additionally, these seasonal patterns may change under a wide variety of factors such as, temperature, latitude, geographic region, race, age, physiological status, presence of stress and disease, body condition, feeding, among others [16,17].

Estrous Cycle in the Mare

The estrous cycle is defined as the interval of time between two consecutive ovulations. The approximate length varies between 18 and 22 days, considering on average a period of 21 days [18,19]. The current nomenclature stipulates that the estrous cycle consists of two clearly differentiated stages: estrus or follicular phase and diestrus or luteal phase. These phases are characterized by internal modifications of the sexual organs and glandular system as well as behavioral alterations based on the dominant levels of E2 and P4 in each of them, respectively [8,9].

Follicular phase

Estrus, heat or follicular phase is characterized by the presence of follicles at different stages of development, and the simultaneous increase in the secretion of E2. It has duration about 5-7 days, with a variability of 3-9 days related to the season. Thus, estrus is extended in autumn (7-10 days) and is shortened considerably, in late spring and early summer (4-5 days). During this period the mare is sexually receptive to the stallion genital tract and is ready to receive and transport of sperm and finally culminates with ovulation [8,19,20].

Follicular dynamics: Follicular growth pattern and ovulation: Ovarian follicular development is a complex dynamic process, characterized by marked proliferation and differentiation of follicular cells, providing an optimal environment for oocyte maturation and preparation for fertilization after ovulation [21]. Among the recruited follicles in each follicular wave, dominance take place and one follicle of the cohort acquires the ability to continue growing while others undergo atresia. The regulation of each wave and follicular selection involves interactions between specific circulating gonadotropins and intrafollicular factors, ensuring that each follicle is properly stimulated to grow or regress at any stage of development [22].

From an experimental point of view, the occurrence of a wave is defined as follicular growth or simultaneous emergence of a variable number of follicles below 6 to 13 mm in diameter [23,24]. In the mare, these follicular waves are classified depending on their ability to develop the dominant follicle (primary waves) or, in contrast, generate only small follicles (smaller waves). Thus, the main waves or greater originate several follicles subordinate and a dominant follicle, while smaller waves, the follicles are not larger than 30 mm in diameter and then regress [10,11,25,26].

During each cycle produces 1 or 2 major follicular waves, differentiated according to time of onset at primary and secondary. The primary major wave occurs near the middle of diestrus, in which the dominant follicle ovulates at the end or near the end of estrus. The largest wave precedes the previous secondary and emerges during late estrus or early diestrus. Basically, there are two anovulatory follicular waves followed by an ovulatory surge during the estrous cycle [14,27]. In horses, there are profound differences in the pattern of follicular waves related to breed. Thus while Quarter Horse mares and ponies usually develops at late diestrus main wave, which culminates with ovulation during estrus in thorough bred mares secondary wave occurs at early diestrus in which the dominant follicle may ovulate, become hemorrhagic or undergo atresia [25,28].

Pierson [13] described the importance of the participation of the gonadotropins FSH and LH in follicular development. Antral follicles acquire receptors for LH and FSH at the level of membranes of granulosa cells and theca, respectively. Theca cells under the prevalence of androgen synthesize LH, which will then be aromatized to estrogen by granulosa cells, previously stimulated by FSH. Increased concentrations of estrogen stimulate the secretion of LH, which in turn induces greater estrogen synthesis. This progressive increase in estrogen also promotes the onset of LH receptors in granulosa cells, which facilitates the transition from the antral stage to preovulatory stage, when the oocyte reaches the final stage of maturation. At 6 days after the emergence of major follicular wave deviation occurs. This event relates to the growth rate difference of the preovulatory follicle size (22.5 mm) compared to the subordinate follicles (19 mm) [11,29,30]. Deviation is related to inhibin secretion [26] and IGF-1 [10,31]. Specifically, inhibin reduces FSH secretion to baseline levels, making it impossible to continue the development of the subordinate follicles [23,25]. However, the dominant follicle continues to grow at a constant rate of 2.3 mm per day until reaching a size of 40 mm in response to the increased sensitivity to FSH. As has been mentioned, at this stage of development, granulosa cells also develop receptors for LH required for final oocyte maturation and ovulation after the LH surge [32,33].

The maximum diameter of the ovulatory follicle usually varies between 40-45 mm in different horse breeds such as Quarter Horse, Arabian, Thoroughbred and Spanish Purebred [34-37], although the range may be higher (30 a 70 mm) [9,37]. However, in breeds with a weight below 350 kg or low height at withers, usually the size of the follicles has a smaller diameter (35-40 mm) [16,38]. Moreover, size differences were established in relation to the breeding season or the presence of multiple ovulations. Therefore, follicles reach a size of 8.5 mm larger in the spring than in summer or autumn and are 4.9 mm smaller in multiple ovulations compared to single [16,37].

The highest concentrations of estrogen secreted by the granulosa cells of the preovulatory follicle also induce the appearance of typical behavioral manifestations of estrus. Estrogens are also responsible for reproductive changes that ensure the reception, transport of sperm and oocyte fertilization [8,18]. After the preovulatory LH surge, ovulation occurs spontaneously 24-48 hours before the end of the follicular phase. The ovulatory process brings rapid evacuation of the oocyte and follicular fluid after follicular rupture at ovulation fossa. Once completed, E2 concentrations return to basal levels and at the same time completing the oestrus behavior in mares [24,28,33,38-40].

Modifications of behavior and reproductive tract during estrus in mares: The predominance of estrogens during the follicular (proliferative phase) is responsible for behavioral changes and reproductive tract during estrus in the mare. Among the external signs of estrus are described, restlessness and irritability, stallion search, lateral tail lift, frequent urination, mucus secretion, vulvar flicker and clitoral eversion. Also they emphasize relaxation of the head and facial muscles, descent of the pelvis and hind limbs separation to address and accommodate the penis at the time of copulation [8,18].

The colposcopic examination can detect longitudinal diameter increase of the vulva, congestion and edema of vulvar and vaginal mucosa [8,18,41]. The cervix is open, relaxed, limp and edematous observing the output of mucus with fluid consistency [8,18]. Increased vascularization under the dominance of estrogen causes absence of tone at cervix, body and uterine horns, detectable by rectal palpation. Follicular growth becomes appreciable by increased ovarian size and tone [41], which during the week prior to ovulation increases linearly at a rate of 2.7 mm per day [12]. However, 24-48 h before ovulation the follicle can lose tone and stop its growth, a fact that occurs in a high percentage of mares (40%) day [12,42]. Uterine tone does not have specific modifications until the time of ovulation [8,18], although the follicular wall collapse after breaking can be identified as a depression in the ovarian surface [43].

Ultrasound examination of the body and uterine horns exhibits a characteristic heterogeneous pattern comprising alternating echogenic and hypoechoic areas, closely related to the increase of estrogen [44]. Echogenic areas correspond to the inner portions of the endometrial folds while echogenic portions are indicative of the presence of edema at the submucosa. From time to time may appear small amount of free fluid intrauterine physiological character. In ponies and mares of various breeds like Appaloosa, Quarter Horse, Thoroughbred, Dutch Warmblood, Standard bred, endometrial folds become visible 7-8 days prior, progressively increasing the day of ovulation. At the level of the uterine horns are characteristic ultrasound images in a "cart wheel "pattern related to the presence of edema and hypertrophy of the endometrial folds [45]. Using ultrasound monitoring can also be detected muscle contraction in cervix, body and uterine horns and fallopian tubes during the estrous [8,18]. After ovulation, endometrial edema disappears and folds are undetectable [12,44-47].

Ovarian ultrasound shows a variable number of follicles from anechogenic consistency that can vary in size according to the time of development [8,18,19,41,48]. Preovulatory follicle exhibits pronounced morphological changes, varying spherical or pear-shaped to conical in 84% of the pre-ovulatory period while the remaining follicles maintained the spherical shape [12]. The follicular wall collapse after the break can also be detected by ultrasound as a hyperechoic irregular area at the cortical region of the ovary [43].

Diestrus or luteal phase

The diestrus or luteal phase begins at the time of ovulation with the formation of CL, which is responsible for the synthesis of progesterone (P_4). Unlike the follicular phase the insensitivity of the CL photoperiod makes the length of this period more constant. In fact, most research estimates an average duration of 14-15 days, but can be more durable in mid-summer (16 days) than in spring or autumn (13 days) [8,19].

Formation of CL: The disorganization of the follicular wall after ovulation allows blood vessels and fibroblasts invade the follicular cavity. Luteinization involves structural and functional changes of granulosa cells. These are the same cells that initially produced E2 and become into luteal cells that produce P_4. The P_4 remains high from day 5 post ovulation until the end of the diestrus and exerts specific functions related to the preparation of the endometrium to accept and maintain pregnancy, endometrial gland development and inhibition of myometrial contractility [38].

Have been described two types of CL regarding the presence or absence of central blood clot. In a high percentage of cases (50-70%) in place of ovulation a core clot develops surrounded by luteal tissue. This type of condition is defined as corpus hemorrhagic. The cavity begins to fill with blood, fibrin and transudate for the first 24 hours, reaching the maximum size at 3 days. Around day 5 post-ovulation CLs that develop central cavity, usually have a significantly higher size (32.8 mm) to those without it (26.0 mm). The ratio of the maximum diameter of the CL is 65 to 80% compared to pre-ovulatory follicle size and has an outer wall thickness of 4-7 mm corresponding to the portion of luteinized tissue. As happens with the size, texture also changes depending on the type of CL. While the corpusluteum that develop central cavity are denser, those who do not have tend to be spongier [49]. Generally, the ratio of non-luteal luteal tissue of the corpus hemorrhagic is minimal during early diestrus and maximum in halfway of diestrus. These events are associated with the gradual decrease of fluid as a result of production and organization of connective tissue associated with the clotting mechanism [50,51]. Notably, the formation of one type or another of CL is a random event. In fact, the morphology luteal repeatability is not always observed in subsequent ovulations [12,50,51].

Additionally, continuous P_4 levels during diestrus reduce the frequency and intensity of GnRH pulses by feedback mechanism. However, because the pulses of FSH are higher than those of LH, a new follicular wave is developed during this period. At the experimental level, cross sections have been made in the ovary in the middle of diestrus, showing alternation of CL and follicles at various stages of development that can reach a variable size (2-30 mm) or return. In the absence of pregnancy the end luteal phase culminates with the lysis of CL induced by the PGF2α of endometrial origin and decreased concentrations of P_4 [8,19]. Luteal regression involves a number of structural and functional events characterized by decreased vascularization, increase of connective tissue, hyalinization, atrophy and fibrosis [43].

Modifications of behavior pattern and reproductive tract during diestrus in mares: During diestrus (secretory phase) the domain of P_4 induces behavioral changes and tubular genitalia, characterized by loss of edema and estrus behavior, characteristic of the follicular phase. During this period there are frequent vocalization reflexes of the mare or I kick attacks to prevent the approach of the stallion [8].

By colposcopic examination, the mucosa of the vulva, vagina and cervix appear pale, dry, with small amount of viscous mucus appearance. The longitudinal diameter of the vulva is shortened and the cervix appears closed, pale and centrally [8,19].

On rectal palpation the cervix, body and uterine horns are firm, narrow and tubular although uterine tone is lower than during gestation. Although it is difficult to explore, the CL could be identified during the first few days post-ovulation, although developing follicles (diameter less than 25 mm) would not be identifiable [43].

The ultrasound of the uterus shows a homogeneous pattern marked by the lack of endometrial folds and the presence of a small amount of intrauterine fluid [46,52,53]. While the luteal tissue is observed hypoechoic, the echogenicity increases in the connective tissue of the ovarian stromal. Although the diameter of the body is higher than hemorrhagic CL without central cavity, the ratio of luteal tissue is similar in both types [46,50-53]. Echogenicity pattern varies according to the period of development and growth or regression of the CL since it is inversely related to the degree of vascularization [37,51]. Furthermore, these changes in the pattern of endometrial and luteal echotexture are closely related to P_4 levels [54]. Thus, the gradual increase in P_4 that characterized the early diestrus is associated with increased diameter and luteal vascularization and decreased echogenicity. The highest concentrations of P_4 that define the half of diestrus are related to the diameter and maximum vascularization and minimum echogenicity. The regression of the CL and P_4 decrease structurally correspond with decreased luteal area and vascularization and increased echogenicity. The corpus luteum is visible by ultrasound until day 17 of the cycle [55]. These structural changes precede functional variations during the maturing period and luteal regression [37,56-58].

Endocrinological Aspects Related with the Estrous Cycle in the Mare

Physiological events that occur during the estrous cycle are regulated by the coordinated interaction of various hormones and releasing factors like GnRH, FSH, LH, E2, P_4 and prostaglandin F-2α (PGF2α), among others [2] (Figure 1). Here are described the most notable changes that everyone has and the physiological involvement during the estrous cycle in the mare.

Gonadotrophin releasing factor

As has been discussed previously, increased photoperiod during spring and summer causes decreased secretion of melatonin. This signal has a positive effect on the pulses of hypothalamic GnRH, which in turn controls the release of gonadotropins [12]. GnRH pulses produced every 45 min originate predominantly LH secretion whereas those occur every 6 h. stimulate the secretion of FSH. The high frequency pulses of GnRH (2 pulses per hour) during estrus favors an increase in LH and FSH decline, while reducing the frequency to 2 pulses per day, leads an increase of FSH and LH inhibition [3]. These endocrine events, allowing the emergence of follicular waves, E2 synthesis and ovulation during estrus and appearance of the CL with P_4 release during diestrus [38].

Follicle stimulating hormone

As has been discussed, FSH describes two types of secretion patterns during the estrous cycle in the mare: uni or bimodal. The bimodal pattern occurs frequently during the spring transition period and ovulatory season. The first peak of FHS appears between the 8th and 14th day of the cycle, moment in which the largest follicle reached a diameter of 13 mm [59]. This initial increase precedes the beginning of the deviation and is associated with increased synthesis of inhibin by the largest follicle [10,11,59-62] and persists until the preovulatory follicle reaches a diameter of 22 mm. The second peak of FSH begins on day 15 of the cycle and it is necessary to complete the development of the preovulatory follicle [23,59,61]. Unlike the bimodal pattern, the first peak of FSH would be absent in the unimodal pattern [63]. In the

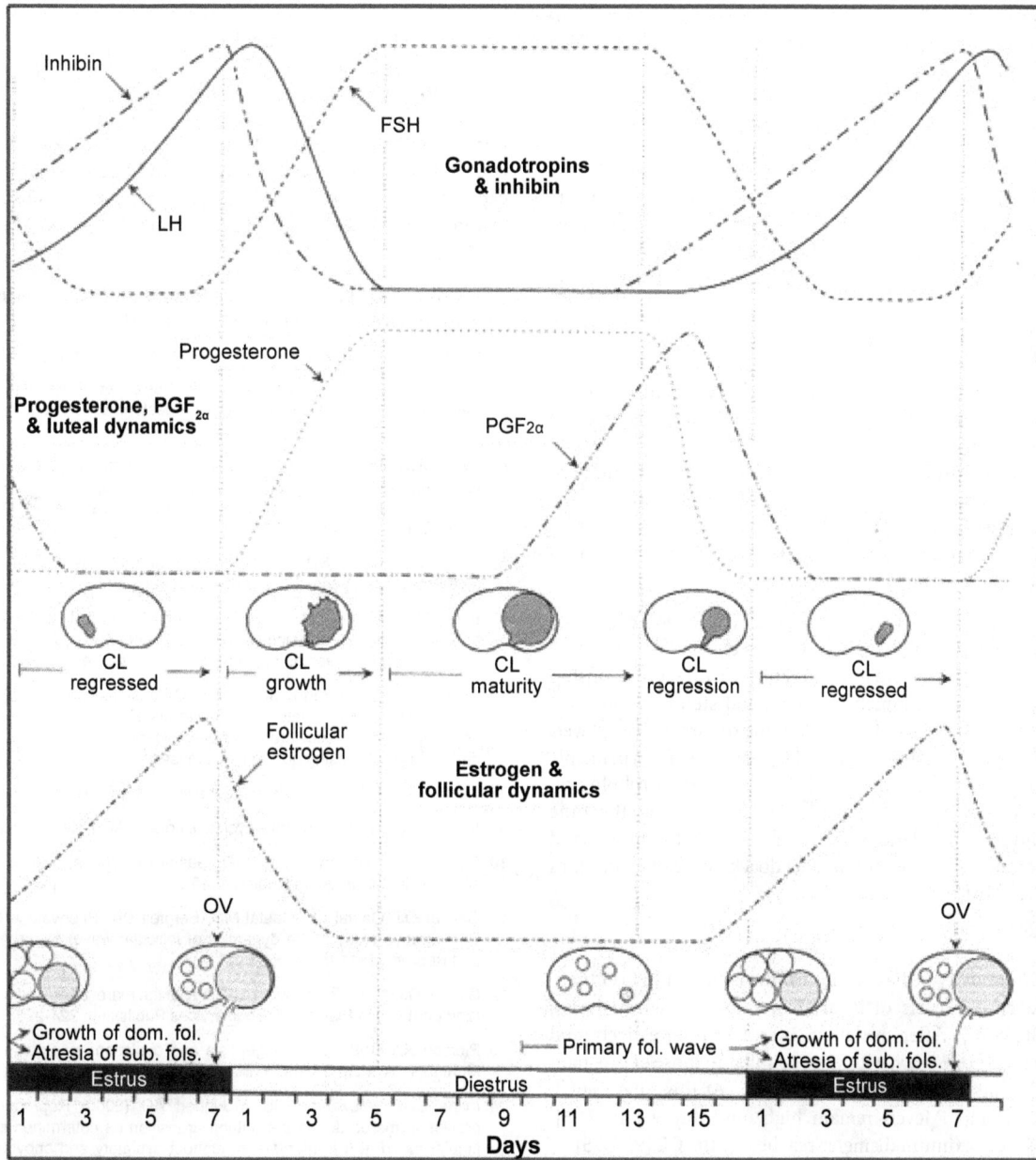

Figure 1: Hormone profiles and temporal relationships with follicular and luteal development during the oestrous cycle in the mare *(Adapted from Ginther OJ (1992) Reproductive Biology of the Mare: Basic and Applied Aspects.(2nd edn). Cross Plains, WI: Equiservices Publishin).*

latter pattern FSH levels remain low during estrus, rise in times around ovulation, maintaining increased during diestrus [61].

FSH is also involved in the development of the LH receptors in the preovulatory follicle [4,64]. At the start of follicular growth, low levels of estradiol exert a negative feedback on HHA controlling the tonic or basal release of gonadotropin. This mechanism controls the follicular growth and E2 synthesis continuously preventing ovarian overstimulation. After the period of follicular growth, once the dominant follicle has been selected, the E2 and inhibin levels are significantly increased. This elevation of E2 is responsible for the characteristic changes of the genital tract and signs of heat during estrus. Furthermore, this response exerts a positive feedback on the HHA, favoring the emergence of preovulatory LH surge, necessary to

produce the ovulation. Additionally, the stimulatory effects of E2 on LH combined to the inhibitory action of inhibin on FSH create the ideal microenvironment for the final maturation of the oocyte, inhibiting the development of immature follicles [18].

Luteinizing hormone

LH levels gradually increases from day -5 to day of ovulation, when it reaches the maximum concentration [9,65]. As already mentioned, the pre-ovulatory LH surge occurs as a result of the positive feedback mechanism exerted by E2 concentrations secreted by the granulosa cells of the preovulatory follicle in the adenohypophysis. However, the peak of E2 is reached 2 days before the LH. During diestrus LH is released in a pulsatile manner, with a frequency of 1.4 pulses per 24 hours and for a period of 20-40 minutes at the central level, or 2-4 h per pulse at the peripheral level [66], therefore P_4 secretion is maintained by basal levels of LH. The decline of LH at the end of diestrus is a result of the combined effect of decreased estrogen positive feedback, and the resurgence of negative feedback induced by P_4 on the HHA. This gonadotropin not only participates in the development and maturation of the primary follicles but also in the development and maintenance of CL during the luteal phase [10,11,19,33,60].

It has been hypothesized that the persistence of high levels of LH after ovulation could induce ovulation in diestrus, which may occur 3-5 days after the first ovulation. However, these ovulations are not accompanied by signs of heat, an event related to the suppressive effects of P_4 on estrous behavior [38,67].

Estradiol-17β

The ability of estrogen synthesis is dependent on the effect of FSH on granulosa cells. In the absence of P_4, estrogens begin to be actively secreted by the preovulatory follicle 5-7 days before ovulation. This event coincides with the time of departure and reaches the peak two days before ovulation [19,33,68], and will be responsible for the preovulatory release of LH. After ovulation, E2 levels begin to decrease gradually after 48 h, reaching basal levels at day 5 post-ovulation [10,11,36,69-71].

Although estrogen levels are directly related to the degree of ovarian activity, sexual receptivity and reproductive tract changes during estrus [8,10,18,44,48,57,61,68,72], there is no evidence of a direct relationship between the intensity of endometrial edema and steroid levels. This situation is much clearer on P_4. In fact, swelling occurs when P_4 levels are less than 1 ng/ml, so this hormone could be responsible in principle on the intensity of edema, among other behavioral and morphological changes of the cervix and uterus [68,72,73]. However, at the time of ovulation inverse correlations are established between E2 and FSH levels associated with the negative feedback effect of inhibin, as previously referred [61].

Progesterone

Steroidogenic activity of P_4 depends on the action of LH on theca cells. As noted above, levels of P_4 are lower than 1 ng/ml during estrus [12,20,36,68,70]. After ovulation, increases progressively and significantly to the 5th or 6th day, with values similar to those of pregnant mares during the first 14 days of gestation [74]. At this time the CL is fully functional and P_4 levels remain high until day 9 [70,72,75], consistent with the maximum diameter reached by the CL [9,37,75].

However, peripheral concentrations of P_4 are highly variable between mares. This variability is associated with secretory capacity CL and hormonal catabolic rate. Perhaps this fact may explain the differences in P_4 levels between ponies and mares during the first 5 days of the luteal period or between Arabian and Spanish Pure bred mares [34], despite the similarity in length of estrous cycles. Among other factors related to variations in levels of P_4 highlights the number of ovulations. In fact, double ovulations induce higher concentrations of P_4 compared to simple ones [75].

P_4 inhibits the secretion and pulsatile release of GnRH and LH, but does not modify the pattern of FSH [8,10,57,73]. This event, unlike what happens in other species, enabling a new wave of follicular growth and in some cases the presence of ovulations during diestrus related to high levels of this hormone [18,33,39,58,76]. After lysis of the CL at the end of diestrus, P_4 is drastically reduced to levels below 1 ng/ml, a fact which promotes the mare returns to estrus [36,70,73,77].

Prostaglandin F2α

In the absence of pregnancy the average life span of the CL is controlled by the release of endometrial PGF2α source, establishing a bimodal pattern of discharge around day 13-16 of diestrus. While the first 4-hour peak precedes the decline of P_4, the second occurs during and after luteolysis. Luteolysis involves decreased blood supply, leukocyte infiltration, cell disruption and loss of lutein steroidogenic capacity by apoptotic or non-apoptotic mechanisms intended to disintegrate the CL and therefore secretion P_4 [58,73,78,79].

References

1. Haimov I, Lavie P (1995) Potential of melatonin replacement therapy in older patients with sleep disorders. Drugs Aging 7: 75-78.

2. Cunningham JG, Klein BG (2009) Veterinary Physiology. (4thedn). Elsevier.

3. Alexander SL, Irvine CH (1991) Control of onset of breeding season in the mare and its artificial regulation by progesterone treatment. J Reprod Fertil Suppl 44: 307-318.

4. Irvine CHG, Alexander SL (1993) Secretory patterns and rates ofgonadotrophin-releasing hormone, follicle-stimulating hormone, and luteinizing hormone revealed by intensive sampling of pituitary venous blood in the luteal phase mare. Endocrinology 132: 212-218.

5. Sharp DC, Davis SD (1993) Vernal transition. In: Equine Reproduction. McKinnon, A.O.; Voss, J.L. (eds.). Lea & Febiger, Philadelphia: 133-143.

6. Evans MJ, Alexander SL, Irvine CH, Kitson NE, Taylor TB (2011) Administration of a gonadotropin-releasing hormone antagonist to mares at different times during the luteal phase of the estrous cycle. Anim Reprod Sci 127: 188-196.

7. Velez IC, Pack JD, Porter MB, Sharp DC, Amstalden M, et al. (2012) Secretion of luteinizing hormone into pituitary venous effluent of the follicular and luteal phase mare: novel acceleration of episodic release during constant infusion of gonadotropin-releasing hormone. Domest Anim Endocrinol 42: 121-128.

8. Crowell-Davis SL (2007) Sexual behavior of mares. Horm Behav 52: 12-17.

9. Aurich C (2011) Reproductive cycles of horses. Anim Reprod Sci 124: 220-228.

10. Ginther OJ, Beg MA, Gastal MO, Gastal EL (2004a) Follicle dynamics and selection in mares. Anim Reprod 1: 45-63.

11. Ginther OJ, Gastal EL, Gastal MO, Bergfelt DR, Baerwald AR, et al. (2004) Comparative study of the dynamics of follicular waves in mares and women. Biol Reprod 71: 1195-1201.

12. Ginther OJ (1992) Reproductive biology of the mare: basic and applied aspects. (2nd edn) Cross Plains, WI: Equiservices Publishing: 224-226.

13. Pierson RA (1993) Folliculogenesis and ovulation. In: Equine Reproduction. McKinnon, A, Voss J (eds.) Williams & Wilkins, Media, PA: 161.

14. Irvine CHG, Alexander SL, Mckinnon AO (2000) Reproductive hormone profiles in mares during the autumn transition as determined by collection of jugular blood at 6 h intervals throughout ovulatory and anovulatory cycles. J Reprod Fertil 118: 101-109.

15. Turner DD, Garcia MC, Ginther OJ (1979) Follicular and gonadotropic changes throughout the year in pony mares. Am J Vet Res 40: 1694-1700.

16. Morel MC, Newcombe JR, Hayward K (2010) Factors affecting pre-ovulatory follicle diameter in the mare: the effect of mare age, season and presence of other ovulatory follicles (multiple ovulation). Theriogenology 74: 1241-1247.

17. Vecchi I, Sabbioni A, Bigliardi E, Morini G, Ferrari L, et al. (2010) Relationship between body fat and body condition score and their effects on estrous cycles of the Standardbred maiden mare. Vet Res Commun 34 Suppl 1: S41-45.

18. Bergfelt DR (2000) Estrous synchronization. In: Equine breeding management and artificial insemination. Samper, JC (ed.) Saunders Company, Philadelphia: 165-177.

19. Ginther OJ, Beg MA, Neves AP, Mattos RC, Petrucci BP, et al. (2008) Miniature ponies: 2. Endocrinology of the oestrous cycle. Reprod Fertil Dev 20: 386-390.

20. Squires EL (1993) Embryo transfer. In: Equine Reproduction. McKinnon AO, Voss, JL (eds.) Lea & Febiger, Philadelphia.

21. Armstrong DG, Webb R (1997) Ovarian follicular dominance: the role of intraovarian growth factors and novel proteins. Rev Reprod 2: 139-146.

22. McMeen SL (2002) Follicular growth and development and gonadotropin response of mares treated with dihidrotestosterone and estradiol benzoate. Thesis of Master of Science. Louisiana State University.

23. Ginther OJ, Bergfelt DR (1993) Growth of small follicles and concentrations of FSH during the equine oestrous cycle. J Reprod Fertil 99: 105-111.

24. Ginther OJ, Beg MA, Bergfelt DR, Donadeu FX, Kot K (2001) Follicle selection in monovular species. Biol Reprod 65: 638-647.

25. Ginther OJ (2000) Selection of the dominant follicle in cattle and horses. Anim Reprod Sci 60-61: 61-79.

26. Donadeu FX, Ginther OJ (2002) Changes in concentrations of follicular fluid factors during follicle selection in mares. Biol Reprod 66: 1111-1118.

27. Ginther OJ (1990) Folliculogenesis during the transitional period and early ovulatory season in mares. J Reprod Fertil 90: 311-320.

28. Stabenfeldt SE, Munglani G, García AJ, LaPlaca MC (2010) Biomimetic microenvironment modulates neural stem cell survival, migration, and differentiation. Tissue Eng Part A 16: 3747-3758.

29. Gastal EL, Gastal MO, Bergfelt DR, Ginther OJ (1997) Role of diameter differences among follicles in selection of a future dominant follicle in mares. Biol Reprod 57: 1320-1327.

30. Watson ED, Thomassen R, Steele M, Heald M, Leask R, et al. (2002) Concentrations of inhibin, progesterone and oestradiol in fluid from dominant and subordinate follicles from mares during spring transition and the breeding season. Anim Reprod Sci 74: 55-67.

31. Ginther OJ, Beg MA, Bergfelt DR, Kot K (2002) Activin A, estradiol, and free insulin-like growth factor I in follicular fluid preceding the experimental assumption of follicle dominance in cattle. Biol Reprod 67: 14-19.

32. Gastal EL, Bergfelt DR, Nogueira GP, Gastal MO, Ginther OJ (1999) Role of luteinizing hormone in follicle deviation based on manipulating progesterone concentrations in mares. Biol Reprod 61: 1492-1498.

33. Gastal EL (2009) Recent advances and new concepts on follicle and endocrine dynamics during the equine periovulatory period. Anim Reprod 6: 144-158.

34. Vivo R, Vinuesa M, Rodriguez I (1992) Valoración del desarrollo folicular preovulatorio en yeguas Pura Raza Española y Árabes. Arch Zootec 41: 19-26.

35. Vinuesa M, Vivo R (1993) Diámetro del folículo preovulatorio y vesícula embrionaria en yeguas árabes y pura raza española. Arch Zootec 42: 263-267.

36. Satué K, Montesinos P, Gardon JC (2013) Influence of oestrogen and progesterone on circulating neutrophils and monocyte during ovulatory and luteal phase in healthy Spanish Purebred mares. Proceeding of XIX Congress of Societa Italiana Veterinari per Equini (SIVE): 383-384.

37. Bergfelt DR, Adams GP (2007) Ovulation and corpus luteum development. In: Current therapy in equine reproduction. Rudolph, P (ed.). Saunders Company Publisher, St. Louis, Missouri: 1-13.

38. Younqquist RS, Threlfall WR (2007) Clinical Reproductive Anatomy and Physiology of the Mare. In: Large Animal Theriogenology. Youngquist RS, Threlfall WR (eds.). Saunders Elsevier, St Louis: 47- 67.

39. Donadeu FX, Pedersen HG (2008) Follicle development in mares. Reprod Domest Anim 43 Suppl 2: 224-231.

40. Gastal EL (2011) Ovulation. Part 1. Follicle development and endocrinology during the periovulatory period. In: Equine Reproduction. McKinnon AO, Squires EL, Vaala WE, Dickson DV (Eds.). (2nd edn). Ames, IA: Wiley-Blackwell: 2020-2031.

41. Samper JC, Pycock JF (2007) The normal uterus in estrous. In: Current therapy in Equine Reproduction. Samper, JC, Pycock, JF, McKinnon AO (eds.). Saunders, St. Louis, Missouri: 32-35.

42. Palmer E, Driancourt MA (1980) Use of ultrasonic echography in equine gynecology. Theriogenology 13: 203-216.

43. Samper JC (2008) Induction of estrus and ovulation: why some mares respond and others do not. Theriogenology 70: 445-447.

44. Pycock JF, Dielman S, Drijhout P, Van der Brug Y, Oei Y, et al. (1995) Correlation of plasma concentrations of progesterone and oestradiol with ultra-sound characteristics of the uterus and duration of oestrous behaviour in the cycling mare. Reprod Dom Anim 30: 224-227.

45. Hayes KE, Pierson RA, Scraba ST, Ginther OJ (1985) Effects of estrous cycle and season on ultrasonic uterine anatomy in mares. Theriogenology 24: 465-477.

46. Ginther OJ, Pierson RA (1984) Ultrasonic anatomy and pathology of the equine uterus. Theriogenology 21: 505-516.

47. Mckinnon AO, Squires EL, Carnevale EM, Harrison LA, Frantz DD, et al. (1987) Diagnostic ultrasonography of uterine pathology in the mare. Proceeding of 33rd Annual Convention of American Association of Equine Practice: 605-622.

48. Bragg Weber ND, Pierson RA, Card CE (2002) Relationship between estradiol 17-ß and endometrial echotexture during natural and hormonally manipulated estrus in Mares. Proceedings A.A.E.P: 41-47.

49. Dickson SE, Fraser HM (2000) Inhibition of early luteal angiogenesis by gonadotropin-releasing hormone antagonist treatment in the primate. J Clin Endocrinol Metab 85: 2339-2344.

50. Bergfelt DR, Ginther OJ (1992) Embryo loss following GnRH-induced ovulation in anovulatory mares. Theriogenology 38: 33-43.

51. Ginther OJ (1995) Ultrasonic imaging and animal reproduction: Fundamentals, Book 1. Ed: Cross Plains, WI: Equiservices Publishing: 27-82.

52. Montavon S (1994) Ultrasonography of the formation and development of the corpus luteum in the mare: review for the practitioner. Schweiz Arch Tierheilkd 136: 91-94.

53. Plata-Madrid H, Younquist RS, Murphy CN, Bennett-Wimbush K, Braun WF, et al. (1994) Ultrasonographic characteristics of the follicular and uterine dynamics in Belgian mares. J Equine Vet Sci 14: 421-423.

54. Ferreira-Dias G, Costa AS, Mateus L, Korzekwa A, Redmer DA, et al. (2006) Proliferative processes within the equine corpus luteum may depend on paracrine progesterone actions. J Physiol Pharmacol 57: 139-151.

55. Burris T (1999) Progestins. In: Encyclopedia of Reproduction. Knobil E, Neill, JD, (eds.) 4, New York: Acedemic Press: 23-30.

56. Bergfelt DR, Brogliatti GM, Adams GP (1998) Gamete recovery and follicular transfer (graft) using transvaginal ultrasonography in cattle. Theriogenology 50: 15-25.

57. Bollwein H, Mayer R, Weber F, Stolla R (2002) Luteal blood flow during the estrous cycle in mares. Theriogenology 57: 2043-2051.

58. Ginther OJ (2012) The end of the tour de force of the corpus luteum in mares. Theriogenology 77: 1042-1049.

59. Gastal EL, Gastal MO, Nogueira GP, Bergfelt DR, Ginther OJ (2000) Temporal interrelationships among luteolysis, FSH and LH concentrations and follicle deviation in mares. Theriogenology 53: 925-940.

60. Ginther OJ, Beg MA, Gastal EL, Gastal MO, Baerwald AR, et al. (2005) Systemic concentrations of hormones during the development of follicular waves in mares and women: a comparative study. Reproduction 130: 379-388.

61. Medan MS, Nambo Y, Nagamine N, Shinbo H, Watanabe G, et al. (2004) Plasma concentrations of Ir-inhibin, inhibin A, inhibin pro-aC, FSH, and estradiol-17ß during estrous cycle in mares and their relationship with follicular growth. Endocrine 25: 7-14.

62. Kenny HA, Woodruff TK (2006) Follicle size class contributes to distinct secretion patterns of inhibin isoforms during the rat estrous cycle. Endocrinology 147: 51-60.

63. Alexander SL, Irvine CH, Livesey JH, Donald RA (1993) The acute effect of lowering plasma cortisol on the secretion of corticotropin-releasing hormone, arginine vasopressin, and adrenocorticotropin as revealed by intensive sampling of pituitary venous blood in the normal horse. Endocrinology 133: 860-866.

64. Reichert LE Jr (1994) The functional relationship between FSH and its receptor as studied by synthetic peptide strategies. Mol Cell Endocrinol 100: 21-27.

65. Evans JW, Hughes JP, Neely DP, Stabenfeldt GH, Winger CM (1979) Episodic LH secretion patterns in the mare during the oestrous cycle. J Reprod Fertil Suppl 143-150.

66. Pantke P, Hyland J, Galloway DB, MacLean AA, Hoppen HO (1991) Changes in luteinizing hormone bioactivity associated with gonadotrophin pulses in the cycling mare. J Reprod Fertil Suppl 44: 13-18.

67. Hughes IA, Dyas J, Robinson J, Walker RF, Fahmy DR (1985) Monitoring treatment in congenital adrenal hyperplasia. Use of serial measurements of

17-OH-progesterone in plasma, capillary blood, and saliva. Ann N Y Acad Sci 458: 193-202.

68. Amer HA, Shawkig G, Ismail R (2008) Profile of steroid hormones during oestrus and early pregnancy in Arabian mares. Slov Vet Res 45: 25-32.

69. Bergfelt DR, Gastal EL, Ginther OJ (2001) Response of estradiol and inhibin to experimentally reduced luteinizing hormone during follicle deviation in mares. Biol Reprod 65: 426-432.

70. Gouraninezhad S, Kohram H, Khajeh GH, Mashhoori M (2006) Estradiol and progesterone changes in estrus cycle of Arabian mare in khouzestan region. Sci Res Ir Vet J 10: 65-71.

71. Ginther OJ, Utt MD, Beg MA (2007) Follicle deviation and diurnal variation in circulating hormone concentrations in mares. Anim Reprod Sci 100: 197-203.

72. Honnens A, Weisser S, Welter H, Einspanier R, Bollwein H (2011) Relationships between uterine blood flow, peripheral sex steroids, expression of endometrial estrogen receptors and nitric oxide synthases during the estrous cycle in mares. J Reprod Dev 57: 43-48.

73. Daels PF, Hughes JP (1993) The normal estrous cycle. In: Equine Reproduction. McKinnon AO, Voss, JL (eds.). Lea & Febiger, Philadelphia: 121-132.

74. Satué K, Domingo R, Redondo JI (2011) Relationship between progesterone, oestrone sulphate and cortisol and the components of renin angiotensin aldosterone system in Spanish purebred broodmares during pregnancy. Theriogenology 76: 1404-1415.

75. Nagy P, Huszenicza G, Reiczigel J, Juhász J, Kulcsár M, et al. (2004) Factors affecting plasma progesterone concentration and the retrospective determination of time of ovulation in cyclic mares. Theriogenology 61: 203-214.

76. Irvine CH, Turner JE, Alexander SL, Shand N, van Noordt S (1998) Gonadotrophin profiles and dioestrous pulsatile release patterns in mares as determined by collection of jugular blood at 4 h intervals throughout an oestrous cycle. J Reprod Fertil 113: 315-322.

77. Kelley D (2009) The effect of moderate exercise on folliculogenesis, cortisol, estradiol and luteinizing hormone in mare. Doctoral Thesis. School of Clemson University:1-119.

78. Shand N, Irvine CH, Turner JE, Alexander SL (2000) A detailed study of hormonal profiles in mares at luteolysis. J Reprod Fertil Suppl : 271-279.

79. Ginther OJ, Beg MA (2011) Hormone concentration changes temporally associated with the hour of transition from preluteolysis to luteolysis in mares. Anim Reprod Sci 129: 67-72.

22

Cholesterol-Binding by the Yeast CAP Family Member Pry1 Requires the Presence of an Aliphatic Side Chain on Cholesterol

Rabih Darwiche and Roger Schneiter*

University of Fribourg, Department of Biology, 1700 Fribourg, Switzerland

Abstract

Pathogen-related yeast protein 1 (Pry1) is a Saccharomyces cerevisiae member of the CAP/SCP/TAPS super-family. Although, CAP proteins have been proposed to be implicated in a number of physiological processes, such as pathogen virulence, sperm maturation and fertilization, host-pathogen interactions and defense mechanisms, the molecular mode of action of these proteins is poorly understood. CAP proteins are mostly secreted and they are stable in the extracellular space over a wide a range of conditions. All members of this superfamily contain a common CAP domain of approximately 150 amino acids, which adopts a unique α-β-α sandwich fold. We have previously shown that the yeast CAP family members act as sterol-binding and -export proteins in vivo and that the Pry proteins bind cholesterol and cholesteryl acetate in vitro. The conserved CAP domain of Pry1 is necessary and sufficient for sterol binding. Based on these observations, it is conceivable that CAP proteins exert their biological function through a common mechanism, such as binding and sequestration of sterols or related small hydrophobic compounds. Here we analyze the ligand specificity of Pry1 in more detail and show that the presence of the aliphatic isooctane side chain of the sterol but not the 3-hydroxyl group is important for binding to Pry1.

Keywords: Pathogen-related yeast 1 (Pry1); CAP/SCP/TAPS super-family; Sterols; Steroids; *In vitro* Ligand-binding assay; *Saccharomyces cerevisiae*

Introduction

The CAP/SCP/TAPS superfamily of proteins (cysteine-rich secretory proteins, antigen 5 (Ag5), pathogenesis related 1 proteins (PR-1)/sperm coating proteins/Tpx-1/Ag5/PR-1/Sc7; Pfam accession number PF00188) comprises more than 4500 members in over 1500 species and family members are found in all kingdoms of life. CAP proteins have been implicated in a wide variety of processes, including immune defense in mammals and plants, pathogen virulence, sperm maturation and fertilization, venom toxicity, and prostate and brain cancers. CAP proteins are mostly secreted and all members of this superfamily share a common CAP domain of approximately 150 amino acids, which adopts a unique α-β-α sandwich fold and is connected by flexible loop regions. The overall structural conservation within the CAP protein family suggests that these proteins exert fundamentally similar functions. However, the molecular mode of action of this protein family has remained enigmatic [1-3].

The genome of the yeast Saccharomyces cerevisiae encodes for three CAP family members, two of which, Pry1 and Pry2, are secreted, whereas Pry3 is a cell wall-associated protein. Pry1 and Pry2 share a redundant function in the export of acetylated cholesterol and cells lacking both PRY1 and PRY2 have a complete block in secretion of the acetylated lipid in vivo [4]. Purified Pry1 and Pry2 bind both free cholesterol and cholesteryl acetate in vitro [4]. The sterol binding and export function maps to the CAP domain, as its expression alone is efficient to rescue sterol export in cells lacking Pry proteins [4]. Additionally, expression of human CAP member, CRISP2 (cysteine- rich secretory protein 2), or the Schistosoma mansoni venom allergen like protein 4, SmVAL4, in yeast rescues the sterol export defect of a pry1Δ pry2Δ double mutant and purified CRISP2 or SmVAL4 proteins bind cholesterol in vitro, indicating that cholesterol binding and export is a conserved function of diverse CAP superfamily members [4-5]. Computational modeling indicates that ligand binding could occur through displacement of a flexible loop, termed the caveolin-binding motif (CBM) that is rich in aromatic side chains [6]. Point mutations within this motif abrogate sterol export and binding while mutations of residues located outside the CBM had no effect on lipid export and binding. The CBM thus appears to play a key role in the ability of CAP proteins to bind cholesterol [5-7].

Results and Discussion

Cells lacking PRY1 and PRY2 are hypersensitive to the plant oil eugenol and this hypersensitivity is rescued by expression of human CRISP2 [3]. To examine whether Pry1 would directly bind the plant oil eugenol (2-methoxy-4-(2-propenyl) phenol), a member of the allylbenzene class of compounds that is present in clove oil, nutmeg, cinnamon, and bay leaf, and is used as local antiseptic and anesthetic [8-12], we performed a competition-binding assay with purified Pry1 and [3H]-cholesterol. Addition of an equimolar amount (50 pmol) of unlabeled eugenol to the labeled cholesterol resulted in a reduction in binding of the radiolabel cholesterol to Pry1. Addition of an excess of eugenol (100-5000 pmol) reduced binding of the radiolabeled cholesterol even further (Figure 1). These experiments reveal that eugenol efficiently competes with [3H]-cholesterol for binding to Pry1 protein, indicating that both cholesterol and eugenol compete for the same or an overlapping binding site. Thus, Pry1 not only binds free sterols but also small hydrophobic compounds and may thereby protect cellular membranes from a potential detrimental action of eugenol and related small membrane perturbing agents.

*Corresponding author: Schneiter R, University of Fribourg, Department of Biology, Chemin du Musée 10, 1700 Fribourg, Switzerland, E-mail: roger.schneiter@unifr.ch

Thus, while sterols and eugenol are ligands that bind CAP family members, there may be other ligands that are potentially more relevant under particular physiological conditions. As part of an ongoing effort to identify endogenous ligand(s) of Pry1, we probe binding of small hydrophobic compounds in vitro using a competition binding assay [9-10].

Therefore, the ability of a variety of unlabeled sterols and steroids to compete with radiolabeled cholesterol for binding to Pry1 was measured [11-12]. Natural phytosterols like stigmasterol and sitosterol and the fungal sterol ergosterol have a chemical structure that is very similar to cholesterol and all three of these sterols competed efficiently with cholesterol for binding to Pry1 (Figure 2). Similarly, epicholesterol, a structural isomer of cholesterol with a 3α, instead of the normal 3b-hydroxyl group, competed efficiently for binding to Pry1. Similarly, precursors in cholesterol biosynthesis, such as lanosterol and desmosterol competed efficiently for binding to Pry1. On the other hand, the cholesterol synthesis inhibitor U18666A failed to compete (Figure 2).

Further analysis of the in vitro substrate specificity of Pry1 indicated that steroids such as pregnenolone, progesterone, and androstenol, which all lack the aliphatic side chain that is present in cholesterol, failed to compete with radiolabeled cholesterol for binding to Pry1 (Figure 3). However, (+)-4-cholesten-3-one, 7-ketocholesterol and epoxycholesterol, which harbor modifications in the ring system, but contain an isooctane side chain, competed for binding to Pry1 (Figure 3). Thus, the presence of the isooctane side chain is crucial for sterol binding to Pry1.

Taken together, our results show that Pry1 is a cholesterol-binding protein that binds natural sterols, sterol precursors and small hydrophobic ligands such as eugenol. The structure of the competing sterols and that of the non-competing steroids further indicates that sterol binding to Pry1 requires the presence of an aliphatic side chain. Different substitutions in the tetracyclic ring structure, particularly in the A and B ring, or modifications on the 3-hydroxyl group, however, do not affect binding to the protein. These results open the possibility that small compounds such as isooctane may be sufficient to block binding of sterols to Pry1 and possibly other CAP superfamily members. Isooctane may thus be sufficient to neutralize the action of CAP proteins under different physiological settings, including venom toxicity or pathogen virulence.

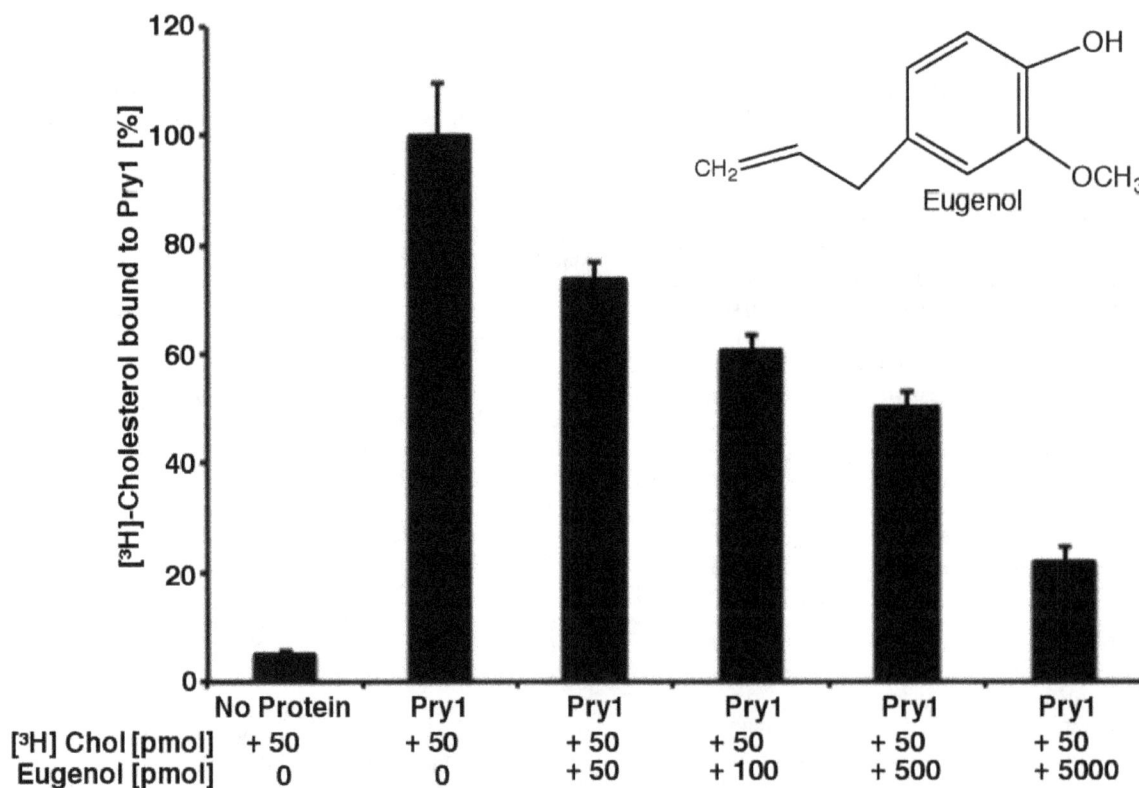

Figure 1: Pry1 protein binds eugenol: Purified Pry1 protein (100 pmol) was incubated with [3H]-cholesterol (50 pmol) as a ligand in the absence (0 pmol), equal amount (50 pmol), or increasing amounts (100-5000 pmol) of eugenol and binding of the radioligand to the protein was measured. The 100% value refers to maximum Pry1 binding capacity in the absence of unlabeled ligand. Values are means ± standard deviations of three independent experiments.

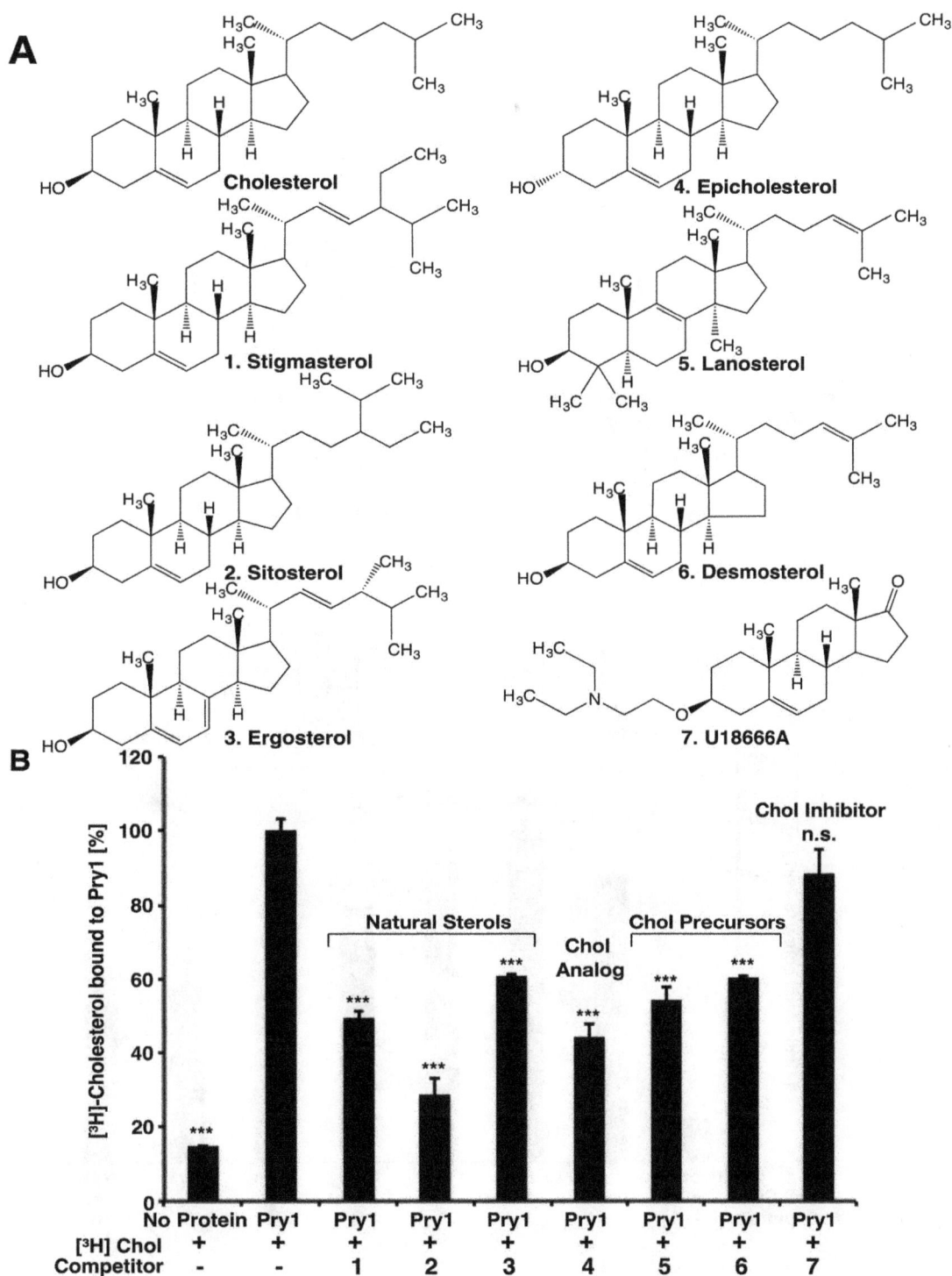

Figure 2: Specificity of sterol binding by Pry1. A) Structures of cholesterol and of the unlabeled sterols tested for their ability to compete with [3H]-cholesterol for binding to Pry1. B) Competitive binding of radiolabeled cholesterol to Pry1 by unlabeled sterol precursors and analogues. Each binding reaction contained 50 pmol of the indicated sterol and an equal amount of [3H]-cholesterol. Values are means ± standard deviations of three independent experiments. Asterisks denote statistical significance (***P<0.0001; n.s. (non-significant)).

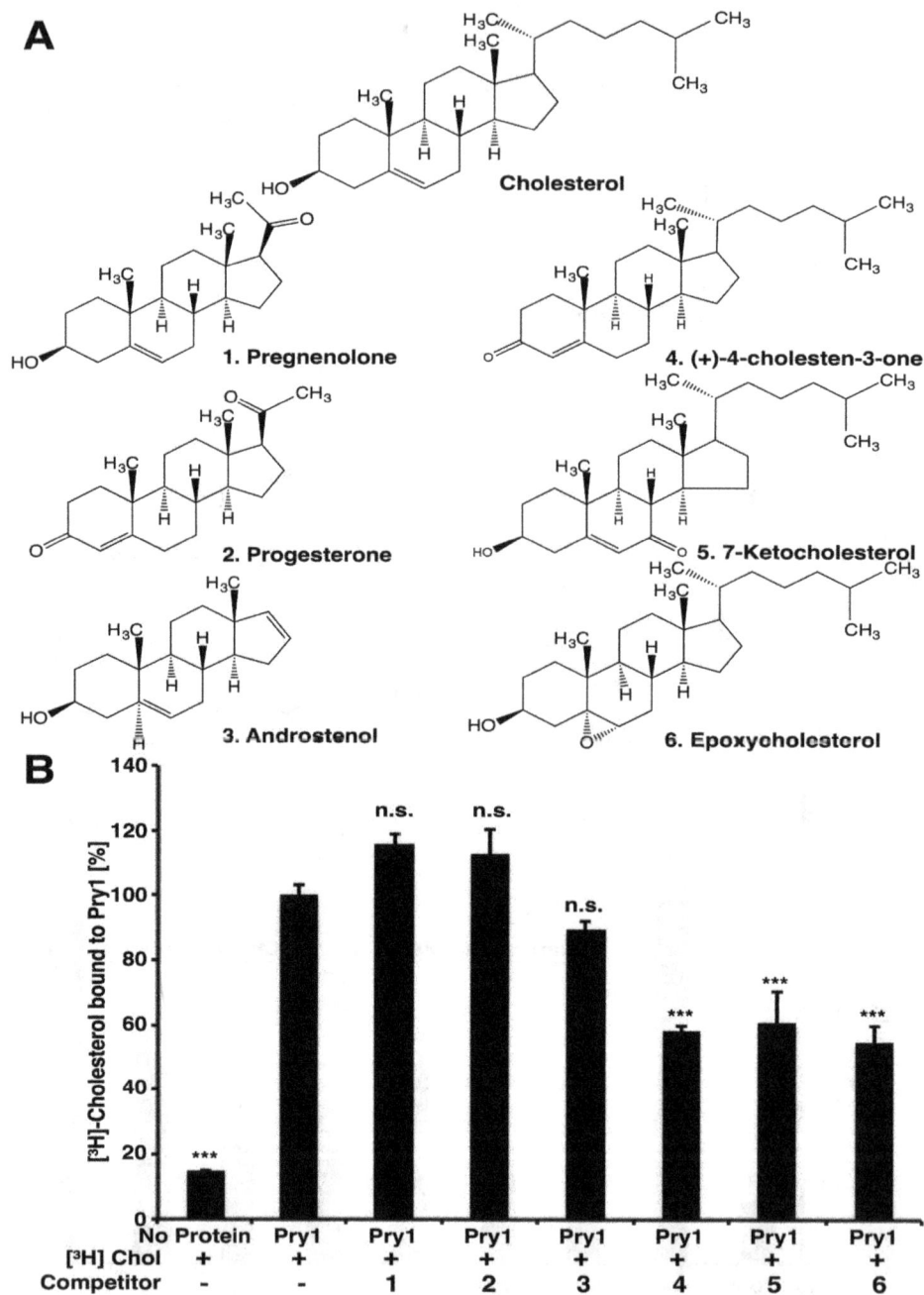

Figure 3: Ligand specificity for Pry1. A) Structures of cholesterol and of unlabeled steroids and sterols tested for their ability to compete with [3H]-cholesterol for binding to Pry1. B) Competitive binding of the indicated ligands. Each reaction contained 50 pmol of the indicated steroid and an equal amount of [3H]-cholesterol. Values are means ± standard deviations of three independent experiments. Asterisks denote statistical significance (***P<0.0001; n.s. (non-significant)).

Acknowledgements

We thank Stéphanie Cottier for critically reading the manuscript. This work was supported by the Swiss National Science Foundation.

References

1. Schneiter R, Di-Pietro A (2013) The CAP protein superfamily: function in sterol export and fungal virulence. Biomol Concepts 4: 519-525.

2. Gibbs GM, Roelants K, O'Bryan MK (2008) The CAP superfamily: cysteine-rich secretory proteins, antigen 5, and pathogenesis-related 1 proteins--roles in reproduction, cancer, and immune defense. Endocr Rev 29:865-897.

3. Cantacessi C, Campbell BE, Visser A, Geldhof P, Nolan MJ, et al. (2009) A portrait of the "SCP/TAPS" proteins of eukaryotes--developing a framework for fundamental research and biotechnological outcomes. Biotechnol Adv 27: 376-388.

4. Choudhary V, Schneiter R (2012) Pathogen-related yeast (PRY) proteins and members of the CAP superfamily are secreted sterol-binding proteins. Proc Natl Acad Sci U S A 109: 16882-16887.

5. Kelleher A, Darwiche R, Rezende WC, Farias LP, Leite LC, et al. (2014) Schistosoma mansoni venom allergen-like protein 4 (SmVAL4) is a novel lipid-binding SCP/TAPS protein that lacks the prototypical CAP motifs. Acta Crystallogr D Biol Crystallogr 70: 2186-2196.

6. Eberle HB, Serrano RL, Fullekrug J, Schlosser A, Lehnmann WD, et al. (2002) Identification and characterization of a novel human plant pathogenesis-related protein that localizes to lipid-enriched microdomains in the Golgi complex. J Cell Sci 115: 827-838.

7. Choudhary V, Darwiche R, Gfeller D, Zoete V, Michielin O, et al. (2014) The caveolin-binding motif of the pathogen-related yeast protein Pry1, a member of the CAP protein superfamily, is required for in vivo export of cholesteryl acetate. J Lipid Res 55: 883-894.

8. Bakkali F, Averbeck S, Averbeck D, Idaomar M (2008) Biological effects of essential oils--a review. Food Chem Toxicol 46: 446-475.

9. Infante RE, Radhakrishnan A, Abi-Mosleh L, Kinch LN, Wang ML (2008) Purified NPC1 protein: II. Localization of sterol binding to a 240-amino acid soluble luminal loop. J Biol Chem 283: 1064-1075.

10. Im YJ, Raychaudhuri S, Prinz WA, Hurley JH (2005) Structural mechanism for sterol sensing and transport by OSBP-related proteins. Nature 437: 154-158.

11. Jacquier N, Schneiter R (2012) Mechanisms of sterol uptake and transport in yeast. J Steroid Biochem Mol Biol 129: 70-78.

12. Tiwari R, Köffel R, Schneiter R (2007) An acetylation/deacetylation cycle controls the export of sterols and steroids from S. cerevisiae. EMBO J 26: 5109-5119.

23

Does Interrelationship of Allopregnanolone and Tetrahydrodeoxycorticosterone during Pregnancy and Postpartum Depression Exist? A Review of the Current Evidence

Mansur A Sandhu[1]*, Muhammad S Anjum[1], Nasir Mukhtar[1], Riaz Hussain[1] and Imtiaz A Khan[2]

[1]Department of Veterinary Biomedical Sciences, PMAS-Arid Agriculture University Rawalpindi, 46300, Shamasabad square, Pakistan
[2]Department of Veterinary Pathobiology, PMAS-Arid Agriculture University Rawalpindi, 46300, Shamasabad square, Pakistan

Abstract

Pregnancy and postpartum changes affect more than a half of women in the world. Neuroactive steroids play a vital role in mental health, behavior, mood development, neuron-protection and memory. This review sums up what is well-known regarding the two types of neuroactive steroids *viz.* allopregnanolone (ALP) and tetrahydrodeoxycorticosterone (THDOC). There is a strong correlation between body progesterone concentration and ALP production. The stage of estrus cycles determines the levels of ALP in body, however, THDOC is a stress induced neuroactive steroid and its level is changeable with the type and severity of stress. The physiological response of stress is affected by THDOC and influences paraventricular nucleus in hypothalamus which in turn controls hypothalamic-pituitary-adrenal and gonadal axis. Both neuroactive steroids are potent endogenous modulators of γ-aminobutyric acid type A ($GABA_A$) receptors and their production gets higher during pregnancy. Now a question arises "do both classes of neuroactive steroids have a potent correlation in their action?" This manuscript will bring you up to date on the interaction and function of these two during pregnancy and postpartum depression.

Keywords: Tetrahydrodeoxycorticosterone; Allopregnanolone; Pregnancy; Postpartum period; Neuroactive steroid; Depression

Introduction

Neurosteroids like tetrahydrodeoxycorticosterone (THDOC) and allopregnanolone (ALP) are metabolites of steroids and formed by the action of 5α-reductase type-1 and 3α-hydroxysteroid dehydrogenase enzymes [1,2]. THDOC and ALP has anticonvulsant, anxiolytic, sedative effects [3,4] and induces behavioural/health changes during pregnancy and menstruation while, anxiety and depression in epilepsy [5-9]. Neuroactive steroids are manufactured in the neurons, astrocytes and glial cells and can be produced from the same tissue [10]. The γ-aminobutyric acid (GABA) system is one of the many inhibitory systems and present in about 25% of the brain receptors [11]. There are three types of GAB_A receptors *viz.* $GABA_A$, $GABA_B$ and $GABA_C$. Both of these neuroactive hormones are $GABA_A$ receptor agonist which is pentameric and has an ion channel in its center [12]. Barbiturates are also GABAA agonist, and these anesthetics inhibit ovulation in rats [13]. There is also a known correlation of ALP and THDOC with GnRH, LH and FSH [14]. Since, there are few studies on the function and working of ALP and THDOC, however, the correlation of neurosteroid influencing the pregnancy and postpartum period is not yet well known. It is likely that GABAergic progesterone metabolites work singularly or coordinal to induce physiological/pathologic effects.

What is allopregnanolone?

ALP is a 3α-hydroxy-A ring-reduced steroid. It is synthesized *de novo* either in brain [15], in the adrenal gland cortex [10,16], and in corpus luteum during the ovulatory menstrual period [17]. The alteration in physiological rhythms of progesterone depends upon stress, stage of menstrual cycle, menopause, and pregnancy. When there is sudden decrease in body progesterone before premenstrual bleeding is the cause of premenstrual syndrome with similar symptoms in the postmenopausal women [18,19]. ALP levels gets higher during

early and postmenopausal women receiving dehydroepiandrosterone and the values get as much higher as are pragmatic in pregnancy [20]. This steroid metabolite exerts neuromodulatory possessions in CNS and is a $GABA_A$ receptor agonist that affects mood, modulating anxiety, and memory [21,22]. There is a positive correlation between body ALP levels and the level of progesterone [23,24]. In estrus cycle, the body ALP level diverges with the change in phases of estrus. During luteal phase the level of ALP is about four times higher than the follicular phase [25] and gets at its peak with the advancement in pregnancy [24]. Animal studies show that the ALP levels remain elevated in the brain than blood circulation [16]. After the exposure to stress there is an increase of circulating ALP [25] than the normal calm and quite state, however, in adrenalectomized rats [10] the concentration of ALP remained undetectable in the plasma.

What is THDOC?

An increased activity of hypothalamic-pituitary-adrenal (HPA)-axis is due to more production of corticotropin releasing hormone (CRH), which is a key arbitrator of CNS stress [26]. After acute stress the hypothalamus production of CRH increases that prompts the discharge of ACTH from the anterior pituitary gland, which ultimately excites cortex of the adrenal for the production of glucocorticoids and neuroactive steroid precursors [27]. There are two types of glucocorticoids present eg. cortisol (human & non-human primates) and corticosterones (rodents); these give negative feedback upon

*Corresponding author: Mansur A Sandhu, Department of Veterinary Biomedical Sciences, Faculty of Veterinary and Animal Sciences, PMAS, Arid Agriculture University, Rawalpindi, Pakistan, E-mail: mansoorsandhu@uaar.edu.pk

the pituitary gland and hypothalamus. To counteract the increase of ACTH or corticosterone in stressed rats 3α, 5α-THDOC come and play its role to decline hypothalamic CRH mRNA levels and vasopressin [28] ultimately ACTH discharge and corticosterone levels of rats. Out of adrenal cortex, the 3α, 5α-THDOC development calls for the accessibility of deoxycorticosterone, and its synthesis is under ACTH control [29]. This decrease of CRH level may has a positive effect to save animal from stressful conditions, returning the body back towards homeostasis and is critical for mental health in premenstrual dysphoric disorders. However, after adrenalactomy the production of THDOC fades away from the brain along with disappearance of 2l-hydroxylase. THDOC synthesis in brain needs deoxycorticosterone production by adrenal cortex. Interestingly THDOC release is more after stress stimuli. During the time of stress there is about 7-8 folds increase in the formation of THDOC from rat adrenal cortex and in plasma [25,30], it takes about 10-30 minutes to get its peak after stress [4] stimuli. Together with adrenal cortex, THDOC is also renewed from its forerunner in the brain neurons [6]. Enzymatic cleavage of deoxycorticosterone is with 5α-reductase and 3α-hydroxysteroid oxidoreductase (Figure 1) to form 5α-DHDOC and 3α, 5α-THDOC increase during depression.

Interaction of THDOC and ALP with other hormones

To exert the effects in brain, cortisol also uses mineralocorticoid receptor and its affinity is 10-folds higher than glucocorticoid receptors. In brain mineralocorticoid receptor is primarily articulated in the hippocampus. Both glucocorticoid and mineralocorticoid receptors are blamed for the production of anxiety and cognitive conditions [31]. Different studies on laboratory animals have confirmed that after stress there is an increase in mineralocorticoid receptor of hippocampus [32,33] and anxiolytic if we block mineralocorticoid receptors [34,35]. On the other hand, Otte et al. [36] demonstrated the inter-relationship of human mineralocorticoid receptor blockage with anxiolytic effects and shown similar results. In human, there is an increased production of plasma cortisol concentration with the use of mineralocorticoid receptor blocking agents as described by Arvat et al. [37] and Wellhoener et al. [38].

The ALP along with THDOC (Figure 2) is potent endogenous modulators of GABA$_A$ receptors having the role of anxiolytic, anticonvulsant, and sedative actions [39]. Evidences show that THDOC has a predisposition to protect neurons of developing brain in opposition to unfavorable emotional conditions. It is important to note down that, GABAergic agonists have the tendency to persuade behavioral modifications for the period of perinatal life [40]. However the mechanism through which THDOC induces gene transcription of corticoids receptor and neuropeptides remain difficult to understand. Thus the hypothesis was put forward that different neuron-hormones

can modulate glucocorticoid receptors and CRH gene transcription [41]. There are strong evidences that neuroactive steroids also interact with steroid receptors, after oxidation THDOC and THP have the tendency to bind with progesterone receptor [42]. With occurrence of catamenial epilepsy seizure there is a sudden decline in progesterone secretion during the premenstrual period [43] and the treatment with progestin is helpful [44]. There may be relationship of seizures attenuation by augmentation of GABA$_A$-mediated inhibition of neural excitability after progestin treatment. Since, progesterone metabolites are potent allosteric modulators of GABA$_A$ receptors [5]. Recent studies have revealed that serum FSH and LH reduces after I/V injection of ALP during the follicular phase and a negative relationship was flanked by ALP and FSH. In an animal model the increased concentration of ALP or it's injection to boost the circulating levels has an opposing effects on the circulating levels of GnRH, LH, FSH and this will ultimately suppress the formation of follicle and release of ova [14,45]. Similar results of delayed follicular phase with THDOC enhancement are present in rats [13] but no effect in primates [46]. These results can be correlated with human where elevated levels of ALP may induce premature ovarian failure [47].

Relationship of THDOC and ALP with pregnancy and postpartum depression

Pregnancy is among the most common physiological condition with lofty levels of steroids in a woman at child bearing age that makes her more prone to depression [48,49]. This postpartum depression (PPD) is a transitory type during pregnancy and after childbirth. Two forms of PPD: either "baby blues" or "late onset". The baby blues type exists as many as 80% of women subsequent to delivery and generally resolves in few weeks devoid of treatment. The later onset form of PPD is more ruthless and is diagnosed after few weeks of delivery and its existence is in about 10-16% of childbearing women. The indications of PPD consist of anxiety, problematic sleep, sadness, memory impairment, mood changes, and tearfulness [50]. An average of 20% women with blues will expand long-term depression. There are evidences that infant-mother bond gets disturbed with PPD [51] and later problems in child's socio-emotional development [52,53]. In adrenal and CNS, neuroactive steroids (THDOC and ALP) are created *de novo* from cholesterol (Figure 2) [54] and the change in levels of steroid hormone ultimately changes the levels of neuroactive steroids [54]. A variety of physiological (pregnancy) and pathological (stress) alterations in the body lead to modify the levels of neuroactive steroids in the CNS. Exogenous administration of steroid hormones results in depression merely among all the women those have the history of postpartum depression [55]. This shows that some women must be predisposed to postpartum depression. Every individual either human or animal are at all times under the challenges of stress. Though, all

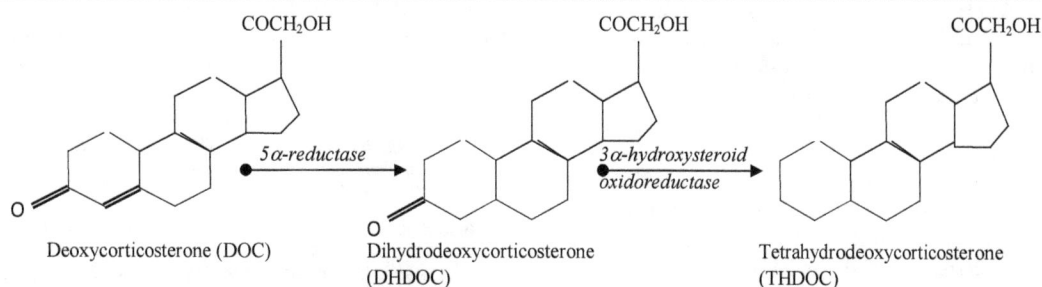

Figure 1: Structural alteration of Deoxycorticosterone (DOC) to 5α-dihydrodeoxycorticosterone (DHDOC) and then Tetrahydrodeoxycorticosterone (THDOC) through enzymes 5α reductase and 3α hydroxysteroid oxidoreductase.

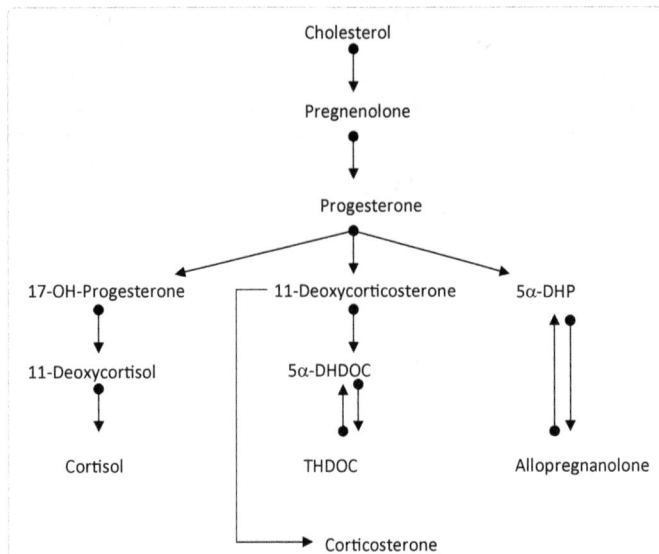

Figure 2: The creation of neurosteroids from cholesterol along with metabolic pathway. DHDOC=Dihydrodeoxycorticosterone, THDOC=Tetrahydrodeoxycorticosterone, DHP=Dihydroprogesterone.

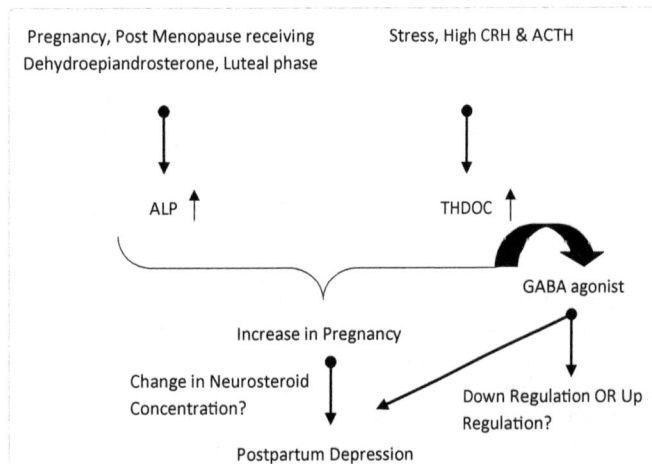

Figure 3: The flow diagram showing events and possible neurosteroids correlations in the creation of pregnancy and postpartum depression. CRH=corticotrophin releasing hormone; ACTH=Adrenocorticotropic hormone; THDOC=tetrahydrodeoxycorticosterone; ALP=allopregnanolone; GABA=aminobutyric acid receptor.

imbalance in these neurostroids was observed with the use of fluoxetine and fluvoxamine and control group got higher levels of neurostroids then clinically depressed patients [62]. During first trimester of gestation noticeable dizziness is pragmatic, which is later decreased in next trimesters of the gestation. This can be correlated with the levels of neuroactive steroids, even in later pregnancy progesterone and ALP gets higher those effects on sedation. In non-pregnant women sedation takes place with lower concentrations of ALP [63]. This may be due to $GABA_A$ tolerance to ALP at some stage in pregnancy. Perhaps, the change in mood and neurological disorders during PPD is due to down regulation of $GABA_A$ receptors during pregnancy, as there is abrupt fall of progesterone and their metabolites. The results of an animal study reveals that, at 18 days of rat pregnancy a decline in the appearance of $GABA_A$ receptor δ subunit in hippocampus was observed, which bounces back to virgin levels within 48 hours postpartum [64]. The eminently high levels of THDOC not only affect $GABA_A$ but also alter neuronal excitability. The psychological health changes of the 'third day blues' and PPD [65,66] are hormone-related indications similarly as premenstrual dysphoric disorder [67]. It is also stated that $GABA_A$ receptors down-regulated is one among all causes of adverse behavior change. However, Sanna et al. [68] stated more complex regulation of $GABA_A$ receptors throughout pregnancy or there may be species differences in steroid hormone-mediated $GABA_A$ receptors regulation. They proposed if there is deficiency of $GABA_A$ receptor regulation in pregnancy and postpartum period, this may influence mood disarray during postpartum such as PPD. The association of mood disorders with postpartum period is particularly related to changing levels of steroid hormone or the site of steroid hormone action namely the $GABA_A$ receptor δ subunit. When the mice are deficient in $GABA_A$ receptor δ subunit (*Gabrd*$^{-/-}$ mice), they show signs of depression within 48 hours postpartum with forced swimming stress. These mice also fail to make nest and keep their pups away from dam those die due to neglecting behavior or cannibalism [63,64]. Based on the presented data we can put forward a hypothesis (Figure 3) that different psychological changes, mood disorders, intolerance, and problematic sleep may be due to the change in neurosteroid (ALP and THDOC) concentration, sensitivity or down/up regulation of the hormone/$GABA_A$ receptors.

Concluding Remarks

The authors have tried to summarize the evidences pertaining THDOC and ALP with pregnancy and postpartum depression (PPD). Though discussion is very brief, still we can state that a strong correlation exists between THDOC and ALP. Both of these neuroactive steroids have anxiolytic, anticonvulsant and other protective properties. Almost all neuroactive steroids share similar receptors for steroid hormones, have an important role in the up-regulation and down-regulations of $GABA_A$ receptors. Further studies are strongly needed before ascertaining any conclusion from the interactions of neuroactive steroids with other endocrine hormones, responses in stress, pregnancy and generation of postpartum depression.

References

1. Hosie AM, Wilkins ME, da Silva HM, Smart TG (2006) Endogenous neurosteroids regulate GABAA receptors through two discrete transmembrane sites. Nature 444: 486-489.

2. Agís-Balboa RC, Pinna G, Zhubi A, Maloku E, Veldic M, et al. (2006) Characterization of brain neurons that express enzymes mediating neurosteroid biosynthesis. Proc Natl Acad Sci U S A 103: 14602-14607.

3. Reddy DS, Rogawski MA (2002) Stress-induced deoxycorticosterone-derived neurosteroids modulate GABA(A) receptor function and seizure susceptibility. J Neurosci 22: 3795-3805.

environments pose its unique set of stresses and the body must be talented for proper response to maintain homeostasis [56]. The stress in pregnancy also activates HPA-axis resulting in overproduction of corticosteroids and high levels in both circulating and brain THDOC (from 1-5 nM to 15-30 nM) as given by Reddy and Rogawski, [3]; Maguire and Mody, [57] and ALP (about 8-folds) as described by Purdy et al. [10]. Another factor of increased ALP during pregnancy is high levels of progesterone (about 200-folds) [58] and exogenous steroids especially in the treatment of preterm labour may results in an increases of neuroactive steroids ALP and THDOC [59]. So, we can state that both THDOC and ALP are important in pregnancy and have a direct role in PPD production. Neuroactive steroids such as 3α, 5α-tetrahydroprogesterone (THP) and THDOC work mutually as positive modulators of $GABA_A$ receptors [60]. With the use of antidepressant medicines the production of THP and THDOC in rat's brain increase with no change in blood levels [61]. In a human study

4. Reddy DS (2003) Pharmacology of endogenous neuroactive steroids. Crit Rev Neurobiol 15: 197-234.

5. Tuveri A, Paoletti AM, Orrù M, Melis GB, Marotto MF, et al. (2008) Reduced serum level of THDOC, an anticonvulsant steroid, in women with perimenstrual catamenial epilepsy. Epilepsia 49: 1221-1229.

6. Reddy DS (2003) Is there a physiological role for the neurosteroid THDOC in stress-sensitive conditions? Trends Pharmacol Sci 24: 103-106.

7. Reddy DS (2006) Physiological role of adrenal deoxycorticosterone-derived neuroactive steroids in stress-sensitive conditions. Neuroscience 138: 911-920.

8. Eser D, Schüle C, Baghai TC, Romeo E, Rupprecht R (2006) Neuroactive steroids in depression and anxiety disorders: clinical studies. Neuroendocrinology 84: 244-254.

9. Maguire J, Mody I (2007) Neurosteroid synthesis-mediated regulation of GABA(A) receptors: relevance to the ovarian cycle and stress. J Neurosci 27: 2155-2162.

10. Purdy RH, Morrow AL, Moore PH Jr, Paul SM (1991) Stress-induced elevations of gamma-aminobutyric acid type A receptor-active steroids in the rat brain. Proc Natl Acad Sci U S A 88: 4553-4557.

11. Hendry SH, Schwark HD, Jones EG, Yan J (1987) Numbers and proportions of GABA-immunoreactive neurons in different areas of monkey cerebral cortex. J Neurosci 7: 1503-1519.

12. Nayeem N, Green TP, Martin IL, Barnard EA (1994) Quaternary structure of the native GABAA receptor determined by electron microscopic image analysis. J Neurochem 62: 815-818.

13. Hagino N, Ramaley JA, Gorski RA (1966) Inhibition of estrogen-induced precocious ovulation by pentobarbital in the rat. Endocrinology 79: 451-454.

14. Timby E, Hedström H, Bäckström T, Sundström-Poromaa I, Nyberg S, et al. (2011) Allopregnanolone, a GABAA receptor agonist, decreases gonadotropin levels in women. A preliminary study. Gynecol Endocrinol 27: 1087-1093.

15. Melcangi RC, Magnaghi V, Martini L (1999) Steroid metabolism and effects in central and peripheral glial cells. J Neurobiol 40: 471-483.

16. Corpéchot C, Young J, Calvel M, Wehrey C, Veltz JN, et al. (1993) Neurosteroids: 3 alpha-hydroxy-5 alpha-pregnan-20-one and its precursors in the brain, plasma, and steroidogenic glands of male and female rats. Endocrinology 133: 1003-1009.

17. Ottander U, Poromaa IS, Bjurulf E, Skytt A, Bäckström T, et al. (2005) Allopregnanolone and pregnanolone are produced by the human corpus luteum. Mol Cell Endocrinol 239: 37-44.

18. Bicíková M, Dibbelt L, Hill M, Hampl R, Stárka L (1998) Allopregnanolone in women with premenstrual syndrome. Horm Metab Res 30: 227-230.

19. Genazzani AR, Petraglia F, Bernardi F, Casarosa E, Salvestroni C, et al. (1998) Circulating levels of allopregnanolone in humans: gender, age, and endocrine influences. J Clin Endocrinol Metab 83: 2099-2103.

20. Luisi S, Petraglia F, Benedetto C, Nappi RE, Bernardi F, et al. (2000) Serum allopregnanolone levels in pregnant women: changes during pregnancy, at delivery, and in hypertensive patients. J Clin Endocrinol Metab 85: 2429-2433.

21. Robel P, Baulieu EE (1994) Neurosteroids Biosynthesis and function. Trends Endocrinol Metab 5: 1-8.

22. Baulieu EE, Robel P, Schumacher M (2001) Neurosteroids: beginning of the story. Int Rev Neurobiol 46: 1-32.

23. Wang M, Seippel L, Purdy RH, Bäckström T (1996) Relationship between symptom severity and steroid variation in women with premenstrual syndrome: study on serum pregnenolone, pregnenolone sulfate, 5 alpha-pregnane-3,20-dione and 3 alpha-hydroxy-5 alpha-pregnan-20-one. J Clin Endocrinol Metab 81: 1076-1082.

24. Parízek A, Hill M, Kancheva R, Havlíková H, Kancheva L, et al. (2005) Neuroactive pregnanolone isomers during pregnancy. J Clin Endocrinol Metab 90: 395-403.

25. Havlíková H, Hill M, Kancheva L, Vrbíková J, Pouzar V, et al. (2006) Serum profiles of free and conjugated neuroactive pregnanolone isomers in nonpregnant women of fertile age. J Clin Endocrinol Metab 91: 3092-3099.

26. Serra M, Pisu MG, Littera M, Papi G, Sanna E, et al. (2000) Social isolation-induced decreases in both the abundance of neuroactive steroids and GABA(A) receptor function in rat brain. J Neurochem 75: 732-740.

27. Holsboer F, Spengler D, Heuser I (1992) The role of corticotropin-releasing hormone in the pathogenesis of Cushing's disease, anorexia nervosa, alcoholism, affective disorders and dementia. Prog Brain Res 93: 385-417.

28. Patchev VK, Montkowski A, Rouskova D, Koranyi L, Holsboer F, et al. (1997) Neonatal treatment of rats with the neuroactive steroid tetrahydrodeoxycorticosterone (THDOC) abolishes the behavioral and neuroendocrine consequences of adverse early life events. J Clin Invest 99: 962-966.

29. Mensah-Nyagan AG, Do-Rego JL, Beaujean D, Luu-The V, Pelletier G, et al. (1999) Neurosteroids: expression of steroidogenic enzymes and regulation of steroid biosynthesis in the central nervous system. Pharmacol Rev 51: 63-81.

30. Barbaccia ML, Concas A, Serra M, Biggio G (1998) Stress and neurosteroids in adult and aged rats. Exp Gerontol 33: 697-712.

31. de Kloet ER, Joëls M, Holsboer F (2005) Stress and the brain: from adaptation to disease. Nat Rev Neurosci 6: 463-475.

32. Ladd CO, Huot RL, Thrivikraman KV, Nemeroff CB, Plotsky PM (2004) Long-term adaptations in glucocorticoid receptor and mineralocorticoid receptor mRNA and negative feedback on the hypothalamo-pituitary-adrenal axis following neonatal maternal separation. Biol Psychiatry 55: 367-375.

33. Sandi C, Touyarot K (2006) Mid-life stress and cognitive deficits during early aging in rats: individual differences and hippocampal correlates. Neurobiol Aging 27: 128-140.

34. Smythe JW, Murphy D, Timothy C, Costall B (1997) Hippocampal mineralocorticoid, but not glucocorticoid, receptors modulate anxiety-like behavior in rats. Pharmacol Biochem Behav 56: 507-513.

35. Bitran D, Shiekh M, Dowd JA, Dugan MM, Renda P (1998) Corticosterone is permissive to the anxiolytic effect that results from the blockade of hippocampal mineralocorticoid receptors. Pharmacol Biochem Behav 60: 879-887.

36. Otte C, Moritz S, Yassouridis A, Koop M, Madrischewski AM, et al. (2007) Blockade of the mineralocorticoid receptor in healthy men: effects on experimentally induced panic symptoms, stress hormones, and cognition. Neuropsychopharmacology 32: 232-238.

37. Arvat E, Maccagno B, Giordano R, Pellegrino M, Broglio F, et al. (2001) Mineralocorticoid receptor blockade by canrenoate increases both spontaneous and stimulated adrenal function in humans. J Clin Endocrinol Metab 86: 3176-3181.

38. Wellhoener P, Born J, Fehm HL, Dodt C (2004) Elevated resting and exercise-induced cortisol levels after mineralocorticoid receptor blockade with canrenoate in healthy humans. J Clin Endocrinol Metab 89: 5048-5052.

39. Reddy DS, Kulkarni SK (2000) Development of neurosteroid-based novel psychotropic drugs. Prog Med Chem 37: 135-175.

40. Schroeder H, Humbert AC, Koziel V, Desor D, Nehlig A (1995) Behavioral and metabolic consequences of neonatal exposure to diazepam in rat pups. Exp Neurol 131: 53-63.

41. Rage F, Jalaguier S, Rougeot C, Tapia-Arancibia L (1993) GABA inhibition of somatostatin gene expression in cultured hypothalamic neurones. Neuroreport 4: 320-322.

42. Rupprecht R, Reul JM, Trapp T, van Steensel B, Wetzel C, et al. (1993) Progesterone receptor-mediated effects of neuroactive steroids. Neuron 11: 523-530.

43. Herzog AG, Klein P, Ransil BJ (1997) Three patterns of catamenial epilepsy. Epilepsia 38: 1082-1088.

44. Herzog AG (1995) Progesterone therapy in women with complex partial and secondary generalized seizures. Neurology 45: 1660-1662.

45. Sullivan SD, Moenter SM (2003) Neurosteroids alter gamma-aminobutyric acid postsynaptic currents in gonadotropin-releasing hormone neurons: a possible mechanism for direct steroidal control. Endocrinology 144: 4366-4375.

46. Hagino N (1979) Effect of nembutal on LH release in baboons. Horm Metab Res 11: 296-300.

47. Bernardi F, Hartmann B, Casarosa E, Luisi S, Stomati M, et al. (1998) High levels of serum allopregnanolone in women with premature ovarian failure. Gynecol Endocrinol 12: 339-345.

48. Myers JK, Weissman MM, Tischler GL, Holzer CE 3rd, Leaf PJ, et al. (1984) Six-month prevalence of psychiatric disorders in three communities 1980 to 1982. Arch Gen Psychiatry 41: 959-967.

49. O'Hara MW, Swain AM (1996) Rates and risk of postpartum depression: a meta-analysis. Int Rev Psychiatry 8: 37-54.

50. Zonana J, Gorman JM (2005) The neurobiology of postpartum depression. CNS Spectr 10: 792-799, 805.

51. Cummings ME, Davies PT (1992) prenatal depression, family functioning, and child adjustment: risk factors, processes, and pathways. In: Cicchetti D, Toth SL, eds. Development Perspectives on Depression. Rochester, NY: University of Rochester Press. 283-322.

52. Downey G, Coyne JC (1990) Children of depressed parents: an integrative review. Psychol Bull 108: 50-76.

53. Patel M, Bailey RK, Jabeen S, Ali S, Barker NC, et al. (2012) Postpartum depression: a review. J Health Care Poor Underserved 23: 534-542.

54. Stoffel-Wagner B (2001) Neurosteroid metabolism in the human brain. Eur J Endocrinol 145: 669-679.

55. Bloch M, Schmidt PJ, Danaceau M, Murphy J, Nieman L, et al. (2000) Effects of gonadal steroids in women with a history of postpartum depression. Am J Psychiatry 157: 924-930.

56. Sandhu MA, Mirza FQ, Afzal F, Mukhtar N (2012) Effect of heat stress on cellular and humoral immunity and its cure with a-tocopherol in meat type birds. Livestock Sci 148: 181-188.

57. Maguire J, Mody I (2009) Steroid hormone fluctuations and GABA(A)R plasticity. Psychoneuroendocrinology 34 Suppl 1: S84-90.

58. Bäckström T, Andersson A, Andreé L, Birzniece V, Bixo M, et al. (2003) Pathogenesis in menstrual cycle-linked CNS disorders. Ann N Y Acad Sci 1007: 42-53.

59. Concas A, Mostallino MC, Porcu P, Follesa P, Barbaccia ML, et al. (1998) Role of brain allopregnanolone in the plasticity of gamma-aminobutyric acid type A receptor in rat brain during pregnancy and after delivery. Proc Natl Acad Sci U S A 95: 13284-13289.

60. Lambert JJ, Belelli D, Hill-Venning C, Peters JA (1995) Neurosteroids and GABAA receptor function. Trends Pharmacol Sci 16: 295-303.

61. Uzunov DP, Cooper TB, Costa E, Guidotti A (1996) Fluoxetine-elicited changes in brain neurosteroid content measured by negative ion mass fragmentography. Proc Natl Acad Sci U S A 93: 12599-12604.

62. Uzunova V, Sheline Y, Davis JM, Rasmusson A, Uzunov DP, et al. (1998) Increase in the cerebrospinal fluid content of neurosteroids in patients with unipolar major depression who are receiving fluoxetine or fluvoxamine. P Natl Acad Sci USA 95: 3239-3244.

63. Timby E, Balgård M, Nyberg S, Spigset O, Andersson A, et al. (2006) Pharmacokinetic and behavioral effects of allopregnanolone in healthy women. Psychopharmacology (Berl) 186: 414-424.

64. Maguire J, Mody I (2008) GABA(A)R plasticity during pregnancy: relevance to postpartum depression. Neuron 59: 207-213.

65. Nemeroff CB (2008) Understanding the pathophysiology of postpartum depression: implications for the development of novel treatments. Neuron 59: 185-186.

66. Pearlstein T, Howard M, Salisbury A, Zlotnick C (2009) Postpartum depression. Am J Obstet Gynecol 200: 357-364.

67. Bloch M, Rotenberg N, Koren D, Klein E (2006) Risk factors for early postpartum depressive symptoms. Gen Hosp Psychiatry 28: 3-8.

68. Sanna E, Mostallino MC, Murru L, Carta M, Talani G, et al. (2009) Changes in expression and function of extrasynaptic GABAA receptors in the rat hippocampus during pregnancy and after delivery. J Neurosci 29: 1755-1765.

24

Effects of Aromatase Inhibition on the Physical Activity Levels of Male Mice

Robert S Bowen[1,2]*, David P Ferguson[2,3] and J Timothy Lightfoot[2,3]

[1]Science and Mathematics Division, Truett-McConnell College, Cleveland, GA 30528, USA
[2]Department of Kinesiology, University of North Carolina Charlotte, Charlotte, NC 28223, USA
[3]Department of Health and Kinesiology, Texas A&M University, College Station, TX 77845, USA

Abstract

Increasing activity levels in an inactive population can lead to associative increases in health and well-being. Both biologic and genetic factors have been identified that alter physical activity levels in humans and rodents with an extensive early literature regarding sex steroid effects on physical activity. Currently, it is suggested that the androgens require conversion to estrogens prior to eliciting any effects on activity patterns. Recent data contradicts this assertion; thus, the purpose of this study was to evaluate the necessity of the aromatase complex in activity regulation. Wheel running was assessed in male C57BL/6J mice under various sex steroid-disrupted and aromatase-inhibited conditions. Inhibition of the aromatase complex was achieved through administration of two different aromatase inhibiting substances—letrozole and exemestane. Wheel running was unaffected by aromatase inhibition in reproductively intact and sex steroid supplemented mice. Orchidectomy significantly reduced wheel running activity. Steroid replacement recovered wheel running to pre-surgical levels; however, aromatase inhibition did not further affect wheel running levels. The recovery of wheel running in mice with androgen supplementation and the further persistence of wheel running in mice with compromised aromatase function suggests that the androgens—testosterone in particular—may directly affect wheel running patterns in male mice.

Keywords: Sex Steroid; Sex Hormone; Locomotion; Exemestane; Letrozole

Introduction

Physical inactivity affects public health and unnecessarily burdens the health care system. The risks of many diseases including obesity, diabetes, heart disease and several types of cancer are enhanced in individuals with habitually low physical activity levels [1]. Although evidence exists suggesting that activity levels are determined by extrinsic and environmental factors, a growing number of scientific studies suggest large genetic and biological influences also exist [2-8]. Androgens and estrogens have been the focus of extensive research relating to activity levels in rodents. Notably, the surgical removal of testes or ovaries results in noted reductions in daily wheel running activity [9-13].

Currently, it is suggested that testosterone requires conversion to an estrogenic compound before any modulatory interactions to the wheel running response will occur. Roy and Wade [14] administered aromatizable and non-aromatizable forms of androgens to orchidectomized rats. The aromatizable androgen notably increased wheel running, but administration of the non-aromatizable molecule resulted in continued quiescence.

Supporting Roy and Wade's earlier study, Watai et al. [15] found that wheel running activity was hindered in an estrogen-deficient aromatase knockout mouse model. Conversely, Hill et al. [16], using a similar aromatase knockout model found that the male knockout animals ran nearly twice as far as wild type animals, an observation that was reversed in three weeks with the administration of 17β-estradiol. While the use of knockout animals can lead to difficulties with interpretation due to issues arising during development [17], it is interesting that the two studies using aromatase knockout animals resulted in completely opposite results.

Thus, other experimental methods, such as the use of aromatase-inhibiting substances to circumvent the issues related to the use of knockout animals, are warranted for further elucidation of the roles of the sex steroids in physical activity regulation. With a pharmacological approach, the functionality of particular physiological pathways can be altered without hindering normal development. Therefore, the purpose of this study was to evaluate wheel running activity in the presence of irreversible and reversible aromatase inhibitors under normal physiological conditions and during artificial manipulation of endogenous sex steroid levels in male mice.

Materials and Methods

Eighty male C57BL/6J mice (Jackson Laboratories, Bar Harbor, ME) were used in three experimental procedures. All mice were housed in an environmentally controlled animal husbandry facility under a 12/12 h light/dark cycle with lights illuminating the housing room at 6:00am daily. After arrival at the research facility, mice were initially housed with six to eight littermates prior to initiating experimental protocols. After acclimation and at approximately eight weeks of age (≈54 days old), the animals were individually housed in standard rat sized cages with metal running wheels during each experiment. The cages were equipped with a stainless metal food hopper and glass water bottle allowing *ad libitum* access to both food and water. Activity data collection began when the mice were 63 days of age. Physical activity levels are near a maximum and demonstrate low levels of variation

---

*Corresponding author: Robert S Bowen, 100 Alumni Drive, Science and Mathematics Division, Truett-McConnell College, Cleveland, GA 30528, USA, E-mail: rbowen@truett.edu

across the ages utilized in this experiment [18] minimizing the effects of age on wheel running indices. This project conformed to the ethical standards set forth by the scientific community and was approved by the UNC Charlotte Institutional Animal Care and Use Committee prior to initiation.

Running wheels (450 mm circumference; Ware Manufacturing, Phoenix, AZ) with a 40 mm wide solid running surface were attached to the metal tops of each cage and were equipped with cycling computers (BC500, Sigma Sport, Olney, IL) to track wheel running distance (km) and duration (min). Average speeds (m·min⁻¹) for each day of analysis was calculated by dividing distance by duration. Each experimental epoch lasted seven days and wheel running data was collected every 24 hours. Average daily distance, duration, and speed were calculated for each seven day experimental epoch. Each computer was calibrated to the running wheel's circumference and was checked for proper connectivity on a daily basis by a research technician. Furthermore, the freeness of the wheel's rotation about the axle was checked daily and lubricated as needed. The wheels were sanitized every two weeks for the length of the experiments and were brushed when needed to keep the running surface free of debris (bedding, food, feces, etc.). The physical activity indices measured in this project have previously been shown to exhibit a high level of repeatability in our hands [19].

During this study, control and experimental injections of aromatase inhibitors were administered. Control injections consisted of 0.3% hydroxypropyl cellulose in phosphate buffered saline (HPC+PBS) and were administered in a 500 μl subcutaneous bolus over a two minute period to ensure full delivery and absorption of the solution. Experimental injections contained the irreversible aromatase inhibitor exemestane (Sigma-Aldrich, St. Louis, MO) suspended in HPC+PBS. Exemestane aggressively inhibits aromatase activity in a wide array of tissues including the brain and adipose tissue [20-21]. The drug was administered subcutaneously at a dosage of 250 mg·kg⁻¹ per 500 μl bolus. This dosing schedule and administration technique has previously been shown to yield maximum inhibition of aromatase activity [22-24]. Prior to administration, steps were taken to maintain the sterility of the injection medium by using a standard liquid autoclave cycle prior to storage in a sterile lab container. The exemestane was dissolved in methanol and passed through a 0.2 micron cellulose filter into a sterile mortar to remove impurities in the drug. The methanol was then evaporated and the residue exemestane was pulverized and added to an aliquot of sterile HPC+PBS to form a dispensable suspension for injection.

Exemestane has both aromatase-inhibiting and androgenic properties. It was speculated that any observed exemestane effect might be due to the androgenic rather than the aromatase inhibiting effects; therefore, the reversible aromatase inhibitor letrozole (Fisher Scientific, Pittsburgh, PA) was used to validate the results achieved in the exemestane phase of the project. Letrozole was administered via sub-cutaneous injections at a concentration of 0.5 μg per 100 μl of 0.3% HPC+PBS for seven days using; the dosing schedule and administration techniques used for letrozole injections followed well established methods [25]. Placebo injections consisted of 0.3% HPC+PBS.

To vary the levels of circulating steroids, two procedures were employed. First, supplementation or replacement of steroids was achieved via silastic (Dow Corning, Midland, MI) implants. Our silastic implant technique has a long established and validated record of supplementation/replacement and has previously been shown to modulate steroid levels in rodents [26-33]. Thus, testosterone and 17β-estradiol (Sigma-Aldrich, St. Louis, MO) were packed into 10 mm

lengths of silastic tubing (Dow Corning, Midland, MI) with an internal diameter of 1.02 mm, external diameter of 2.16 mm, and wall thickness of 0.56 mm. The ends of the tubing were capped with clear silicone glue. Placebo implants were left empty. The implants were surgically inserted under isoflurane anesthesia in a small subcutaneous pocket on the lateral aspect of the neck/back between the skin and the muscle fascia. A two day recovery after the silastic implant surgery was allowed prior to reintroduction of running wheels.

The second technique for altering the levels of circulating steroids was the completion of bilateral orchidectomy surgeries to remove the testes, the major sex steroid producing tissue in male mammals. The surgeries were performed under isoflurane anesthesia after preemptive administration of the analgesic carprofen (5 mg·kg⁻¹). A small incision was made in the midline of the scrotum just inferior to the penis. Each testis was exposed through the incision and was removed along with the epididymis. The incision was closed with a sterile wound clip and the animal was allowed to recover under a heating lamp. Placebo animals received a sham procedure; the testis were exposed but were not excised. The surgical procedures were followed by ten days of recovery without access to running wheels.

Experiment One (Figure 1): Twenty mice, stratified by original group housing, were randomly assigned to a placebo (n=10) or experimental (n=10) group. In both groups, wheel running was monitored under three conditions. First, both groups underwent baseline screening for seven days to assess normal wheel running activity. Next, each mouse received either placebo or exemestane injections; wheel running was monitored for an additional seven days. Lastly, mice were allowed three days of unmonitored wheel running followed by a final seven days to assess wheel running during drug clearance.

To verify the results of experiment one, twenty untreated C57BL/6J mice were used in a confirmatory study with methodological techniques identical to experiment one. In brief, placebo (n=10) or letrozole (n=10) injections were given to reproductively intact mice. Wheel running indices were monitored prior to injections, during injections, and after cessation of injections—each phase lasting seven days. Upon confirmation, further experiments were conducted utilizing exemestane because the androgenic effects of the drug were considered negligible.

Experiment Two (Figure 1): Thirty mice were used in experiment two to evaluate the effects of supplemented sex steroids on wheel running activity during exemestane injections in mice with fully functional reproductive organs. One mouse was euthanized at the onset of the experiment due to an injury sustained during the preliminary group housing phase. The mice were randomly divided into control (n=9), experimental A (n=10), and experimental B (n=10) groups. Wheel running was again assessed at baseline under normal physiological conditions for seven days. During the next seven days of wheel running activity, the mice received exemestane (experimental A and B groups) or placebo (control) injections. In the final seven days of this experiment, the mice received silastic implants containing testosterone (experimental A group) or 17β-estradiol (experimental B group). The control animals received empty implants. After a brief two day recovery, exemestane and control injections were resumed and wheel running was evaluated for seven additional days.

Experiment Three (Figure 1): The third experimental procedure utilized thirty mice and evaluated the effects of orchidectomy and aromatase inhibition on wheel running activity. Replacement strategies (via silastic implants) were employed to reintroduce the sex steroids

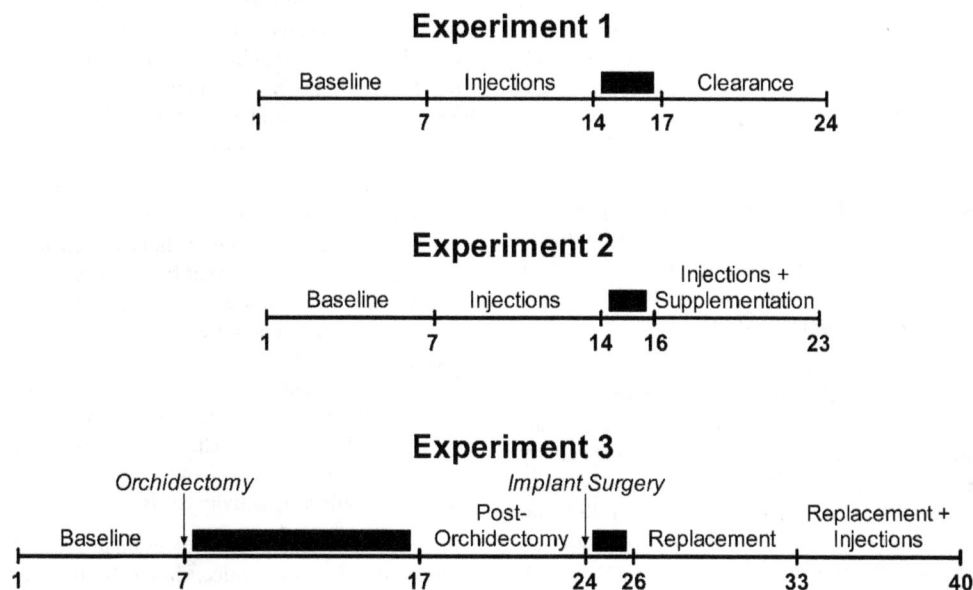

Figure 1: The experimental timelines (days) for assessing physical activity levels in aromatase inhibited and sex steroid modified mice. Black bars represent recovery periods—after surgeries and after cessation of injections—in which running wheels were not in the cages.

after removal of the gonads. The experimental groupings were the same as experiment two. Baseline data was collected at the onset of the experiment over a seven day period. Double and sham orchidectomies were performed and were followed by a ten day recovery period. Wheel running was evaluated at the end of the orchidectomy recovery period for seven days. Silastic implant surgeries were performed followed by two days of recovery. Seven more days of wheel running was assessed following the recovery period. Testosterone, 17β-estradiol, and blank implants were again utilized during this period. A final seven days of wheel running was assessed while placebo or exemestane injections were administered every 24 hours. The silastic capsules remained in place.

The physical activity data collected during each of the four experiments were analyzed using individual two-way (group by condition) analysis of variance (ANOVA) tests for each wheel running indices (distance, duration, or speed). A Tukey's *post-hoc* test was used to assess significant main effects or interactions. The alpha level was set *a priori* at 0.05.

Results

Wheel running indices (experiment one) for male C57BL/6J mice at baseline, receiving exemestane or placebo injections, and during a 10-day clearance period are shown in Figure 2a-c. Blocking aromatase did not inhibit activity and did not significantly alter any of the wheel running indices (distance: $p=0.61$, duration: $p=0.38$, or speed: $p=0.69$) at the administered dosage (250 mg·kg^{-1}).

The wheel running response under a reversible aromatase inhibitor was similar to the response observed with exemestane inhibition. All wheel running parameters were unaffected by letrozole administration and did not deviate from the levels measured in the control animals (distance: $p=0.24$, duration: $p=0.11$, or speed: $p=0.34$). The data for wheel running distance are depicted in Figure 2d; trends for the duration and speed indices were similarly non-significant.

Running distance, duration, and speed for experiment two are shown in Figure 3. Wheel running was assessed at baseline, with exemestane injections, and after implantation of testosterone or 17β-estradiol containing capsules. The difference across experimental conditions and groups were non-significant (distance: $p=0.66$, duration: $p=0.61$, speed: $p=0.56$) with neither testosterone nor 17β-estradiol altering the running response.

Wheel running indices (experiment three) at baseline, after surgical or sham orchidectomies, with placebo, testosterone, or 17β-estradiol implants, and with injections of placebo vehicle or exemestane are shown in Figure 4. Wheel running was significantly altered by these experimental interventions (distance: $F=4.65$, $p=0.0001$, duration: $F=4.82$, $p=0.0001$, speed: $F=6.63$, $p=0.0001$) and Tukey's HSD *post-hoc* tests revealed that several interventions altered the three wheel running activity indices measured (Figure 4). Orchidectomies significantly reduced all three indices of wheel running and testosterone replacement recovered wheel running back to baseline levels; however, 17β-estradiol failed to engender the same level of recovery. There was no significant alteration to activity with administration of exemestane in orchidectomized mice receiving either steroid.

Discussion

Our results demonstrate that activity remains unaffected by the administration of aromatase inhibitors at a dosage of 250 mg·kg^{-1}. The results of this study call into question the limited data that has generated the hypothesis of a primary estrogen-derived activity regulating mechanism. These data add additional impetus for further investigation into the effect of sex-steroids on physical activity in both rodent and human populations, with a needed subsequent focus on pathway identification and molecular mechanisms. Additional studies that focus on the effects the aromatase complex has on activity level regulation is warranted. The current project represents a seminal *modus operandi* in this new avenue of hormonal and steroidal research.

A physiologically normal C57BL/6J mouse runs vigorously when exposed to a running wheel (see Figures 2-4; baseline running data). Alterations to circulating sex steroid concentrations interrupt this normal running pattern [34-37], an effect postulated to occur through the modulation of estrogen levels via the aromatase complex; an assertion primarily based on limited previous research [14]. However, inhibition of the aromatase complex did not significantly alter wheel running activity indicating that a functional aromatase complex may not be required for activity levels to be modulated or maintained at normal levels in the reproductively intact rodent. While contradictory to previous speculations, other than Roy and Wade's [14] data, little direct evidence exists that indicates activity regulation—via the sex steroids—requires the presence of estrogenic compounds.

Roy and Wade [14] assessed the ability of testosterone propionate (an aromatizable androgen) and dihydrotestosterone propionate (a non-aromatizable androgen) to affect activity levels in castrated male rats. Administration of the aromatizable androgen increased activity to the levels observed in estrogen treated animals, but the non-aromatizable androgen had little effect on activity level [14]. Roy and Wade [14] noted only a partial (~ 45%) recovery of wheel running with testosterone administration (~4000 revolutions) compared to estradiol benzoate administration (~9000 revolutions). With testosterone administration, we observed that wheel running not only returned to the levels observed at baseline, but also was notably elevated above the levels induced by 17β-estradiol administration (Figure 4). The difference in testosterone-driven activity between our and Roy and Wade's study may be accounted for by the modes of steroid delivery used. The steroidal compounds were delivered via silastic implants in the current project, but Roy and Wade [14] delivered the steroids via daily injections in sesame oil. The injection methods employed by Roy and Wade [14] required daily contact with the animals, which has been

shown to induce higher levels of stress with resultant decreases in wheel running activity [38]. However, the effects of human interaction on wheel running behavior observed by Richter [38] were not as dramatic as the differences noted between our results and Roy and Wade's [14]. Therefore, though this certainly may explain some of the differences between our study and Roy and Wade's [14], it is likely that other mechanisms also exist that account for this discrepancy.

Watai et al. [15] evaluated activity in an aromatase (Cyp19) knockout mouse model and observed very low activity levels in these mice. Replacement of 17β-estradiol elevated activity in male knockout mice suggesting a requirement for estrogens to be present in order for activity levels to match those observed in normal animals [15]. The use of gene knockout models are not without adversity as developmental differences in mice can result in an obscured representation of reality [17] as well as potential elimination of neighboring regulatory genomic regions in the knockouts [39]. Thus, the results of Watai et al. [15] may be due to such unintended effects and therefore the result of abnormal physiological phenomenon rather than relevant deviations in the mechanisms affecting activity levels.

Conversely, Hill et al. [16] evaluated wheel running activity in estrogen deficient male mice, similar to the mice utilized by Watai et al. [15] and observed compulsory wheel running activity that exceeded the levels observed in wild type controls suggesting that estrogen was inhibiting activity in this model. Interestingly, this effect was not observed in female Cyp19 (aromatase) knockout animals. In addition, compulsory wheel running was ameliorated after the administration of 17β-estradiol in the male, but not female knockout mice [16]. The non-essential need for a functional aromatase complex to maintain normal activity levels observed in the present study and by Hill et al. [16] is contrary to the observations of Roy and Wade [14] and Watai et al. [15]. The technical difference noted in these studies may account

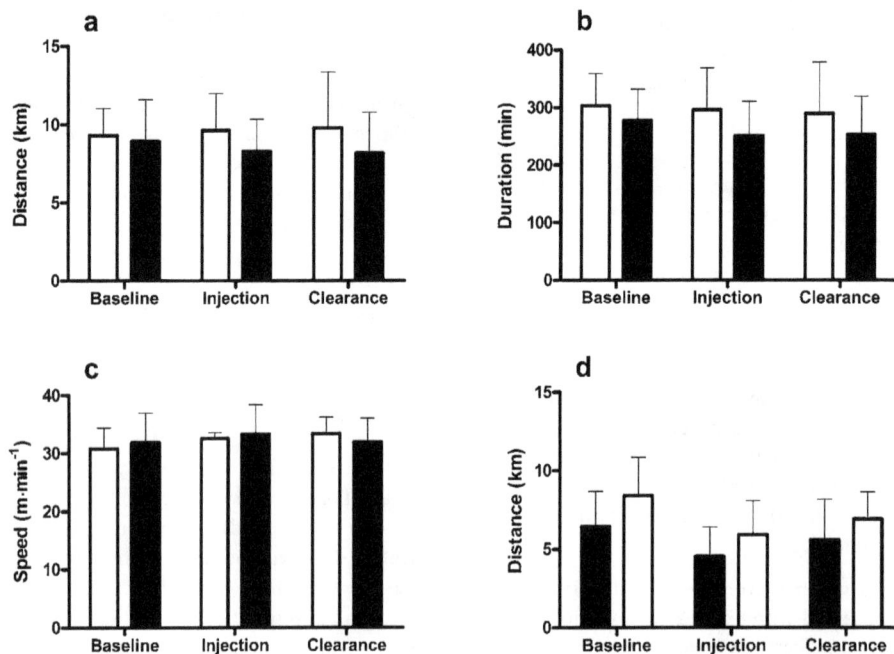

Figure 2: Wheel running indices for male C57BL/6J mice at baseline, during injections, and during post-injection clearance. White bars denote control mice (n=10) that received vehicle injections and black bars denote experimentally treated mice (n=10) that received exemestane (panels a-c; distance, duration, speed) or letrozole (panel d; distance) injections.

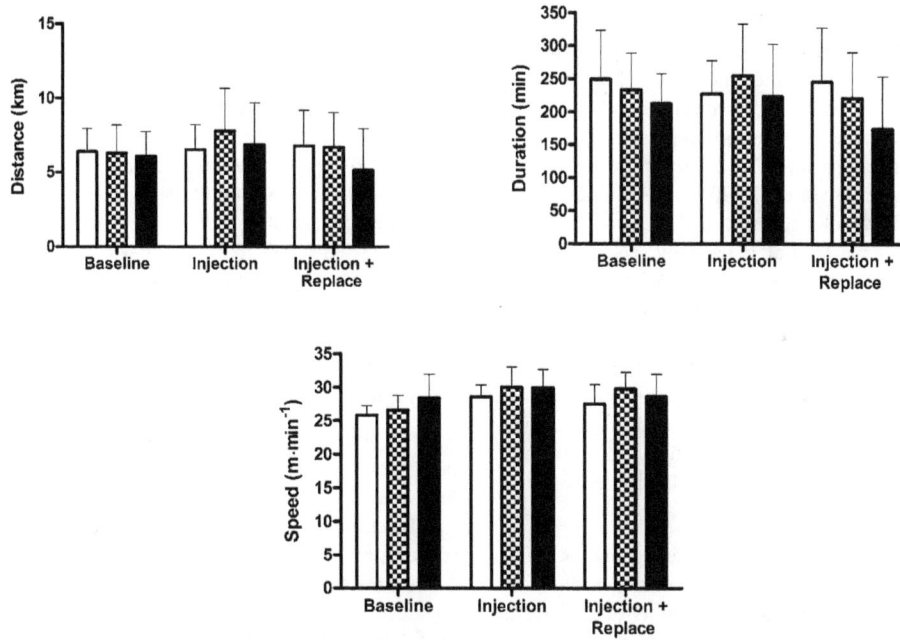

Figure 3: Wheel running indices (distance, duration, and speed) for male C57BL/6J mice at baseline, during injections, and during injections supplemented with either testosterone or 17β-estradiol. White bars denote control mice (n=9) that received vehicle injections and empty silastic implants. Checkered bars denote experimentally treated mice (n=10) that received exemestane injections and silastic implants containing testosterone. Black bars denote experimentally treated mice (n=10) that received exemestane injections and silastic implants containing 17β-estradiol.

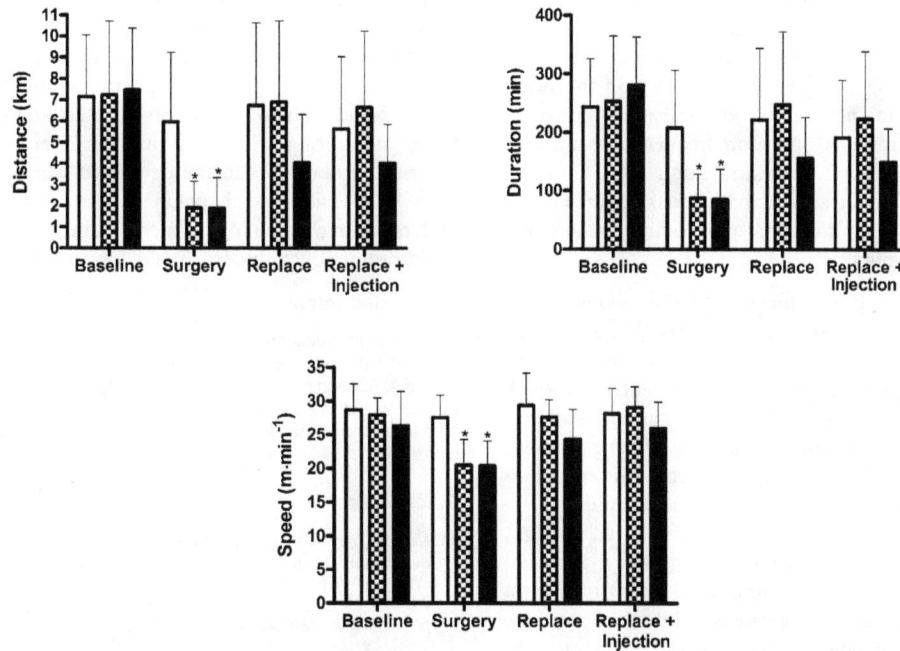

Figure 4: Wheel running indices (distance, duration, and speed) for male C57BL/6J mice at baseline, during injections, during steroid replacement, and during steroid replacement with injections. White bars denote control mice (n=10) that received vehicle injections and empty silastic implants. Checkered bars denote experimentally treated mice (n=10) that received silastic implants containing testosterone and exemestane injections. Black bars denote experimentally treated mice (n=10) that received silastic implants containing 17β-estradiol and exemestane injections. *=significantly different from controls and baseline values.

for some of the observational disparities; however, it is obvious that testosterone may have a stronger effect on physical activity than previously understood thus justifying further study detailing the underlying estrogenic and androgenic mechanisms.

The potential identity of the androgenic steroid mechanisms modulating physical activity remains unclear. Two primary lines of evidence from the current project support the presence of an androgenic activity regulator. First, blockade of the aromatase complex via either reversible or irreversible aromatase inhibiters did not significantly reduce wheel running in reproductively intact or sex steroid treated orchidectomized male mice. Second, testosterone replacement in orchidectomized male mice increased wheel running activity back to baseline levels, while 17β-estradiol increased wheel running to only 50% of baseline levels. Our data represent the second study to suggest the existence of a direct androgenic mechanism in non-genetically modified mice. Flynn et al. [40] exposed mice to the anti-androgenic fungicide vinclozolin at gestational age seven in dam's milk and continued exposure via food after weaning. With exposure to vinclozolin and the resultant androgenic-inhibition, both males and females exhibited decreased wheel running levels; however, only the females reached a statistically significant decrease in wheel running activity at the highest dose of the chemical. The authors [40] concluded that the depressive effects of vinclozolin on activity levels were caused by an inhibitory interaction between the fungicide and the androgen receptor. Thus, the data of Flynn et al. [40] partially supports our hypothesis regarding the existence of an androgenic physical-activity regulating mechanism.

While several authors [41-45] have suggested that the high malleability of the activity response in animals treated with estrogens is a centrally-located (i.e. brain) function, the permeability of the rodent brain to androgens is also high [46] suggesting a potential pathway through which testosterone affects physical activity. To date, only one paper [47] has evaluated brain morphology in aromatase compromised mice and noted lower levels of dopaminergic neurons in the medial preoptic area and arcuate nucleus of male knockout mice. This response would tentatively explain the noted increased activity levels of the aromatase knockout mice based on recent work from Knab et al. [7] that suggested an increased activity level was due to down-regulated dopamine 1 receptor levels. It is hypothesized by Knab et al. [7] that dopamine receptor reward signaling is decreased due to the lower number of receptor containing neurons and to compensate, mice run more, thus initiating a reward signal on a more frequent basis through the reduced number of receptor containing neurons. Therefore, we speculate that testosterone influences activity levels in male mice through interactions with the androgen receptor leading to alteration of central dopamine functioning.

The injection and sampling techniques employed in this project required close contact with the mice several times throughout the study. Interactions between animal handlers and small rodents have been shown to induce a stress response in small rodents [38] which could artificially alter sex steroid levels and wheel running patterns. Steps were taken to minimize stress in this study for humane purposes and to limit the potential to induce aberrant sex steroid concentrations and unnatural running patterns. During all procedures, animals were handled using controlled and secure techniques, monitored for signs of elevated stress (vocalizations, biting, increased mobility, etc.), and directly exposed to technicians for a minimal amount of time. Most contact from initial immobilization to release back into the home cage was less than three minutes. The effectiveness of drug administration to reduce aromatase activity in the study's mouse population was assured through use of routine and previously described techniques. As stated before, the dosage and technique used in this project are a common methodology to reduce aromatase activity in rodents [22-24]. The only major concern was a potential bias induced by multiple handlers during injection events. To circumvent these issues, an individual technician prepared and performed delivery of both pharmaceutical agents using the described simple, effective methods. This well-trained technician is a highly proficient animal handler.

Exemestane is an irreversible aromatase inhibiting drug. In addition to its inhibitory effects, exemestane has been shown to possess androgenic characteristics in clinical situations including an affinity to bind the androgen receptor [48]. The dosage used in this project was previously shown to have physiological effects on bone characteristics, tumor morphology, and estrogen production. These effects could have been due to the androgenic rather than the aromatase inhibitory nature of exemestane. In order to parse the androgenicity and aromatase inhibitory effects of the drug, the results from the first experiment were repeated using letrozole, a reversible aromatase inhibitor that does not have androgenic effects. Using letrozole, similar results were observed as with exemestane indicating that the aromatase inhibiting effects of the drugs did not alter wheel running behavior and that physical activity regulation via estrogenic sources was not an absolute requirement in our model.

The present study evaluated the effects of two aromatase inhibitors on wheel running activity in male C57BL/6J mice. Neither aromatase inhibitor altered wheel running activity in intact, supplemented, or orchidectomized animals. These data, in conjunction with wheel running measures in aromatase knockout mice [16] and vinclozolin treated mice [40], suggests that aromatization of testosterone is not an absolute requirement for activity regulation as has been earlier postulated [14] and that a direct androgenic mechanism regulates activity levels in mice. This proposed androgenic mechanism is likely an additional effect supplementing and/or offsetting the effects of the estrogenic compounds. The complexity of such regulatory mechanisms and the low number of available research studies provide ample basis for reinvigoration of this research area. In particular, studies that partition the androgenic and aromatase inhibitory effects of the irreversible aromatase inhibitors will provide valuable insight into this mechanism. Future research should also utilize pharmacological and chemical methods to manipulate the function of the aromatase complex and androgen receptors of intact and gonadectomized mice while monitoring wheel running. Physical inactivity has reached epidemic proportions in the developed world leading to increasing rates of obesity and hypokinetic diseases; thus identifying and understanding the biological mechanisms that regulate activity levels could profoundly influence human health worldwide.

Acknowledgments

The project described was supported by grants from the National Institutes of Health (NIAMS AR050085), the American College of Sports Medicine Foundation (Doctoral Research Grant Award), and Sigma Xi (Grants-in-Aid of Research). The authors would like to thank the UNC Charlotte Vivarium staff for assistance with animal husbandry needs and Ms. Alicia T. Hamilton for assistance with laboratory techniques.

References

1. Mokdad AH, Marks JS, Stroup DF, Gerberding JL (2004) Actual causes of death in the United States, 2000. JAMA 291: 1238-1245.

2. Joosen AM, Gielen M, Vlietinck R, Westerterp KR (2005) Genetic analysis of physical activity in twins. Am J Clin Nutr 82: 1253-1259.

3. Stubbe JH, Boomsma DI, Vink JM, Cornes BK, Martin NG, et al. (2006) Genetic influences on exercise participation in 37,051 twin pairs from seven countries. PLoS ONE 1: 22.

4. Lightfoot JT, Turner MJ, Daves M, Vordermark A, Kleeberger SR (2004) Genetic influence on daily wheel running activity level. Physiol Genomics 19: 270-276.

5. Leamy LJ, Pomp D, Lightfoot JT (2008) An epistatic genetic basis for physical activity traits in mice. J Hered 99: 639-646.

6. Lightfoot JT, Turner MJ, Pomp D, Kleeberger SR, Leamy LJ (2008) Quantitative trait loci for physical activity traits in mice. Physiol Genomics 32: 401-408.

7. Knab AM, Bowen RS, Hamilton AT, Gulledge AA, Lightfoot JT (2009) Altered dopaminergic profiles: implications for the regulation of voluntary physical activity. Behav Brain Res 204: 147-152.

8. Lightfoot JT, Leamy L, Pomp D, Turner MJ, Fodor AA, et al. (2010) Strain screen and haplotype association mapping of wheel running in inbred mouse strains. J Appl Physiol 109: 623-634.

9. Ogawa S, Chan J, Gustafsson JA, Korach KS, Pfaff DW (2003) Estrogen increases locomotor activity in mice through estrogen receptor alpha: specificity for the type of activity. Endocrinology 144: 230-239.

10. Morgan MA, Schulkin J, Pfaff DW (2004) Estrogens and non-reproductive behaviors related to activity and fear. Neurosci Biobehav Rev 28: 55-63.

11. Gorzek JF, Hendrickson KC, Forstner JP, Rixen JL, Moran AL, et al. (2007) Estradiol and tamoxifen reverse ovariectomy-induced physical inactivity in mice. Med Sci Sports Exerc 39: 248-256.

12. Hydock DS, Lien CY, Schneider CM, Hayward R (2007) Effects of voluntary wheel running on cardiac function and myosin heavy chain in chemically gonadectomized rats. Am J Physiol Heart Circ Physiol 293: 3254-3264.

13. Lightfoot JT (2008) Sex hormones' regulation of rodent physical activity: a review. Int J Biol Sci 4: 126-132.

14. Roy EJ, Wade GN (1975) Role of estrogens in androgen-induced spontaneous activity in male rats. J Comp Physiol Psychol 89: 573-579.

15. Watai K, Tsuda M, Nakata M, Toda K, Ogawa S (2007) Analyses of running wheel activity (RWA) in aromatase-knockout (ArKO) mice. Neurosci Res 58: 108.

16. Hill RA, McInnes KJ, Gong EC, Jones ME, Simpson ER, et al. (2007) Estrogen deficient male mice develop compulsive behavior. Biol Psychiatry 61: 359-366.

17. Chapman PF (2002) Giving drugs to knockout mice: can they do that? Trends Neurosci 25: 277-279.

18. Swallow JG, Garland T, Jr., Carter PA, Zhan WZ, Sieck GC (1998) Effects of voluntary activity and genetic selection on aerobic capacity in house mice (Mus domesticus). J Appl Physiol 84: 69-76.

19. Knab AM, Bowen RS, Moore-Harrison T, Hamilton AT, Turner MJ, et al. (2009) Repeatability of exercise behaviors in mice. Physiol Behav 98: 433-440.

20. Santen RJ, Brodie H, Simpson ER, Siiteri PK, Brodie A (2009) History of Aromatase: Saga of an Important Biological Mediator and Therapeutic Target. Endocr Rev 30: 343-375.

21. Attar E, Bulun SE (2006) Aromatase inhibitors: the next generation of therapeutics for endometriosis? Fertil Steril 85: 1307-1318.

22. Goss PE, Qi S, Cheung AM, Hu H, Mendes M, et al. (2004) Effects of the steroidal aromatase inhibitor exemestane and the nonsteroidal aromatase inhibitor letrozole on bone and lipid metabolism in ovariectomized rats. Clin Cancer Res 10: 5717-5723.

23. Jelovac D, Macedo L, Handratta V, Long BJ, Goloubeva OG, et al. (2004) Effects of exemestane and tamoxifen in a postmenopausal breast cancer model. Clin Cancer Res 10: 7375-7381.

24. di Salle E, Briatico G, Giudici D, Ornati G, Zaccheo T (1989) Aromatase inhibition and experimental antitumor activity of FCE 24304, MDL 18962 and SH 489. J Steroid Biochem 34: 431-434.

25. Luthra R, Kirma N, Jones J, Tekmal RR (2003) Use of letrozole as a chemopreventive agent in aromatase overexpressing transgenic mice. J Steroid Biochem Mol Biol 86: 461-467.

26. Bowman RE, Ferguson D, Luine VN (2002) Effects of chronic restraint stress and estradiol on open field activity, spatial memory, and monoaminergic neurotransmitters in ovariectomized rats. Neuroscience 113: 401-410.

27. Broida J, Svare B (1983) Genotype modulates testosterone-dependent activity and reactivity in male mice. Horm Behav 17: 76-85.

28. Cohen PE, Milligan SR (1993) Silastic implants for delivery of oestradiol to mice. J Reprod Fertil 99: 219-223.

29. Daan S, Damassa D, Pittendrigh CS, Smith ER (1975) An effect of castration and testosterone replacement on a circadian pacemaker in mice (Mus musculus). Proc Natl Acad Sci U S A 72: 3744-3747.

30. Ellis GB, Turek FW (1983) Testosterone and photoperiod interact to regulate locomotor activity in male hamsters. Horm Behav 17: 66-75.

31. Garey J, Morgan MA, Frohlich J, McEwen BS, Pfaff DW (2001) Effects of the phytoestrogen coumestrol on locomotor and fear-related behaviors in female mice. Horm Behav 40: 65-76.

32. Morin LP, Cummings LA (1982) Splitting of wheelrunning rhythms by castrated or steroid treated male and female hamsters. Physiol Behav 29: 665-675.

33. Pieper DR, Lobocki CA, Lichten EM, Malaczynski J (1999) Dehydroepiandrosterone and exercise in golden hamsters. Physiol Behav 67: 607-610.

34. Hoskins RG (1925) Studies on vigor. II. The effect of castration on voluntary activity. Am J Physiol 72: 324-330.

35. Hoskins RG (1925) Studies on vigor. VI. The effects of starvation on the spontaneous activity of castrated rats. Endocrinology 9: 403-406.

36. Wang GH, Richter CP, Guttmacher AF (1925) Activity studies on male castrated rats with ovarian transplants and correlation of the activity with the histology of the grafts. Am J Physiol 73: 581-599.

37. Richter CP (1933) The effect of early gonadectomy on the gross body activity of rats. Endocrinology 17: 445-450.

38. Richter CP (1976) Artifactual seven-day cycles in spontaneous activity in wild rodents and squirrel monkeys. J Comp Physiol Psychol 90: 572-582.

39. Osokine I, Hsu R, Loeb GB, McManus MT (2008) Unintentional miRNA ablation is a risk factor in gene knockout studies: a short report. PLoS Genet 4: 34.

40. Flynn KM, Delclos KB, Newbold RR, Ferguson SA (2001) Behavioral responses of rats exposed to long-term dietary vinclozolin. J Agric Food Chem 49: 1658-1665.

41. Kennedy GC (1964) Hypothalamic control of the endocrine and behavioural changes associated with oestrus in the rat. J Physiol 172: 383-392.

42. Colvin GB, Sawyer CH (1969) Induction of running activity by intracerebral implants of estrogen in overiectomized rats. Neuroendocrinology 4: 309-320.

43. Hitt JC, Gerall AA (1969) Effect of brain stimulation on estrous activity cycles. Psychol Rep 24: 59-68.

44. Wade GN, Zucker I (1970) Modulation of food intake and locomotor activity in female rats by diencephalic hormone implants. J Comp Physiol Psychol 72: 328-336.

45. Gentry RT, Wade GN, Roy EJ (1976) Individual differences in estradiol-induced behaviors and in neural 3H-estradiol uptake in rats. Physiol Behav 17: 195-200.

46. Pardridge WM, Mietus LJ (1979) Transport of steroid hormones through the rat blood-brain barrier. Primary role of albumin-bound hormone. J Clin Invest 64: 145-154.

47. Hill RA, Pompolo S, Jones ME, Simpson ER, Boon WC (2004) Estrogen deficiency leads to apoptosis in dopaminergic neurons in the medial preoptic area and arcuate nucleus of male mice. Mol Cell Neurosci 27: 466-476.

48. Johannessen DC, Engan T, Di Salle E, Zurlo MG, Paolini J, et al. (1997) Endocrine and clinical effects of exemestane (PNU 155971), a novel steroidal aromatase inhibitor, in postmenopausal breast cancer patients: a phase I study. Clin Cancer Res 3: 1101-1108.

25

Endocrine Immune Interactions in the Host-Parasite Relationship: Steroid Hormones as Immune Regulators in Parasite Infections

Aguilar-Díaz H[1], Nava-Castro KE[2], Cerbón-Cervantes MA[1], Meneses-Ruiz DM[3], Ponce-Regalado MD[4] and Morales-Montor J[3*]

[1]Facultad de Química, Departamento de Biología, Universidad Nacional Autónoma de México, México
[2]Departamento de Ciencias Ambientales, Centro de Ciencias de la Atmósfera, Universidad Nacional Autónoma de México, México
[3]Departamento de Inmunología, Instituto de Investigaciones Biomédicas, Universidad Nacional Autónoma de México, México
[4]Universidad de Guadalajara, Centro Universitario de los Altos-Departamento de clínicas, México

Abstract

There is a close relationship between hormones, cytokines, neuropeptides, and neurotransmitters that modulate the host immune response by several effector mechanisms, including both cellular and humoral immunity. Disruption of this communication balance results in disease or in a higher susceptibility to infections. The relationships between parasites and hosts are complex and there is substantial interaction, communication and biochemical co-evolution. The role of certain hormones in parasitic infections has been demonstrated, and there are documented direct effects of hormones on parasites. Many parasites induce the secretion of molecules that influence the physiological and immunological responses in hosts, including intermediaries and vectors. Conversely, the parasites secrete many factors that alter hormone host levels. In some cases, hormones have positive or negative effects on the parasites status. In other cases, effects are mediated indirectly via the host's immune system. In vertebrates, the parasite presence also has a major influence on the host's endocrine status and the normal suite of processes governed by hormones. These processes include host development, establishment, metamorphosis, and reproduction. Thus, understanding the mechanisms involved in immunoendocrine modulation and its effects on parasites is essential for developing new drugs, finding vaccine targets and devising new therapies for several infectious diseases.

Keywords: Sexual steroids; Hormones; Parasites; Immune system

Introduction

Hormones and parasites

Parasites comprise a group of organisms that cause a massive infectious disease problem for humans and several animals of veterinary importance. These organisms are major causes of mortality and morbidity and are detrimental to both the social and economic progress of the developing world. Sex differences in parasitic infections are a biological phenomenon of considerable significance for individual health and disease. The general rule is that females are more resistant to infectious diseases than males [1,2]. However, there are many notable exceptions to this rule and illustrate a female bias in susceptibility to infection [3]. This paradigm implies that the sexual dimorphism in response to parasites is mediated primarily by the immune system of the host, which disregards the ability of some parasites to directly respond to the distinct sex steroid hormone profiles of their female and male hosts [2,4]. Sex hormones play an influential role in the control of parasitic infection by modulating different components of both the innate and adaptive immune responses. Conversely, parasites themselves are phylogenetically diverse, target a range of different tissues, and have evolved numerous alternative strategies to evade or inhibit protective immune responses by strategies, such as antigenic variation, molecular mimicry or affecting antigen processing and presentation. Moreover, parasites exploit host systems for their benefit during establishment, growth, or reproduction [4]. Consequently, the influence of sex hormones on these infective agents can be complex. Sex hormones also exert their effects through genomic and non-genomic mechanisms by interacting with cell cytoplasmic or surface receptors and triggering signaling pathways. The main biological activity occurs by the activation of specific intracellular receptors that function as ligand-activated transcription factors and coordinates the expression of target genes [5]. Our current understanding of the relationship between hormones and parasite infection suggests that parasites can synthesize proteins, such as receptors with the ability to bind host hormones, and cause downstream transcriptional gene activation. As a result, parasites can positively or negatively affect the course of infection [6,7]. Based on the above data, this review examines how hormones effect on the immune system and their implications in parasite infections.

Immune response and hormones

The immune cells: Parasite-induced host response is orchestrated by the complex interactions of molecular and cellular effectors. The innate immune system is the first line of defense that is activated soon after parasite exposure. The cells involved in the host defense are neutrophils, macrophages, natural killer cells (NK) and dendritic cells (DCs) [8]. However, the primary response is performed by neutrophils using two basic mechanisms involving phagocytosis and the release of potent and toxic oxygen-free radicals (respiratory burst) [9]. Macrophages also participate in phagocytosis and respiratory bursts. These cells have the additional ability to present antigens and secrete cytokines, growth factors, and tissue-remodeling agents to alter tissue development [10,11]. DCs are professional antigen presenting cells that function by antigen-presentation on the cell surface to activate T lymphocytes. Finally, NK cells have a cytotoxic phenotype and secrete

*Corresponding author: Jorge Morales Montor, Departamento de Inmunología, Instituto de Investigaciones Biomédicas, Universidad Nacional Autónoma de México. AP 70228, México, E-mail: Jmontor66@biomedicas.unam.mx

small proteins called perforins and proteases known as granzymes. These proteins are involved in the host-rejection of tumors and virally infected cells. In general terms, these responses do not require prior exposure and can be initiated immediately following exposure to a novel parasite. Interestingly, the activity and number of cells associated with innate immunity could differ between the sexes. In females, professional antigen presenting cells (APC) are more efficient at presenting peptides than APC from males. Additionally, the phagocytic activity of macrophages and neutrophils is higher in females than males [12-14]. After parasitic or antigenic stimulation, the production of prostaglandin, thromboxane, and nitric oxide (NO) is higher in females than males [15]. In contrast, other studies demonstrate that several pro-inflammatory cytokines (including IL-6 and TNF-α) are higher in males following trauma [15]. Women with regular menstrual cycles and women during the luteal phase exhibit lower NK cell activity than men. These results correlate with experimental work in mice that demonstrated estradiol could reduce both the number and activity of NK cells [16-18]. However, males and females differ in their innate immune responses. This finding suggests there are sex differences. Previous studies of both humans and rodents have shown that inflammatory immune responses are generally higher in females than males. Thus, these results could explain the higher female susceptibility to developing inflammatory rheumatic diseases, such as rheumatoid arthritis and systemic lupus erythematous [19].

The acquired immune response after parasitic infection is mediated by humoral and cellular activation that includes an antigen-specific mechanism. Antigen presenting cells (macrophages and DCs) have a critical role in this response and stimulate B cells and T cell subsets [20]. B cells are grouped into B1 and B2 cells and are responsible for antibody secretion [21]. T cells are categorized into four distinct subtypes based on transcriptional factors, cytokine production, and function. These subtypes include Th1, Th2, Th17 and regulatory T cells (Treg) [22]. In this cell-mediated immune response there is a marked difference between males and females. Thus, T-cells (particularly CD4 T-cells) can be differentiated depending of the cytokine release and are functionally and phenotypically heterogeneous. Similarly, T cells present different subsets (i.e., Th1 or Th2 cells) to overcome infection and differ between males and females. Females have stronger Th2 responses (i.e., higher IL-4, IL-5, IL-6, and IL-10 production) than males [23]. There are also reports that females have a higher Th1 response (i.e., higher concentrations of IFN-γ) than males. In rodent models, females show higher mitogen-stimulated lymphocyte proliferation, faster wound healing, and increased immunological intolerance to foreign substances than males [15,24,25].

Hormones

Estrogens: Estrogens (E2) are predominantly produced in gonadal tissue and are principally produced by theca and granulosa cells in the ovary and mesenchymal cells [26]. The E2 immunomodulatory role enables the autoimmune disease incidence and age-associated diseases such as hormone-dependent cancer, osteoporosis, and cardiovascular diseases [27]. It has been observed that E2 has immunological roles and suppresses bone marrow leukocyte production, including neutrophils [28]. Estrogens also modulate leukocyte chemotaxis during ischemia and myocardium reperfusion in rat by inhibiting TNF-α production and limiting the binding of deleterious ICAM-1 leukocytes to injured myocardium. Therefore, estrogens protect against myocardial ischemia-reperfusion injury [29]. Previous in *vitro studies* have shown antioxidant effects by limiting superoxide anion production in human neutrophils [30]. E2 administration in mice before spinal

cord injury reduces the production of tissue associated cytokines, such as TNF-α, IL-6, and IL- 1β (Table 1) [31].

During the first week of pregnancy in mice when E2 peak occurs, there is an increase of peritoneal macrophage phagocytic activity [32]. Additionally, exogenous *in vivo* E2 replacement significantly elevates sera lipopolysaccharide-binding protein levels and the cell surface expression of Toll-like receptor 4 (TLR-4) and CD14 (Table 1) [33].

In other murine model studies, exposure to E2 *in vitro* promotes differentiation into functional CD11c[+] and CD11b[+] DCs from bone marrow precursor cells. However, this differentiation is inhibited in E2-deficient medium and also, by estrogen receptor (ER) antagonists (ICI 182, 780 and tamoxifen). The differentiation can be restored by E2 addition in physiological amounts [34]. Moreover, E2 increases DC activation marker expression, including the expression of major histocompatibility complex II (MHCII), CD80 (B7.1), CD86 (B7.2), CD40, CD14, CXCL8 and CCL2 in murine bone marrow-derived DCs (Table 1) [35].

Conversely, the exposure of bone marrow-derived dendritic cells (BMDCs) to E2 enhances IL-12 production in response to the TLR ligands (as CpG and LPS) and induces killer DCs (IKDCs) activity and IFN-γ production. However, there is no difference between the number and function of DCs isolated from spleens of female C57BL/6 mice ovariectomized and ovariectomized mice with E2 replacement (Table 1) [36]. The DCs and monocytes derived from rat spleens with experimental autoimmune encephalomyelitis and differentiated with IL-4 and GM-CSF produce more NO when incubated with E2 (Table 1) [37].

The results of *in vitro* experiments show that NK and NKT cell numbers are increased by E2 stimulation [38]. The cell increase is probably caused by the up regulation of MCM7 and MCM10, which control cell proliferation [39]. However, E2 stimulation reduced NK and NKT cytotoxicity by decreasing the expression of soluble factors, such as granzyme B and FasL. Additionally, CD69, NKp46, NKG2DL and 2B4 receptors were downregulated, which inhibited NK cell activation (Table 1) [40].

In general, E2 exerts different effects on T-lymphocytes by altering cytokine production and modulating cell proliferation. Thus, low E2 concentrations can promote the Th1 response and cell-mediated immunity. However, high concentrations augment Th2 responses and humoral immunity [41]. The splenic lymphocytes and T cells purified from mice treated with E2 show upregulation of the transcription factor T-bet, and this causes IFN-γ production and Th1 cell migration (Table 1) [42]. In several models, increased IL-4 expression from Th2 cells positively correlates with cyclical variations in estrogen levels in humans [43]. Moreover, mice treated with high doses of estrogen have decreased IL-17 production by Th17 cells [44]. Treg cell frequency increases in pregnant mice exposed to E2 through the transcriptional induction of Foxp3, IL-10, and PD-1 overexpression in both lymphoid organs and blood compared to non-estrogen treated or non- pregnant mice (Table 1) [45,46]. In other mouse models, long-term exposure to exogenous high doses of E2 enhances polyclonal B cell activation [47]. Physiological concentrations of E2 stimulate B antibody production by B lymphocytes in the genital tract and systemic lymphoid tissues of normal cycling female macaques during the menstrual cycle periovulatory period [48]. In male and female humans, E2 enhances IgG and IgM production by peripheral blood mononuclear cells (PBMCs) without altering cell viability, proliferation, or non-specific differentiation (Table 1) [49].

Hormones	Immune cells	Effect	References
Estradiol (E2)	Neutrophils	Regulate the number and function Decrease chemotaxis by altering the expression of ICAM-1 Decrease superoxide anion production Produce cytokines TNF-α, IL-6, and IL-1beta	[28-31]
	Macrophages	Increase macrophage phagocytic activity Increase CD14, LBP and TLR42	[32,33]
	Dendritic cells	Promote functional differentiation Increase the expression of MHC II, CD14, CD40, CD80, CD86, CXCL8 and CCL2 Induce IKDCs and increase nitric oxide	[34-36]
	NK cells	Decrease cytotoxicity Upregulate the number of cells and expression of CD69, NKp46, NKG2DL, CD244, granzyme B and FasL	[39,40]
	Lymphocytes	Upregulate T-bet expression (Th1 and proinflammatory cytokines) Increase IL-4 production from CD4+ T cells Decrease production of IL-17 Upregulate Treg cells (expression of Foxp3, IL-10 and PD-L1) Stimulate antibody production	[42-49]
Progesterone (P4)	Macrophages	Inhibition classical pathway activation (iNOS and arginase activity)	[61]
	Dendritic cells	Inhibit the activity of mature DCs Down-regulate TNF-α, IL-1β, MHC II, CD80 Inhibit DC-stimulated proliferation of T cells	[62]
	NK cells	Regulate differentiation (Hox A10) Reduce in cytotoxicity (HLA-G) Inhibit of perforin release (PIBF) Th2 differentiation and cytokine production (PIBF)	[13,14,63,66]
	Lymphocytes	Promote differentiation of Th2 Induce migration of Treg cells to the pregnant uterus	[13,181]
Testosterone	Macrophages	Inhibit the function of macrophages	[12]
(T4)		Reduce TLR4 expression Inhibit NO production	
	APC's	Down-regulate IL-1β, IL-6 and TNF-α	[70]
	Lymphocytes	Reduce Th1 cytokine release Induce Th2 profile Maintain Treg cells	[72,73]
DHEA	Neutrophil	Increase superoxide generation	[75]
	Dendritic cells	Induce mature DCs	[76]
	Lymphocytes	Enhance IL-2 secretion of Th1 cells and cytotoxicity function of T cells Induce apoptosis pathway Fas/Fas-L	[77,78]

Table 1: Effects of steroids hormones on immune response.

One remarkable effect that E2 can exert (concentration-dependent) is a proinflammatory or anti-inflammatory response. Low levels of E2 induce TNF-α, IL-6, and IL-1β. E2 also inhibits Th2-type cytokines and increases leukocyte migration to sites of inflammation [41]. However, at high levels, E2 inhibits cell-mediated immunity and decreases the expression of activation markers [50,51]. E2 inhibits TNF-α, IL-1β, and IL-6 production by T cells, macrophages, and DCs. Conversely, E2 induces Th2-type cytokines, such as IL-4, IL-10, and TGF-β, that results in anti-inflammatory effects [52]. E2 peak levels reduce Th1-type cytokine production (TNF-α and IFN-γ) by T cells, macrophages, and DCs [41,53,54]. E2 also enhances antibody production by enhancing IL-10 in human peripheral blood mononuclear cells (Table 1) [49]. In the female genital tract, E2 elevates IgG, IgA, and SC levels in ovariectomized rat uterus [55,56]. However, E2 action on cervicovaginal IgA, IgG, and SC is independent of the uterine influence because the E2 treatment of rats with ligated uterocervical junctions had decreased cervicovaginal IgA and SC levels. This is an important finding if the uterus is the main antibody source in genital tract secretions. After hysterectomy, the levels of IgG are reduced by one half and the levels of IgA are decreased by 15-fold [56]. E2 also affects lymphocytes, macrophages, NK cells and the migration and infiltration of other cells into the female genital tract. Additionally, E2 inhibits MCP-1 expression in endometrial stromal cells by controlling endometrial macrophage migration [57]. Furthermore, high E2 levels decrease macrophage and inflammatory T cell recruitment through ICAM-1, E-selectin, and VCAM-1 downregulation [58]. In contrast, E2 increases CD56+ NK cell recruitment to human endometrium by CXCL10 and CXCL11 chemokine upregulation [59]. Finally, E2-mediates the inhibition of antigen presentation and CTL activity in the female reproductive tract through the induction of TGF-β production by the uterine epithelial cells (Table 1) [60].

Progesterone: The hormone progesterone (P4) is secreted by the *corpus luteum* in the ovary and placenta. Principally, P4 is involved in the regulation of the female menstrual cycle and in pregnancy and embryogenesis of humans and other species. During early pregnancy, P4 recruits macrophages into the endometrium. The macrophages contribute to embryo implantation and pregnancy initiation by altering the remodeling process, uterine decidual response and placental trophoblast invasion. In mice, P4 negatively regulates macrophage activation of innate and classical pathways associated with NO and IL-12 production by down regulating inducible nitric oxide synthase 2 (iNOS) and arginase (Table 1) [61].

DCs derived from LPS-activated rat bone marrow cells treated with P4 have suppressed pro-inflammatory cytokine secretion (TNF-α, IL-1β). Additionally, the expression of activation markers, such as MHC class II and CD80, are downregulated. This causes reduced stimulation and T lymphocyte proliferation (Table 1) [62]. Moreover, P4 suppresses several innate immune responses including macrophage and NK cell activity and NF-κB signal transduction [63]. Activated lymphocytes express P4 receptors during pregnancy and high levels can stimulate the synthesis of progesterone-induced binding factor (PIBF) [14]. P4 also increases Th2 type cytokine production by IL-4 receptor stimulation and subsequent activation of the Jak/STAT pathway (Table 1) [13]. This activation results in inflammatory Th1 responses both at the maternal fetal interface and systemically [64,65].

Previous studies have demonstrated that P4 exerts a strong immunosuppressive effect on the production and transepithelial transport of IgG and IgA [56]. Studies of ovariectomized rats treated with P4 showed a significant decline in IgA and IgG cervicovaginal

expression. In monocytes, P4 inhibits NK cell activity and FcγR expression and reduces antibody-dependent cell cytotoxicity mediated by the progesterone-induced blocking factor (PIBF) [66]. Finally, membrane-associated and intracellular progesterone receptors are expressed by a number of immune cells including macrophages, NK cells, and γδ-T cells [62,67].

Testosterone: Testosterone (T4) is the main androgen secreted by testicular Leydig cells in males. It is also produced in small quantities by ovarian theca cells in females in response to the luteinizing hormone [68]. T4 inhibits histamine and serotonin release by mast cells after stimulation by compound 48/80 or neuropeptide P [69]. *In vitro* studies with macrophage (RAW 264.7 cells) cell lines treated with T4 showed decreased TLR-4 expression and TLR-4 specific ligand sensitivity. Furthermore, orchidectomized mice are more susceptible to lethal LPS challenge *in vivo*. Interestingly, significantly higher TLR-4 cell surface expression was observed in macrophages isolated from these animals (Table 1) [12]. Moreover, treating a group of diabetic men with T4 decreased IL-1β, IL-6, and TNF-α production *ex vivo* by APCs (Table 1) [70]. Further evidence of the role for T4 in regulating immunity is obtained from studies of male medical castration, which decreases Treg cell levels. In contrast, androgen therapy replenishes the Treg cell numbers (Table 1) [71].

Female *SJL* mice are more susceptible than males to experimental autoimmune encephalomyelitis (EAE) induced by myelin basic protein (MBP) specific T lymphocytes. However, the females implanted with dihydrotestosterone exhibited a significantly less severe EAE course (Table 1) [72]. Finally, T4 inhibits immunoglobulin IgM and IgG production. A recent study using human peripheral blood mononuclear cells (PBMC) demonstrated this effect is mediated indirectly by T4 inhibition of monocyte-derived IL-6 production (Table 1) [73].

Dehydroepiandrosterone: Dehydroepiandrosterone (DHEA) is a pregnenolone-derived C-19 steroid that is predominantly synthesized in the adrenal cortex cells [74]. DHEA sulfate ester (DHEAS) activates recombinant protein kinase C-beta (PKC-beta), which results in amplified phosphorylation of p47 (phox). Phosphorylated p47 is an active component of the reduced nicotinamide adenine dinucleotide phosphate complex responsible for neutrophil superoxide generation (Table 1) [75]. Additionally, DHEAS synergizes with GM-CSF and IL-4 to generate mature DCs from monocytes (Table 1) [76]. Moreover, DHEAS regulates cytokine production by both myeloid and lymphoid cells. Thus, most reports suggest this steroid is a potent inducer of IL-2 secretion by Th1 cells and human T cell cytotoxic function (Table 1) [77]. Finally, DHEA enhances Fas and Fas-L expression to induce thymocyte apoptosis [78].

Hormones, immune response and parasitic infection

In helminths infections: Protective immunity against helminth parasites is generally dependent on the development of a strong Th2 response involving IL-4 and IL-13. In general, females are more resistant than males. This is particularly true for gut parasitic helminth infections. There are many examples (*Strongyloides ratti*) where gonadectomy significantly reduces worm burdens in male rats but ovariectomy has no effect on parasite burdens in females [79]. Thus, increased male susceptibility to gut parasitic nematodes may be a direct result of androgenic as opposed to estrogenic influences on immunity. As a result, ovariectomy of females has no effect, but injection of testosterone into females or males increases gut worm burdens [79]. *Nippostrongylus brasiliensis* infection of Indian soft-furred rats reveals that males are more susceptible to infection since parasite burdens are higher in males than in females after 4 weeks of infection [80]. According to this, orchidectomy reduced parasite burdens in males while ovariectomy had no effect in females [80]. The intestinal parasite *Trichuris muris* is a significant example illustrating how sex hormones influence mast cell activity in female mice by favoring gut parasitic nematode expulsion [81]. Studies utilizing cytokine deficient mice might reveal underlying mechanisms modulating sex hormone influences on immunity and outcomes of parasite infection. Female C57BL/6, BALB/c IL-4 -/- and BALB/c mice showed *T. muris* infection resistance; however, male C57BL/6, IL-4 -/- and BALB/c are susceptible. This observation reflects the female ability to generate IL-13 [82,83]. In experimental assays, the administration of recombinant IL-13 to male BALB/c IL-4 -/- induces worm expulsion, while IL-13 neutralization in BALB/c IL-4 -/- inhibited expulsion [82,83]. These results suggest there is a possible link between E2 and the ability to produce IL-13 or IL-4 as mediators of resistance against this parasite and the infection susceptibility is a consequence of inadequate TH2 cells production [82,83].

In the case of the intracellular parasite *Trichinella spiralis*, estrogens can increase the resistance of male CD1 mice to parasites, as measured both by adult worm burdens and tissue larvae [84]. Gonadectomy also increases male resistance and T4 treatment increases female susceptibility. Consequently, both T4 and E2 influence *T. spiralis* control in a reciprocal manner, and this control is Th2 dependent [84]. Mast cells also play a crucial role in worm expulsion as in the case of *T. muris* [85]. These results suggest that sex hormones influence the Th2 response during gut parasitic infections and demonstrate the invariable female resistance to helminthic parasites (including filarial nematodes, in which Th2 responses promote resistance to infection). *Litomosoides sigmodontis* filarial survival is reduced in males compared to female BALB/c mice and the microfilariae prevalence and density are higher in females [86]. The susceptibility of BALB/c mice to *L. sigmodontis* is caused by the generation of potent regulatory T cell responses that overcome Th2 effector functions and permit survival of the adult parasite [87]. It is important to emphasize that E2 at physiological levels expands $CD4^+CD25^+FoxP3^+$ regulatory T cells expressing IL-10 [87,88] and that IL-10 is essential for microfilariae persistence [89].

Several groups have demonstrated that *in vitro* culture of *Taenia solium* cysticerci in the presence of sex steroid (P4) induces evagination in 100% of treated cysticerci [90]. In contrast, T4 and DHEA induce the opposite effect and inhibits 85% to 90% of evagination events [5]. The use of the P4 competitive antagonist RU486 inhibits the evagination process in cysticerci, and this effect is mediated by a classical steroid receptor that is able to block the transcription of some genes [90]. The use of flutamide (androgen antagonist) does not reverse the T4 and the DHEA effect [5]. These results suggest the cysticerci evagination process could be mediated by a specific P4-receptor present on the parasite (Figure 1) [90]. In contrast, host treatment with P4 reduces the number of parasitic worms [91]. The effect of E2 on *T. crassiceps* cysticerci showed that the hormone is able to induce budding and increase the parasite infective capacity to 200% [5]. The effect could be mediated through a specific estrogen receptor that promotes the expression of *c-fos* and *c-jun* (AP-1 transcriptional complex) and suggests that E2 has proliferative effects on the parasite [92]. Our laboratory also demonstrates that exposure of T. crassiceps cysticerci to E2 and P4 induced differential protein expression patterns regarding to changes in actin, tubulin and myosin expression altering flame cells at the level of the ciliary tuft [93]. In contrast T4 and DHT induced 90% of mortality caused by an alteration in the function of flame cells, without changes in actin, tubulin or myosin expression [94].

DHEA has been shown to affect different stages of *Schistosoma mansoni in vitro*. The treatment with DHEA decreases adult worm oviposition and increases the cercariae mortality rate to 100% [95]. In mouse models of *S. mansoni* infection, the sex difference is reversed and the female mice are more susceptible to infection because they develop higher inflammatory responses as measured by organ weights and delayed type hypersensitivity responses [96]. In mice, adrenalectomy exacerbates disease, as measured by worm burden and host mortality following inoculation with *S. mansoni* parasites [97]. In contrast, human males are more susceptible to *S. mansoni* infection than females [98]. In the case of *Schistosoma hematobium*, the treatment with T4 decreases the adult parasite reproductive capacity and reduces its fecundity through sexual hormone interaction with a glutathione S-tranferase (Sh28GST) to inhibit parasite metabolism [99]. A stimulant effect of murine epidermal growth factor (EGF) has been found on *Brugia malayi* microfilariae *in vitro*. EGF induces overexpression of *Raf* and *Ran* transcriptional levels and causes microfilariae growth and differentiation [100]. These experimental reports suggest that some human helminth and nematode parasites have molecular structures analogous to the classic hormone receptors. These receptors have similar functions as in mammals (Figure 1) [4,5,101].

In protozoa infections: In parasitic protozoa, some hormonal effects have also been reported on different morphologic stages. In *Toxoplasma gondii* murine infection models, females develop severe brain inflammation and are more likely to die following infection than males [102]. Male mice produce higher concentrations of TNF-α, IL-12, and IFN-γ than females during acute infection [102,103]. In female mice, ovariectomy reduces and administration of E2 exacerbates tissue cyst development caused by *T. gondii* infection [104,105]. The ovariectomized female mice treated with pharmacological doses of potent E2 compounds including 17β-estradiol, diethylstilbestrol, or alpha-dienestrol, renders mice more susceptible to disease as measured by brain cyst formation [105]. The host treatment with T4 reduces the parasite number and pathology [104,106]. *T. gondii* infection in rodents results in pronounced behavioral alterations including increased exploratory behavior and aggression. These changes may make the infected animal more conspicuous to and reduces definitive host fear (the cat) [107,108]. However, different studies with genetically engineered mice have shown that *T. gondii* stimulates the innate immune response during the initial parasite establishment and growth. During chronic infection, the disease state can be maintained directly by adaptive immune responses to control and benefit both host and parasite survival [109]. To achieve this outcome, *T. gondii* express a number of TLR ligands, including GPI-anchors [110], HSP70 [111,112] and profilin [113]. The parasite also induces IL-12 production through CCR5 receptor ligation [114]. These processes result in the activation of macrophages, DCs, and NK cells that produce IL-12, TNF-α, and IFN-γ. The production of cytokines can control parasite growth, induce Th1 cell expansion and facilitate the cytotoxic $CD8^+$ T cell development [115,116]. *Plasmodium sp.* infection is similar between males and females [117], however, previous studies suggested that males have higher parasitic burdens [118,119], but females have higher mortality rates [120]. It has been observed that cortisol treatment *in vitro* in *P. falciparum* merozoites increases the size and number of gametocytes produced. E2 treatment increases parasite growth and reproduction [121,122]. In contrast, prolactin can mediate lethal effects on various parasite stages [123]. In diseased rodent models using *Plasmodium chabaudi* female C57BL/10 [119,120] and C57BL/6 [124] mice, there was less

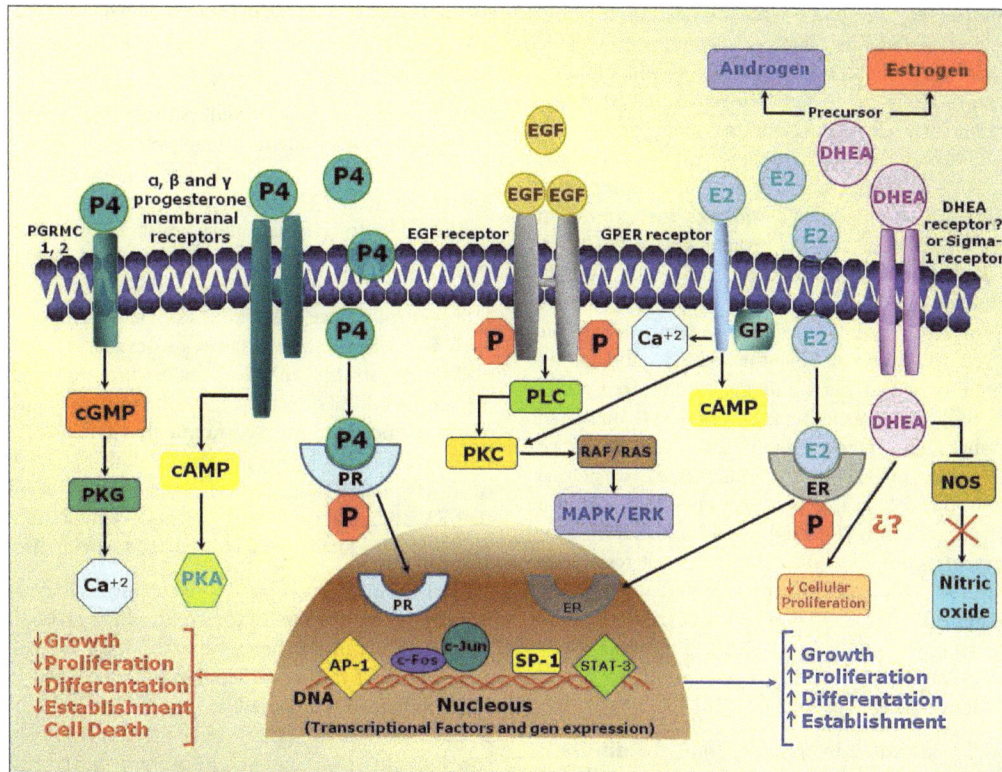

Figure 1. Signaling pathways and positive or negative effects of different hormones on the growth, differentiation, proliferation and establishment of parasitic cells. Some hormone signals are involved in the expression of transcription factors in the cell nucleus (genomic effects). These factors regulate the gene expression or the second messenger expression (no genomic effects), which results in the activation and/or inhibition of signaling cascades. DHEA: dehydroepiandrosterone; P4: Progesterone; EGF: murine epidermal growth factor; E2: 17-β-Estradiol.

parasitic induced mortality compared with male mice. Moreover, during *P. chabaudi* infection, T4 is a key modulator in the sexual dimorphism exhibited. Hormonal treatment in females can prevent self-healing, whereas male castration leads to self-healing [125,126]. Interestingly, in this disease model T4 is not signaling through classical androgen or estrogen receptor [125-128]. *In vivo* assays showed that female C57BL/10 mice orally administered T4 had increased mortality rates and death was associated with a decreased peritoneal cell generation of reactive oxygen species [129].However, in *P. falciparum* T4 and DHEA increase the growth and parasite reproduction [123]. Finally, T4 treatment of females results in CD8$^+$ T cell increases in the spleen and decreases in numbers of overall splenocytes [130]. Conversely, P4 treatment in mice increases growth and reproduction and favored parasite establishment [122]. Recent data showed that gonadectomy of increased T and B splenic cells in both sexes, increased macrophages cells and decreased the NK subpopulation only in male mice infected with *Plasmodium berghei ANKA*. Gonadectomy also induced an increase in the synthesis of IgG1, IgG2b, IgG3, and total IgG; the pro-inflammatory cytokines TNF-α and IL-6 and induced higher levesl of NO only in female mice. This suggest that female sex hormones have anti- inflammatory properties in malaria [131,132].

The intestinal protozoans *Entamoeba sp.* and *Giardia sp.* are transmitted fecal-orally and cause amoebiasis and giardiasis, respectively. During infection neutrophils play an important role in both diseases. For example, the alpha-defensins secreted by neutrophils *in vitro* have anti-giardial properties [133] and neutrophil-depleted mice have more severe amoebic liver abscess (ALA) and intestinal amoebiasis [134]. Macrophages produced NO is involved in protection of invasive amoebiasis [135]. Additionally, mast cells play a critical role in controlling giardiasis [136]. Studies performed using C57BL/6 mice infected with *Giardia muris* showed that male mice have higher parasite burdens in their gut [137,138], and more prolonged disaccharidase deficiency [138] than females. Moreover, infected female C57BL/6 mice had elevated levels of parasite-specific IgG and stronger IgG2b and IgG3 responses than males [139]. In *E. histolytica* human infection the invasive disease predominates in males compared to females [140]. Studies in mice have demonstrate that females show a significantly early IFN-γ production and the presence of Natural Killer T-cells (NKT) cells compared with male mice, which have higher levels of IL-4-producing cells. This cytokine and NKT cells seem to be important in the control of the disease since the use of IFN-gamma-neutralizing monoclonal antibodies or NKT-deficient female mice showed an exacerbated amoebic liver absses (ALA) [141]. *In vitro* exposure to DHEA and cortisol increase *E. histolytica* trophozoite proliferation and DNA synthesis. DHEA also induces a progressive loss of adherence capacity, which is crucial during intestinal infection [134] (Figure 1). In contrast, during intestinal infection treatment with testosterone (T 4) stimulated trophozoites migration from intestine to liver and increased ALA infections [141].

Trypanosoma spp. is the causal agent to Chagas´ disease in America and sleeping sickness in Africa. Chagas´ disease consists of acute and chronic phases. Although the role of the immune system during disease clearance and pathogenesis is not well understood, studies have shown sex hormones play a role in disease modulation. It is well documented that male mice and rats are more susceptible to disease than females in *T. cruzi* experimental infection [142-145]. In addition, males are clinically more likely to develop severe cardiomyopathies [146] and exhibit abnormal electrocardiograms more often than females [147]. Data indicates that EGF induces an increase in the growth, metabolic activity, and DNA synthesis of *Trypanosoma cruzi* trypomastigotes *in vitro*. Additionally, EGF induces the expression of receptors with tyrosine kinase activity, protein kinase C (PKC), and mitogen-activated protein kinases (MAPK) [148]. Susceptibility and/or resistance could be directly linked to the presence of female sex hormones, and ovariectomized females are more susceptible to disease [142,145,148]. However, a role for male sex hormones in mediating susceptibility is less clear, and gonadectomized males are reported to have reduced parasite burdens [145] and unaltered parasitemia and mortality [142]. Interestingly, female mice treated with high pharmacological doses of 17β-estradiol increases parasitemia and mortality. The low physiological doses have either no effect or reduced parasite burden and death [143]. DHEA administration after *T. cruzi* infection plays an essential role in enhancing host resistance. The macrophages infected with *T. cruzi* express different hormonal receptors and secrete more TNF-α, IL-12 and NO after treatment with DHEA. This cytokine secretion results in a decreased trypomastigote load in blood and suggests its protective role is a result of potent immunoregulatory actions during infection [149,150].

In the sleeping sickness caused by *T. brucei spp.*, the disease is characterized by two distinct stages; an early hemolytic stage followed by a late meningoencephalitic stage. This last phase is characterized by leukocyte infiltration into the central nervous system, astrocyte and microglial activation, and acute neuroinflammation that ultimately results in coma and death [151]. African trypanosomes have developed many mechanisms to evade host immune response. However, most important is their ability to switch immunodominant variant surface glycoprotein (VSG´s), exchange the antigen surface and always avoid the immune response [152,153]. In this case, sex hormones play a role in modulating immunity to African trypanosomes. Researchers have found that female mice have lower parasitemia and survive longer than their male counterparts [154]. During human disease, males have trypanosomes in their cerebral spinal fluid more often than females and males have more relapses following treatment [155]. Unfortunately, no further research has determined the roles of specific sex hormones during disease. It has been shown that infection can result in hypogonadism and decreased T4 and E2 levels in both clinical and experimental studies [156-159].

Human babesiosis is caused by the intraerythrocytic protozoan parasite called *Babesia microti*. Researchers studying this infection have found that male mice are more susceptible to disease [160]. However, studies of WA1-type babesial report that female mice are more susceptible [160]. While the mechanisms behind female susceptibility to WA1-type babesial are unclear, research into male susceptibility to *B. microti* indicates that T4 causes longer and more severe infections in mice that have been castrated and implanted with T4 compared to mice castrated and implanted with inert oil [161,162]. Additionally, higher-ranking mice within a home cage have higher T4 higher levels, and these higher levels are associated with depressed levels of serum immunoglobulin and reduced resistance to infection with *B. microti* [163]. Interestingly, ixodidae ticks preferentially attach to rodents with high T4 levels [162]. Although T4 exacerbates disease, E2 does not confer resistance to *B. microti* disease [164]. More research is required

to examine both the basic immune responses against *Babesia* parasites and the role that sex hormones play during disease. Additional studies investigating differences between parasite species and mouse strains are also needed.

The sexually transmitted parasite *Trichomonas vaginalis* is an extracellular mucosal protozoan with a progressive growth. Several studies show that *T. vaginalis* has androgen and estrogen receptors on its cell surface (Figure 1) [165]. Interestingly, to study *T. vaginalis* in the laboratory, female mice must receive estrogen treatments to establish disease [166,167]. Similarly, in clinical studies, female volunteers also require estrogen treatment to establish the disease [168]. Furthermore, conditions associated with high levels of estrogen, such as menses and pregnancy, can exacerbate *T. vaginalis* infections [169]. 17β-estradiol enhances the *in vitro* growth of parasites, whereas T4 and P4 inhibit growth at early phases. Other studies using euthymic and athymic BALB/c mice found that females are more susceptible than males at developing abscesses following subcutaneous injections of *T. vaginalis* [170]. Conversely, some *in vitro* studies have found that E2 inhibits *T. vaginalis* growth [171] and both virulence factor and cell-detaching factor, which are correlated with disease severity [172].

Leishmania spp. is an obligate intracellular protozoan parasite transmitted by the bite of certain sandfly species. In humans infected with *L. mexicana*, females generally have increased Th1 responses, as measured by DTH reactions and decreased Th2 responses and IgE production compared to males [173]. In *L. major* infections, gonadectomy increases male resistance and T4 implants increase female susceptibility [174]. Similarly, E2 promotes macrophage mediated killing of *L. mexicana* at physiological levels through increased NO production independent of proinflammatory cytokine expression [175]. During *L. donovani* infection, T4 regulates murine bone marrow-derived macrophage p38 MAPK activation in a negative manner, and this promotes parasite survival [176]. *L. mexicana* infection is more severe than *L. major* infection because virulence is based on downregulation of macrophage function and IFN-γ induced Jak1, Jak2, and STAT1 activation [177,178]. E2 upregulates IFN-γ mRNA expression by T cells [39] whereas T4 inhibits production of this cytokine [71]. The IL-10 cellular sources are potentially subject to sex hormone control [179]. Thus, the Th1/Th2 paradigm of resistance/susceptibility to intracellular parasites is a gross oversimplification of a far more complicated network of regulatory/counter-regulatory interactions that are also subject to further modulation by sex hormones.

Conclusion

As previously mentioned, during many parasitic infections, there is a reciprocal relationship amongst sex steroids, the immune system, and the eventual elimination or establishment of the parasites in humans. In certain cases, hormones can regulate the innate immune response and the subsequent adaptive immune response [180].

The hormonal microenvironment may favor or inhibit the survival of parasites differentially between the sexes. This result may represent a highly evolved host-parasite relationship in which certain hormones appear to serve as proliferation or death factors that influence the establishment of infection and are independent of the host immune response. All of to the data suggest the parasites exploit endocrine mechanisms developed by the host for its own advantage.

The elucidation of neuroimmunoendocrine interactions during parasite infections is fundamental to understand the mechanisms involved in parasite establishment, growth, and reproduction in human hosts. A deeper comprehension of this complex relationship could have implications in the control and treatment of various infections throughout the world. The physiologic elements that are essential in the network of neuroimmunoendocrine interactions during parasite infection could have a deep biological and physiopathological impact. Thus, a better understanding could be extremely valuable in designing vaccines and new antiparasitic drugs and in controlling various human and veterinary parasitosis. It may also lead to the development of new therapies for autoimmune diseases.

Acknowledgements

Financial support: Grant #176803 was obtained from Programa de Fondos Sectoriales CB-SEP, Consejo Nacional de Ciencia y Tecnología (CONACyT) and Grant IN208715 was obtained from Programa de Apoyo a Proyectos de Innovacion Tecnologica, Direccion General de Asuntos del Personal Academico, Universidad Nacional Autonoma de Mexico, both provided to Jorge Morales-Montor. Hugo Aguilar-Díaz had a posdoctoral fellowship from Programa de Becas Posdoctorales Dirección General de Asuntos de Personal Académico (DGAPA) UNAM, and Dulce María Meneses Ruiz was a recipient of a posdoctoral fellowship from CB-2010/151747 CONACYT, UNAM

References

1. Nacher M, Singhasivanon P, Treeprasertsuk S, Silamchamroon U, Phumratanaprapin W, et al. (2003) Gender differences in the prevalences of human infection with intestinal helminths on the Thai-Burmese border. Ann Trop Med Parasitol 97: 433-435.

2. Nava-Castro K, Hernández-Bello R, Muñiz-Hernández S, Camacho-Arroyo I, Morales-Montor J (2012) Sex steroids, immune system, and parasitic infections: facts and hypotheses. Ann N Y Acad Sci 1262: 16-26.

3. Poulin R (1996) Helminth growth in vertebrate hosts: does host sex matter? Int J Parasitol 26: 1311-1315.

4. Escobedo G, Roberts CW, Carrero JC, Morales-Montor J (2005) Parasite regulation by host hormones: an old mechanism of host exploitation? Trends Parasitol 21: 588-593.

5. Escobedo G, Larralde C, Chavarria A, Cerbón MA, Morales-Montor J (2004) Molecular mechanisms involved in the differential effects of sex steroids on the reproduction and infectivity of Taenia crassiceps. J Parasitol 90: 1235-1244.

6. Ibarra-Coronado EG, Escobedo G, Nava-Castro K, Jesus Ramses CR, Hernandez-Bello R, et al. (2011) A helminth cestode parasite express an estrogen-binding protein resembling a classic nuclear estrogen receptor. Steroids 76: 1149-1159.

7. Taubert S, Ward JD, Yamamoto KR (2011) Nuclear hormone receptors in nematodes: evolution and function. Mol Cell Endocrinol 334: 49-55.

8. Magor BG, Magor KE (2001) Evolution of effectors and receptors of innate immunity. Dev Comp Immunol 25: 651-682.

9. Faurschou M, Borregaard N (2003) Neutrophil granules and secretory vesicles in inflammation. Microbes Infect 5: 1317-1327.

10. Sindrilaru A, Scharffetter-Kochanek K (2013) Disclosure of the Culprits: Macrophages-Versatile Regulators of Wound Healing. Adv Wound Care (New Rochelle) 2: 357-368.

11. Sunderkötter C, Steinbrink K, Goebeler M, Bhardwaj R, Sorg C (1994) Macrophages and angiogenesis. J Leukoc Biol 55: 410-422.

12. Rettew JA, Huet-Hudson YM, Marriott I (2008) Testosterone reduces macrophage expression in the mouse of toll-like receptor 4, a trigger for inflammation and innate immunity. Biol Reprod 78: 432-437.

13. Szekeres-Bartho J, Faust Z, Varga P, Szereday L, and Kelemen K (1996) The immunological pregnancy protective effect of progesterone is manifested via controlling cytokine production. American journal of reproductive immunology 35, 348-351.

14. Szekeres-Bartho J, Polgar B (2010) PIBF: the double edged sword. Pregnancy and tumor. Am J Reprod Immunol 64: 77-86.

15. Klein SL (2004) Hormonal and immunological mechanisms mediating sex differences in parasite infection. Parasite Immunol 26: 247-264.

16. Miller L, Hunt JS (1996) Sex steroid hormones and macrophage function. Life Sci 59: 1-14.

17. Roberts CW, Walker W, Alexander J (2001) Sex-associated hormones and immunity to protozoan parasites. Clin Microbiol Rev 14: 476-488.

18. Robinson DP, Klein SL (2012) Pregnancy and pregnancy-associated hormones alter immune responses and disease pathogenesis. Horm Behav 62: 263-271.

19. Pennell LM, Galligan CL, Fish EN (2012) Sex affects immunity. J Autoimmun 38: J282-291.

20. Schlitzer A, McGovern N, Ginhoux F (2015) Dendritic cells and monocyte-derived cells: Two complementary and integrated functional systems. Semin Cell Dev Biol 41: 9-22.

21. Allman D, Pillai S (2008) Peripheral B cell subsets. Curr Opin Immunol 20: 149-157.

22. Raphael I, Nalawade S, Eagar TN, Forsthuber TG (2015) T cell subsets and their signature cytokines in autoimmune and inflammatory diseases. Cytokine 74: 5-17.

23. Girón-González JA, Moral FJ, Elvira J, García-Gil D, Guerrero F, et al. (2000) Consistent production of a higher TH1:TH2 cytokine ratio by stimulated T cells in men compared with women. Eur J Endocrinol 143: 31-36.

24. Blankenhorn EP, Troutman S, Clark LD, Zhang XM, Chen P, et al. (2003) Sexually dimorphic genes regulate healing and regeneration in MRL mice. Mamm Genome 14: 250-260.

25. Krzych U, Strausser HR, Bressler JP, and Goldstein AL (1981) Effects of sex hormones on some T and B cell functions as evidenced by differential immune expression between male and female mice and cyclic pattern of immune responsiveness during the estrous cycle. Prog Clin Biol Res 70: 145-150.

26. Simpson ER (2003) Sources of estrogen and their importance. J Steroid Biochem Mol Biol 86: 225-230.

27. Ansar Ahmed S, Penhale WJ, Talal N (1985) Sex hormones, immune responses, and autoimmune diseases. Mechanisms of sex hormone action. Am J Pathol 121: 531-551.

28. Gaunt SD, Pierce KR (1985) Myelopoiesis and marrow adherent cells in estradiol-treated mice. Vet Pathol 22: 403-408.

29. Squadrito F, Altavilla D, Squadrito G, Campo GM, Arlotta M, et al. (1997) 17Beta-oestradiol reduces cardiac leukocyte accumulation in myocardial ischaemia reperfusion injury in rat. Eur J Pharmacol 335: 185-192.

30. Bekesi G, Tulassay Z, Racz K, Feher J, Szekacs B, et al. (2007) The effect of estrogens on superoxide anion generation by human neutrophil granulocytes: possible consequences of the antioxidant defense. Gynecological endocrinology : the official journal of the International Society of Gynecological Endocrinology 23: 451-454.

31. Cuzzocrea S, Genovese T, Mazzon E, Esposito E, Di Paola R, et al. (2008) Effect of 17beta-estradiol on signal transduction pathways and secondary damage in experimental spinal cord trauma. Shock 29: 362-371.

32. Baranao RI, Tenenbaum A, Sales ME, and Rumi LS (1992) Functional alterations of murine peritoneal macrophages during pregnancy. American journal of reproductive immunology 27: 82-86.

33. Rettew JA, Huet YM, Marriott I (2009) Estrogens augment cell surface TLR4 expression on murine macrophages and regulate sepsis susceptibility in vivo. Endocrinology 150: 3877-3884.

34. Paharkova-Vatchkova V, Maldonado R, and Kovats S (2004) Estrogen preferentially promotes the differentiation of CD11c+ CD11b(intermediate) dendritic cells from bone marrow precursors. Journal of immunology 172: 1426-1436.

35. Bengtsson AK, Ryan EJ, Giordano D, Magaletti DM, Clark EA (2004) 17beta-estradiol (E2) modulates cytokine and chemokine expression in human monocyte-derived dendritic cells. Blood 104: 1404-1410.

36. Siracusa MC, Overstreet MG, Housseau F, Scott AL, Klein SL (2008) 17beta-estradiol alters the activity of conventional and IFN-producing killer dendritic cells. J Immunol 180: 1423-1431.

37. Zhang QH, Hu YZ, Cao J, Zhong YQ, Zhao YF, et al. (2004) Estrogen influences the differentiation, maturation and function of dendritic cells in rats with experimental autoimmune encephalomyelitis. Acta Pharmacol Sin 25: 508-513.

38. Baral E, Nagy E, Berczi I (1995) Modulation of natural killer cell-mediated

cytotoxicity by tamoxifen and estradiol. Cancer 75: 591-599.

39. Nakaya M, Tachibana H, Yamada K (2006) Effect of estrogens on the interferon-gamma producing cell population of mouse splenocytes. Biosci Biotechnol Biochem 70: 47-53.

40. Hao S, Zhao J, Zhou J, Zhao S, Hu Y, et al. (2007) Modulation of 17beta-estradiol on the number and cytotoxicity of NK cells in vivo related to MCM and activating receptors. Int Immunopharmacol 7: 1765-1775.

41. Straub RH (2007) The complex role of estrogens in inflammation. Endocr Rev 28: 521-574.

42. Karpuzoglu E, Phillips RA, Gogal RM Jr, Ansar Ahmed S (2007) IFN-gamma-inducing transcription factor, T-bet is upregulated by estrogen in murine splenocytes: role of IL-27 but not IL-12. Mol Immunol 44: 1808-1814.

43. Faas M, Bouman A, Moesa H, Heineman MJ, de Leij L, et al. (2000) The immune response during the luteal phase of the ovarian cycle: a Th2-type response? Fertil Steril 74: 1008-1013.

44. Wang C, Dehghani B, Li Y, Kaler LJ, Vandenbark AA, et al. (2009) Oestrogen modulates experimental autoimmune encephalomyelitis and interleukin-17 production via programmed death 1. Immunology 126: 329-335.

45. Polanczyk MJ, Hopke C, Vandenbark AA, and Offner H (2007) Treg suppressive activity involves estrogen-dependent expression of programmed death-1 (PD-1). International immunology 19: 337-343.

46. Tai P, Wang J, Jin H, Song X, Yan J, et al. (2008) Induction of regulatory T cells by physiological level estrogen. J Cell Physiol 214: 456-464.

47. Nilsson N, Carlsten H (1994) Estrogen induces suppression of natural killer cell cytotoxicity and augmentation of polyclonal B cell activation. Cell Immunol 158: 131-139.

48. Lü FX, Abel K, Ma Z, Rourke T, Lu D, et al. (2002) The strength of B cell immunity in female rhesus macaques is controlled by CD8+ T cells under the influence of ovarian steroid hormones. Clin Exp Immunol 128: 10-20.

49. Kanda N, Tamaki K (1999) Estrogen enhances immunoglobulin production by human PBMCs. J Allergy Clin Immunol 103: 282-288.

50. Attanasio R, Gust DA, Wilson ME, Meeker T, and Gordon TP (2002) Immunomodulatory effects of estrogen and progesterone replacement in a nonhuman primate model. Journal of clinical immunology 22: 263-269.

51. Enomoto LM, Kloberdanz KJ, Mack DG, Elizabeth D, and Weinberg A (2007) Ex vivo effect of estrogen and progesterone compared with dexamethasone on cell-mediated immunity of HIV- infected and uninfected subjects. Journal of acquired immune deficiency syndromes 45: 137-143.

52. Zang YC, Halder JB, Hong J, Rivera VM, Zhang JZ (2002) Regulatory effects of estriol on T cell migration and cytokine profile: inhibition of transcription factor NF-kappa B. J Neuroimmunol 124: 106-114.

53. Härkönen PL, Väänänen HK (2006) Monocyte-macrophage system as a target for estrogen and selective estrogen receptor modulators. Ann N Y Acad Sci 1089: 218-227.

54. Salem ML, Hossain MS, and Nomoto K (2000) Mediation of the immunomodulatory effect of beta- estradiol on inflammatory responses by inhibition of recruitment and activation of inflammatory cells and their gene expression of TNF-alpha and IFN-gamma. International archives of allergy and immunology 121: 235-245.

55. Jalanti R, Isliker H (1977) Immunoglobulins in human cervico-vaginal secretions. Int Arch Allergy Appl Immunol 53: 402-408.

56. Wira CR, Sandoe CP (1989) Effect of uterine immunization and oestradiol on specific IgA and IgG antibodies in uterine, vaginal and salivary secretions. Immunology 68: 24-30.

57. Kaushic C, Frauendorf E, Rossoll RM, Richardson JM, Wira CR (1998) Influence of the estrous cycle on the presence and distribution of immune cells in the rat reproductive tract. Am J Reprod Immunol 39: 209-216.

58. Nakagami F, Nakagami H, Osako MK, Iwabayashi M, Taniyama Y, et al. (2010) Estrogen attenuates vascular remodeling in Lp(a) transgenic mice. Atherosclerosis 211: 41-47.

59. Sentman CL, Meadows SK, Wira CR, Eriksson M (2004) Recruitment of uterine NK cells: induction of CXC chemokine ligands 10 and 11 in human endometrium by estradiol and progesterone. J Immunol 173: 6760-6766.

60. Wira CR, and Rossoll RM (2003) Oestradiol regulation of antigen presentation by uterine stromal cells: role of transforming growth factor-ß production by epithelial cells in mediating antigen- presenting cell function. Immunology 109: 398-406.

61. Menzies FM, Henriquez FL, Alexander J, Roberts CW (2011) Selective inhibition and augmentation of alternative macrophage activation by progesterone. Immunology 134: 281-291.

62. Butts CL, Shukair SA, Duncan KM, Bowers E, Horn C, et al. (2007) Progesterone inhibits mature rat dendritic cells in a receptor-mediated fashion. Int Immunol 19: 287-296.

63. Su L, Sun Y, Ma F, Lü P, Huang H, et al. (2009) Progesterone inhibits Toll-like receptor 4-mediated innate immune response in macrophages by suppressing NF-kappaB activation and enhancing SOCS1 expression. Immunol Lett 125: 151-155.

64. Krishnan L, Guilbert LJ, Russell AS, Wegmann TG, Mosmann TR, et al. (1996) Pregnancy impairs resistance of C57BL/6 mice to Leishmania major infection and causes decreased antigen-specific IFN-gamma response and increased production of T helper 2 cytokines. Journal of immunology 156: 644-652.

65. Sacks GP, Clover LM, Bainbridge DR, Redman CW, Sargent IL (2001) Flow cytometric measurement of intracellular Th1 and Th2 cytokine production by human villous and extravillous cytotrophoblast. Placenta 22: 550-559.

66. Szekeres-Bartho J, Par G, Szereday L, Smart CY, and Achatz I (1997) Progesterone and non-specific immunologic mechanisms in pregnancy. American journal of reproductive immunology 38: 176-182.

67. Arruvito L, Giulianelli S, Flores AC, Paladino N, Barboza M, et al. (2008) NK cells expressing a progesterone receptor are susceptible to progesterone-induced apoptosis. J Immunol 180: 5746-5753.

68. Kumar P1, Sait SF (2011) Luteinizing hormone and its dilemma in ovulation induction. J Hum Reprod Sci 4: 2-7.

69. Muñoz-Cruz S, Mendoza-Rodríguez Y, Nava-Castro KE, Yepez-Mulia L, Morales-Montor J (2015) Gender-related effects of sex steroids on histamine release and FcÎµRI expression in rat peritoneal mast cells. J Immunol Res 2015: 351829.

70. Corrales JJ, Almeida M, Burgo R, Mories MT, Miralles JM, et al. (2006) Androgen-replacement therapy depresses the ex vivo production of inflammatory cytokines by circulating antigen- presenting cells in aging type-2 diabetic men with partial androgen deficiency. J Endocrinol 189: 595-604.

71. Page ST, Plymate SR, Bremner WJ, Matsumoto AM, Hess DL, et al. (2006) Effect of medical castration on CD4+ CD25+ T cells, CD8+ T cell IFN-gamma expression, and NK cells: a physiological role for testosterone and/or its metabolites. Am J Physiol Endocrinol Metab 290: E856-863.

72. Dalal M, Kim S, and Voskuhl RR (1997) Testosterone therapy ameliorates experimental autoimmune encephalomyelitis and induces a T helper 2 bias in the autoantigen-specific T lymphocyte response. Journal of immunology 159: 3-6.

73. Kanda N, Tsuchida T, and Tamaki K (1996) Testosterone inhibits immunoglobulin production by human peripheral blood mononuclear cells. Clinical and experimental immunology 106: 410-415.

74. Mesiano S, Jaffe RB (1997) Developmental and functional biology of the primate fetal adrenal cortex. Endocr Rev 18: 378-403.

75. Radford DJ, Wang K, McNelis JC, Taylor AE, Hechenberger G, et al. (2010) Dehydroepiandrosterone sulfate directly activates protein kinase C-beta to increase human neutrophil superoxide generation. Mol Endocrinol 24: 813-821.

76. Canning MO, Grotenhuis K, de Wit HJ, and Drexhage HA (2000) Opposing effects of dehydroepiandrosterone and dexamethasone on the generation of monocyte-derived dendritic cells. European journal of endocrinology / European Federation of Endocrine Societies 143: 687-695.

77. Suzuki T, Suzuki N, Daynes RA, Engleman EG (1991) Dehydroepiandrosterone enhances IL2 production and cytotoxic effector function of human T cells. Clin Immunol Immunopathol 61: 202-211.

78. Liang J, Yao G, Yang L, Hou Y (2004) Dehydroepiandrosterone induces apoptosis of thymocyte through Fas/Fas-L pathway. Int Immunopharmacol 4: 1467-1475.

79. Kiyota M, Korenaga M, Nawa Y, Kotani M (1984) Effect of androgen on the expression of the sex difference in susceptibility to infection with Strongyloides

ratti in C57BL/6 mice. Aust J Exp Biol Med Sci 62 : 607-618.

80. Tiuria R, Horii Y, Tateyama S, Tsuchiya K, and Nawa Y (1994) The Indian soft-furred rat, Millardia meltada, a new host for Nippostrongylus brasiliensis, showing androgen-dependent sex difference in intestinal mucosal defence. Int J Parasitol 24: 1055-1057.

81. Hepworth MR, Hardman MJ, Grencis RK (2010) The role of sex hormones in the development of Th2 immunity in a gender-biased model of Trichuris muris infection. Eur J Immunol 40: 406-416.

82. Bancroft AJ, Artis D, Donaldson DD, Sypek JP, Grencis RK (2000) Gastrointestinal nematode expulsion in IL-4 knockout mice is IL-13 dependent. Eur J Immunol 30: 2083-2091.

83. Bancroft AJ, McKenzie AN, Grencis RK (1998) A critical role for IL-13 in resistance to intestinal nematode infection. J Immunol 160: 3453-3461.

84. Reddington JJ, Stewart GL, Kramar GW, Kramar MA (1981) The effects of host sex and hormones on Trichinella spiralis in the mouse. J Parasitol 67: 548-555.

85. Knight PA, Brown JK, and Pemberton AD (2008) Innate immune response mechanisms in the intestinal epithelium: potential roles for mast cells and goblet cells in the expulsion of adult Trichinella spiralis. Parasitology 135: 655-670.

86. Graham AL, Taylor MD, Le Goff L, Lamb TJ, Magennis M, et al. (2005) Quantitative appraisal of murine filariasis confirms host strain differences but reveals that BALB/c females are more susceptible than males to Litomosoides sigmodontis. Microbes and infection / Institut Pasteur 7: 612-618.

87. Taylor MD, LeGoff L, Harris A, Malone E, Allen JE, et al. (2005) Removal of regulatory T cell activity reverses hyporesponsiveness and leads to filarial parasite clearance in vivo. J Immunol 174: 4924-4933.

88. Taylor MD, Harris A, Babayan SA, Bain O, Culshaw A, et al. (2007) CTLA-4 and CD4+ CD25+ regulatory T cells inhibit protective immunity to filarial parasites in vivo. J Immunol 179: 4626-4634.

89. Hoffmann WH, Pfaff AW, Schulz-Key H, Soboslay PT (2001) Determinants for resistance and susceptibility to microfilaraemia in Litomosoides sigmodontis filariasis. Parasitology 122: 641-649.

90. Escobedo G, Camacho-Arroyo I, Hernandez-Hernandez OT, Ostoa-Saloma P, Garcia-Varela M, et al. (2010) Progesterone induces scolex evagination of the human parasite Taenia solium: evolutionary implications to the host-parasite relationship. J Biomed Biotechnol 591079.

91. Escobedo G, Camacho-Arroyo I, Nava-Luna P, Olivos A, Pérez-Torres A, et al. (2011) Progesterone induces mucosal immunity in a rodent model of human taeniosis by Taenia solium. Int J Biol Sci 7: 1443-1456.

92. Morales-Montor J, Escobedo G, Rodriguez-Dorantes M, Téllez-Ascencio N, Cerbón MA, et al. (2004) Differential expression of AP-1 transcription factor genes c-fos and c-jun in the helminth parasites Taenia crassiceps and Taenia solium. Parasitology 129: 233-243.

93. Ambrosio JR, Ostoa-Saloma P, Palacios-Arreola MI, Ruíz-Rosado A, Sánchez-Orellana PL, et al. (2014) Oestradiol and progesterone differentially alter cytoskeletal protein expression and flame cell morphology in Taenia crassiceps. International Journal for Parasitology 44: 687-696.

94. Ambrosio JR, Valverde-Islas L, Nava-Castro KE, Palacios-Arreola MI, Ostoa-Saloma P, et al. (2015) Androgens Exert a Cysticidal Effect upon Taenia crassiceps by Disrupting Flame Cell Morphology and Function. PLoS One 10: e0127928.

95. Morales-Montor J, Mohamed F, Ghaleb AM, Baig S, Hallal-Calleros C, et al. (2001) In vitro effects of hypothalamic-pituitary-adrenal axis (HPA) hormones on Schistosoma mansoni. J Parasitol 87: 1132-1139.

96. Eloi-Santos S, Olsen NJ, Correa-Oliveira R, Colley DG (1992) Schistosoma mansoni: mortality, pathophysiology, and susceptibility differences in male and female mice. Exp Parasitol 75: 168-175.

97. Morales-Montor J, Mohamed F, Damian RT (2004) Schistosoma mansoni: the effect of adrenalectomy on the murine model. Microbes Infect 6: 475-480.

98. Degu G, Mengistu G, Jones J (2002) Some factors affecting prevalence of and immune responses to Schistosoma mansoni in schoolchildren in Gorgora, northwest Ethiopia. Ethiop Med J 40: 345-352.

99. Remoué F, Mani JC, Pugnière M, Schacht AM, Capron A, et al. (2002) Functional specific binding of testosterone to Schistosoma haematobium 28-kilodalton glutathione S-transferase. Infect Immun 70: 601-605.

100. Dissanayake S (2000) Upregulation of a raf kinase and a DP-1 family transcription factor in epidermal growth factor (EGF) stimulated filarial parasites. Int J Parasitol 30: 1089-1097.

101. Gomez Y, Valdez RA, Larralde C, and Romano MC (2000) Sex steroids and parasitism: Taenia crassiceps cisticercus metabolizes exogenous androstenedione to testosterone in vitro. The Journal of steroid biochemistry and molecular biology 74: 143-147.

102. Walker W, Roberts CW, Ferguson DJ, Jebbari H, Alexander J (1997) Innate immunity to Toxoplasma gondii is influenced by gender and is associated with differences in interleukin-12 and gamma interferon production. Infect Immun 65: 1119-1121.

103. Roberts CW, Cruickshank SM, Alexander J (1995) Sex-determined resistance to Toxoplasma gondii is associated with temporal differences in cytokine production. Infect Immun 63: 2549-2555.

104. Liesenfeld O, Nguyen TA, Pharke C, Suzuki Y (2001) Importance of gender and sex hormones in regulation of susceptibility of the small intestine to peroral infection with Toxoplasma gondii tissue cysts. J Parasitol 87: 1491-1493.

105. Pung OJ, Luster MI (1986) Toxoplasma gondii: decreased resistance to infection in mice due to estrogen. Exp Parasitol 61: 48-56.

106. Kaňková S, Kodym P, Flegr J (2011) Direct evidence of Toxoplasma-induced changes in serum testosterone in mice. Exp Parasitol 128: 181-183.

107. Arnott MA, Cassella JP, Aitken PP, Hay J (1990) Social interactions of mice with congenital Toxoplasma infection. Ann Trop Med Parasitol 84: 149-156.

108. Webster JP, Brunton CF, MacDonald DW (1994) Effect of Toxoplasma gondii upon neophobic behaviour in wild brown rats, Rattus norvegicus. Parasitology 109 : 37-43.

109. Yap GS, Shaw MH, Ling Y, Sher A (2006) Genetic analysis of host resistance to intracellular pathogens: lessons from studies of Toxoplasma gondii infection. Microbes Infect 8: 1174-1178.

110. Debierre-Grockiego F, Campos MA, Azzouz N, Schmidt J, Bieker U, et al. (2007) Activation of TLR2 and TLR4 by glycosylphosphatidylinositols derived from Toxoplasma gondii. J Immunol 179: 1129-1137.

111. Aosai F, Rodriguez Pena MS, Mun HS, Fang H, Mitsunaga T, et al. (2006) Toxoplasma gondii-derived heat shock protein 70 stimulates maturation of murine bone marrow-derived dendritic cells via Toll-like receptor 4. Cell Stress Chaperones 11: 13-22.

112. Mun HS, Aosai F, Norose K, Piao LX, Fang H, et al. (2005) Toll-like receptor 4 mediates tolerance in macrophages stimulated with Toxoplasma gondii-derived heat shock protein 70. Infect Immun 73: 4634-4642.

113. Lauw FN, Caffrey DR, Golenbock DT (2005) Of mice and man: TLR11 (finally) finds profilin. Trends Immunol 26: 509-511.

114. Aliberti J, Valenzuela JG, Carruthers VB, Hieny S, Andersen J, et al. (2003) Molecular mimicry of a CCR5 binding-domain in the microbial activation of dendritic cells. Nat Immunol 4: 485-490.

115. Parker SJ, Roberts CW, and Alexander J (1991) CD8+ T cells are the major lymphocyte subpopulation involved in the protective immune response to Toxoplasma gondii in mice. Clinical and experimental immunology 84: 207-212.

116. Combe CL, Curiel TJ, Moretto MM, Khan IA (2005) NK cells help to induce CD8(+)-T-cell immunity against Toxoplasma gondii in the absence of CD4(+) T cells. Infect Immun 73: 4913-4921.

117. Venugopalan PP, Shenoy DU, Kamath A, Rajeev A (1997) Distribution of malarial parasites: effect of gender of construction workers. Indian J Med Sci 51: 89-92.

118. Landgraf B, Kollaritsch H, Wiedermann G, Wernsdorfer WH (1994) Parasite density of Plasmodium falciparum malaria in Ghanaian schoolchildren: evidence for influence of sex hormones? Trans R Soc Trop Med Hyg 88: 73-74.

119. Wildling E, Winkler S, Kremsner PG, Brandts C, Jenne L, et al. (1995) Malaria epidemiology in the province of Moyen Ogoov, Gabon. Trop Med Parasitol 46: 77-82.

120. Kochar DK, Thanvi I, Joshi A, Shubhakaran, Agarwal N, et al. (1999) Mortality trends in falciparum malaria--effect of gender difference and pregnancy. J Assoc Physicians India 47: 774-778.

121. Maswoswe SM, Peters W, Warhurst DC (1985) Corticosteroid stimulation of

the growth of Plasmodium falciparum gametocytes in vitro. Ann Trop Med Parasitol 79: 607-616.

122. Lingnau A, Margos G, Maier WA, Seitz HM (1993) The effects of hormones on the gametocytogenesis of Plasmodium falciparum in vitro. Appl Parasitol 34: 153-160.

123. Bayoumi NK, Elhassan EM, Elbashir MI, Adam I (2009) Cortisol, prolactin, cytokines and the susceptibility of pregnant Sudanese women to Plasmodium falciparum malaria. Ann Trop Med Parasitol 103: 111-117.

124. Cernetich A, Garver LS, Jedlicka AE, Klein PW, Kumar N, et al. (2006) Involvement of gonadal steroids and gamma interferon in sex differences in response to blood-stage malaria infection. Infect Immun 74: 3190-3203.

125. Benten WP, Wunderlich F, Mossmann H (1992) Testosterone-induced suppression of self-healing Plasmodium chabaudi malaria: an effect not mediated by androgen receptors? J Endocrinol 135: 407-413.

126. Benten WP, Wunderlich F, Mossmann H (1992) Plasmodium chabaudi: estradiol suppresses acquiring, but not once-acquired immunity. Exp Parasitol 75: 240-247.

127. Benten WP, Wunderlich F, Herrmann R, and Kuhn-Velten WN (1993) Testosterone-induced compared with oestradiol-induced immunosuppression against Plasmodium chabaudi malaria. J Endocrinol 139: 487-494.

128. Wunderlich F, Benten WP, Lieberherr M, Guo Z, Stamm O, et al. (2002) Testosterone signaling in T cells and macrophages. Steroids 67: 535-538.

129. Mossmann H, Benten WP, Galanos C, Freudenberg M, Kühn-Velten WN, et al. (1997) Dietary testosterone suppresses protective responsiveness to Plasmodium chabaudi malaria. Life Sci 60: 839-848.

130. Benten WP, Bettenhaeuser U, Wunderlich F, Van Vliet E, Mossmann H (1991) Testosterone-induced abrogation of self-healing of Plasmodium chabaudi malaria in B10 mice: mediation by spleen cells. Infect Immun 59: 4486-4490.

131. Legorreta-Herrera M, Mosqueda-Romo NA, Nava-Castro KE, Morales-Rodríguez AL, Buendía-González FO, et al. (2015) Sex hormones modulate the immune response to Plasmodium berghei ANKA in CBA/Ca mice. Parasitol Res 114: 2659-2669.

132. Mosqueda-Romo NA, Rodríguez-Morales AL, Buendía-González FO, Aguilar-Sánchez M, Morales-Montor J, et al. (2014) Gonadal steroids negatively modulate oxidative stress in CBA/Ca female mice infected with P. berghei ANKA. Biomed Res Int 2014: 805495.

133. Aley SB, Zimmerman M, Hetsko M, Selsted ME, Gillin FD (1994) Killing of Giardia lamblia by cryptdins and cationic neutrophil peptides. Infect Immun 62: 5397-5403.

134. Carrero JC, Cervantes C, Moreno-Mendoza N, Saavedra E, Morales-Montor J, et al. (2006) Dehydroepiandrosterone decreases while cortisol increases in vitro growth and viability of Entamoeba histolytica. Microbes and infection / Institut Pasteur 8: 323-331.

135. Seydel KB, Smith SJ, Stanley SL Jr (2000) Innate immunity to amebic liver abscess is dependent on gamma interferon and nitric oxide in a murine model of disease. Infect Immun 68: 400-402.

136. Li E, Zhou P, Petrin Z, Singer SM (2004) Mast cell-dependent control of Giardia lamblia infections in mice. Infect Immun 72: 6642-6649.

137. Daniels CW, Belosevic M (1995) Comparison of the course of infection with Giardia muris in male and female mice. Int J Parasitol 25: 131-135.

138. Daniels CW, Belosevic M (1995) Disaccharidase activity in male and female C57BL/6 mice infected with Giardia muris. Parasitol Res 81: 143-147.

139. Daniels CW, Belosevic M (1994) Serum antibody responses by male and female C57Bl/6 mice infected with Giardia muris. Clin Exp Immunol 97: 424-429.

140. Acuna-Soto R, Maguire JH, Wirth DF (2000) Gender distribution in asymptomatic and invasive amebiasis. Am J Gastroenterol 95: 1277-1283.

141. Lotter H, Jacobs T, Gaworski I, Tannich E (2006) Sexual dimorphism in the control of amebic liver abscess in a mouse model of disease. Infect Immun 74: 118-124.

142. Chapman WL Jr, Hanson WL, Waits VB (1975) The influence of gonadectomy of host on parasitemia and mortality of mice infected with Trypanosoma cruzi. J Parasitol 61: 213-216.

143. de Souza EM, Rivera MT, Araújo-Jorge TC, de Castro SL (2001) Modulation induced by estradiol in the acute phase of Trypanosoma cruzi infection in mice. Parasitol Res 87: 513-520.

144. dos Santos CD, Toldo MP, do Prado Júnior JC (2005) Trypanosoma cruzi: the effects of dehydroepiandrosterone (DHEA) treatment during experimental infection. Acta Trop 95: 109-115.

145. D'Ambrosio Fernandes R, Caetano LC, dos Santos CD, Abrahao AA, Pinto AC, et al. (2008) Alterations triggered by steroid gonadal hormones in triglycerides and the cellular immune response of Calomys callosus infected with the Y strain of Trypanosoma cruzi. Vet Parasitol 152: 21-27.

146. Basquiera AL, Sembaj A, Aguerri AM, Omelianiuk M, Guzman S, et al. (2003) Risk progression to chronic Chagas cardiomyopathy: influence of male sex and of parasitaemia detected by polymerase chain reaction. Heart 89: 1186-1190.

147. Brabin L, Brabin BJ (1992) Parasitic infections in women and their consequences. Adv Parasitol 31: 1-81.

148. Ghansah TJ, Ager EC, Freeman-Junior P, Villalta F, and Lima MF (2002) Epidermal growth factor binds to a receptor on Trypanosoma cruzi amastigotes inducing signal transduction events and cell proliferation. J Eukaryot Microbiol 49: 383-390.

149. Kuehn CC, Oliveira LG, Santos CD, Augusto MB, Toldo MP, et al. (2011) prior and concomitant dehydroepiandrosterone treatment affects immunologic response of cultured macrophages infected with Trypanosoma cruzi in vitro? Vet Parasitol 177: 242-246.

150. Santos CD, Toldo MP, Santello FH, Filipin Mdel V, Brazão V, et al. (2008) Dehydroepiandrosterone increases resistance to experimental infection by Trypanosoma cruzi. Vet Parasitol 153: 238-243.

151. Bisser S, Ouwe-Missi-Oukem-Boyer ON, Toure FS, Taoufiq Z, Bouteille B, et al. (2006) Harbouring in the brain: A focus on immune evasion mechanisms and their deleterious effects in malaria and human African trypanosomiasis. Int J Parasitol 36: 529-540.

152. Barry JD, McCulloch R (2001) Antigenic variation in trypanosomes: enhanced phenotypic variation in a eukaryotic parasite. Adv Parasitol 49: 1-70.

153. Vanhamme L, Pays E, McCulloch R, Barry JD (2001) An update on antigenic variation in African trypanosomes. Trends Parasitol 17: 338-343.

154. Greenblatt HC, Rosenstroich DL (1984) Trypanosoma rhodesiense infection in mice: sex dependence of resistance. Infect Immun 43: 337-340.

155. Pépin J, Milord F, Khonde A, Niyonsenga T, Loko L, et al. (1994) Gambiense trypanosomiasis: frequency of, and risk factors for, failure of melarsoprol therapy. Trans R Soc Trop Med Hyg 88: 447-452.

156. Hublart M, Tetaert D, Croix D, Boutignon F, Degand P, et al. (1990) Gonadotropic dysfunction produced by Trypanosoma brucei brucei in the rat. Acta Trop 47: 177-184.

157. Soudan B, Tetaert D, Hublart M, Racadot A, Croix D, et al. (1993) Experimental „chronic" African trypanosomiasis: endocrine dysfunctions generated by parasitic components released during the tryptanolytic phase in rats. Exp Clin Endocrinol 101: 166-172.

158. Soudan B, Tetaert D, Racadot A, Degand P, and Boersma A (1992) Decrease of testosterone level during an experimental African trypanosomiasis: involvement of a testicular LH receptor desensitization. Acta Endocrinol (Copenh) 127: 86-92.

159. Boersma A, Noireau F, Hublart M, Boutignon F, Lemesre JL, et al. (1989) Gonadotropic axis and Trypanosoma brucei gambiense infection. Ann Soc Belg Med Trop 69: 127-135.

160. Aguilar-Delfin I, Homer MJ, Wettstein PJ, Persing DH (2001) Innate resistance to Babesia infection is influenced by genetic background and gender. Infect Immun 69: 7955-7958.

161. Hughes VL, Randolph SE (2001) Testosterone increases the transmission potential of tick-borne parasites. Parasitology 123: 365-371.

162. Hughes VL, Randolph SE (2001) Testosterone depresses innate and acquired resistance to ticks in natural rodent hosts: a force for aggregated distributions of parasites. J Parasitol 87: 49-54.

163. Barnard CJ, Behnke JM, and Sewell J (1994) Social behaviour and susceptibility to infection in house mice (Mus musculus): effects of group size, aggressive behaviour and status-related hormonal responses prior to infection

on resistance to Babesia microti. Parasitology 108: 487-496.

164. Wood PR, Clark IA (1982) Apparent irrelevance of NK cells to resolution of infections with Babesia microti and Plasmodium vinckei petteri in mice. Parasite Immunol 4: 319-327.

165. Ford LC, Hammill HA, DeLange RJ, Bruckner DA, Suzuki-Chavez F, et al. (1987) Determination of estrogen and androgen receptors in Trichomonas vaginalis and the effects of antihormones. Am J Obstet Gynecol 156: 1119-1121.

166. Cappuccinelli P, Lattes C, Cagliani I, Negro Ponzi A (1974) Features of intravaginal Trichomonas vaginalis infection in the mouse and the effect of oestrogen treatment and immunodepression. G Batteriol Virol Immunol 67: 31-40.

167. Van Andel RA, Kendall LV, Franklin CL, Riley LK, Besch-Williford CL, et al. (1996) Sustained estrogenization is insufficient to support long-term experimentally induced genital Trichomonas vaginalis infection in BALB/c mice. Lab Anim Sci 46: 689-690.

168. Azuma T (1968) A study on the parasiting condition of trichomonas vaginalis with special reference to the relationship between estrogen and the growth of trichomonas vaginalis. J Jpn Obstet Gynecol Soc 15: 168-172.

169. Brown MT (1972) Trichomoniasis. Practitioner 209: 639-644.

170. Landolfo S, Martinotti MG, Martinetto P, Forni G, Rabagliati AM (1981) Trichomonas vaginalis: dependence of resistance among different mouse strains upon the non-H-2 gene haplotype, sex, and age of recipient hosts. Exp Parasitol 52: 312-318.

171. Sugarman B, Mummaw N (1988) The effect of hormones on Trichomonas vaginalis. J Gen Microbiol 134: 1623-1628.

172. Garber GE, Lemchuk-Favel LT, Rousseau G (1991) Effect of beta-estradiol on production of the cell-detaching factor of Trichomonas vaginalis. J Clin Microbiol 29: 1847-1849.

173. Lynch NR, Yarzábal L, Verde O, Avila JL, Monzon H, et al. (1982) Delayed-type hypersensitivity and immunoglobulin E in American cutaneous leishmaniasis. Infect Immun 38: 877-881.

174. Mock BA, Nacy CA (1988) Hormonal modulation of sex differences in resistance to Leishmania major systemic infections. Infect Immun 56: 3316-3319.

175. Lezama-Dávila CM, Isaac-Márquez AP, Barbi J, Cummings HE, Lu B, et al. (2008) Role of phosphatidylinositol-3-kinase-gamma (PI3Kgamma)-mediated pathway in 17beta-estradiol-induced killing of L. mexicana in macrophages from C57BL/6 mice. Immunol Cell Biol 86: 539-543.

176. Liu L, Wang L, Zhao Y, Wang Y, Wang Z, et al. (2006) Testosterone attenuates p38 MAPK pathway during Leishmania donovani infection of macrophages. Parasitol Res 99: 189-193.

177. Nandan D, and Reiner NE (1995) Attenuation of gamma interferon-induced tyrosine phosphorylation in mononuclear phagocytes infected with Leishmania donovani: selective inhibition of signaling through Janus kinases and Stat1. Infection and immunity 63: 4495-4500.

178. Bhardwaj N, Rosas LE, Lafuse WP, and Satoskar AR (2005) Leishmania inhibits STAT1-mediated IFN-gamma signaling in macrophages: increased tyrosine phosphorylation of dominant negative STAT1beta by Leishmania mexicana. Int J Parasitol 35: 75-82.

179. Bhardwaj S, Srivastava N, Sudan R, Saha B (2010) Leishmania interferes with host cell signaling to devise a survival strategy. J Biomed Biotechnol 2010: 109189.

180. Hernandez-Bello R, Escobedo G, Guzman C, Ibarra-Coronado EG, Lopez-Griego L, et al. (2010) Immunoendocrine host-parasite interactions during helminth infections: from the basic knowledge to its possible therapeutic applications. Parasite immunology 32: 633-643.

181. Mao G, Wang J, Kang Y, Tai P, Wen J, et al. (2010) Progesterone increases systemic and local uterine proportions of CD4+CD25+ Treg cells during midterm pregnancy in mice. Endocrinology 151: 5477-5488.

26

Fluticasone Induces Epithelial Injury and Alters Barrier Function in Normal Subjects

Ruth E. MacRedmond[1], Gurpreet K. Singhera[1], Samuel J. Wadsworth[1], Susan Attridge[1], Mohammed Bahzad[1], Kristy Williams[1], Harvey O. Coxson[1], Steven R. White[2] and Delbert R. Dorscheid[1]*

[1]Centre for Heart Lung Innovation, St. Paul's Hospital, University of British Columbia, Vancouver, Canada
[2]Department of Medicine, University of Chicago, Chicago, Illinois, USA

Abstract

Objective: The airway epithelium has a number of roles pivotal to the pathogenesis of asthma, including provision of a physical and immune barrier to the inhaled environment. Dysregulated injury and repair responses in asthma result in loss of airway epithelial integrity. Inhaled corticosteroids are a corner stone of asthma treatment. While effective in controlling asthma symptoms, they fail to prevent airway remodeling. Direct cytopathic effects on the airway epithelium may contribute to this.

Methods: This study examined the effects of a 4-week treatment regimen of inhaled fluticasone 500 µg twice daily in healthy human subjects. Induced sputum was collected for cell counts and markers of inflammation. Barrier function was examined by diethylenetriaminepentacetic acid (DTPA) clearance measured by nuclear scintillation scan, and albumin concentration in induced sputum.

Results: Steroid exposure resulted in epithelial injury as measured by a significant increase in the number of airway epithelial cells in induced sputum. There was no change in airway inflammation by induced sputum inflammatory cell counts or cytokine levels. Epithelial shedding was associated with an increase in barrier function, as measured by both a decrease in DTPA clearance and decreased albumin in induced sputum. This likely reflects the normal repair response.

Conclusion: Inhaled corticosteroids cause injury to normal airway epithelium. These effects warrant further evaluation in asthma, where the dysregulated repair response may contribute to airway remodeling.

Keywords: Airway epithelial cell; Asthma; Asthma-medication; corticosteroids

Introduction

Asthma is a chronic inflammatory disease of the airways characterized by reversible airflow obstruction, airway hyper reactivity and airways remodeling [1-4]. Complex interactions between environmental insults and genetically determined host factors generate abnormal injury/repair responses in the airway, resulting in persistent inflammation, epithelial damage and ultimately in the structural changes of airway remodeling. Previously considered a bystander in what was designated primarily an immunological disorder, the role of the epithelium in the pathogenesis of asthma is increasingly recognized [5]. The bronchial epithelium provides chemical, physical, and immunologic barriers to the inhaled environment [6], and has a critical role in orchestrating the inflammatory response to inhaled allergens and pathogens [4]. Loss of epithelial integrity is a hallmark of asthma [7-10]. The potential mechanisms to explain damaged airway epithelium remain unclear and likely are multifactorial, including repetitive exposure to allergic insults (environmental, infectious, inflammatory agents), inflammatory processes [11], a predisposing epithelial dysfunction [5,12] and sub-optimal control with recommended treatment regimens.

Corticosteroids have been the foundation of the pharmaceutical treatment of asthma since the early 1990's and are used currently as the first line and initial maintenance treatment ("controller") in patients with recurrent symptoms [1,13]. Corticosteroids are powerful anti-inflammatory agents with a number of cellular targets which reduce recruitment and activation of inflammatory cells in the airway [14]. The glucocorticoid receptor is expressed in airway epithelium [15], and recent work has demonstrated a wide range of additional mechanisms including regulation of epithelial innate and adaptive immune responses [16]. Inhaled corticosteroids have been demonstrated to improve symptoms, exacerbation frequency, and overall quality of life in most patients with asthma [17,18]. However, corticosteroid treatment does not reliably reverse or prevent airway remodeling [19] or alter the natural history of the disease even when therapy is started in childhood [20]. In addition, there is a substantial subset of asthmatics (10-25%) that are resistant to corticosteroid therapy with ongoing symptoms and airway inflammation [21].

Th2-mediated inflammation, which is responsive to inhaled corticosteroid (ICS) therapy, contributes to the pathogenesis and clinical syndrome of asthma, and may have a role in airway remodeling. Abnormalities in the airway epithelium resulting in dysregulated injury, inflammation and repair are recognized to be equally important [22], however in the context of airway remodeling, the anti-inflammatory benefits of corticosteroids may be offset by direct toxic effects on the airway epithelium. Using a variety of in vitro and animal models and clinically relevant doses of corticosteroid, we have previously shown

---

*Corresponding author: Delbert R. Dorscheid, Centre for Heart Lung Innovation, St. Paul's Hospital, Rm. 166, 1081 Burrard Street, Vancouver, B.C. V6Z 1Y6, Canada, E-mail: del.dorscheid@hli.ubc.ca

that corticosteroids have adverse effects on airway health, increasing epithelial apoptosis, slowing repair and impairing immune responses to viral and bacterial pathogens [23-30]. These adverse effects on the epithelium may occur in parallel with the beneficial anti-inflammatory effects of corticosteroids in asthma, and thus be masked. By studying the effects of inhaled corticosteroids on healthy adults without asthma/airway inflammation, any adverse effects of corticosteroids on the epithelium will be more evident.

The aim of this study was to examine the effect of a 4 week treatment regimen of inhaled corticosteroids on the airway epithelium in healthy human subjects. Damage to the airway epithelium was measured by number of epithelial cells shed into induced sputum. We used two measures of barrier function, examining both bulk diffusive flows as reflected by albumin concentration in the induced sputum and DTPA clearance, which is thought to be a more sensitive measure of tight junction integrity [31]. Differential cell counts and cytokine levels in the induced sputum were measured to reflect airway inflammation.

Materials and Methods

Subjects

Healthy subjects aged 18 years and above with no history of smoking, asthma/allergy or other respiratory condition were recruited by newspaper advertising. Subjects were excluded on the basis of abnormal spirometry at baseline screening. The study was approved by the Research Ethics Board (REB) of University of British Columbia/ Providence Healthcare REB# P01-0095. All subjects gave written consent to participate in the study.

Study Protocol

This was an uncontrolled before and after observational study (Figure 1). At visit zero [V0] (screening visit), baseline spirometric lung function was obtained in accordance to the standards of the American Thoracic Society (ATS). Only the subjects with an FEV1 of > 80% and with normal lung function were eligible for enrollment into the study. At visit one [V1], a baseline nuclear medicine scintillation scan (DTPA) was performed, and subjects returned the following day for sputum induction. Each subject was then instructed on the proper technique for the delivery of fluticasone via a metered dose inhaler (MDI) with a spacer device. Each subject inhaled fluticasone 250 µg (Flovent, Glaxo SmithKline Inc, Canada) two puffs twice a day (a daily total of 1000 µg daily) for four weeks. Each subject was contacted weekly by the research coordinator to monitor compliance and assess for any adverse events. At visit two [V2] at the conclusion of the inhaled steroid treatment, each subject returned for assessment including symptom review and spirometry and completed a nuclear medicine scintillation scan and a sputum induction following the same protocol as V1.

99mTc-DTPA lung clearance test

Transepithelial clearance of DTPA was measured using a nuclear medicine scintillation scan [31]. Subjects inhaled an aeorosolized mist of Technetium-labeled diethylenetriaminepentacetic acid (99mTc-DTPA) via a Fisoneb Ultrasonic nebulizer. Each subject inhaled a dosage of 185 MBq of DTPA for 5 minutes while lying supine on a Siemens PHO/gamma scintillation camera. Subjects were instructed to make rapid inspiratory efforts to ensure central deposition of the particles in the upper airways. Immediately after the delivery of the aerosolized DTPA 30-second image counts were performed for a total of 30 minutes. Anterior and posterior images were taken with a dual headed camera. The region of interest (ROI) was drawn over the central portions of each lung and time-activity curves were derived from the counts per frame computed in the ROI. The T½ value (time required for clearance of 50% of the activity from lung fields) was calculated with the help of the established formula [32]. Decreased T½ denotes faster clearance.

Sputum induction and processing

Sputum samples were obtained by inhaling increasing concentrations of hypertonic saline solutions (3%, 4%, and 5%) using an ultrasonic nebulizer (Univerisal III model, FLAEM Nuova; Brescia, Italy). The whole sputum sample was collected in a plastic container, weighed, and incubated in 3 volumes of dithiothreitol (DTT) 5 mmol/L (Sputolysin; Calbiochem Corp; San Diego, CA) for 15 minutes at room temperature. An equal volume of phosphate-buffered saline (PBS) was then added to the solution and vortexed for 30 seconds. Cell viability was checked by Trypan blue exclusion. The differential cell count was performed on cytospin products that were stained (Diff-Quick stain; Fisher Scientific; Springfield, NJ). Specimens were considered adequate where viability was >80% and squamous cell contamination was <50%. The bronchial epithelial cells were identified by their columnar shape, round nucleus and cilia on the broad end of the cell. A total of 300 non-squamous cells were counted by two independent blinded observers. Results were averaged and bronchial epithelial cells were expressed as percentage of the total non-squamous cells, and differential counts of inflammatory cells were expressed as a percentage of total inflammatory cells. Following centrifugation at 800 g for 10 min at 4°C, the supernatant was separated from the cell pellet and immediately stored at -80°C for batch analysis.

Measurement of airway inflammation

The concentrations of inflammatory mediators IL-6 and IL-8 and the repair marker Heparin-binding EGF- like factor (HB-EGF) [33] were measured in induced sputum cell free supernatant in duplicate by standard ELISA. Induced sputum albumin concentration was measured in unprocessed sputum by ELISA and expressed as µg albumin / mg sputum.

Statistical analysis

Statistical software Graphpad Prism 5 was used for the analysis. Mann-Whitney U test was used for comparison of groups (median values) as the sample size was small and normal distribution could not be assumed. Paired t-test (Wilcoxen) was used to test for effect of treatment between week 0 and week 4. Statistical significance was defined as p-value < 0.05.

Results

Study population

Thirty-eight patients were enrolled of which 36 completed the study, two subjects failing to return for the V2 assessment. The 36 consisted of 18 males and 18 females with mean age of 30.9 years (24 - 43) years and average FEV1 of 100 (13.2)% predicted. Paired data for DTPA clearance are presented for all 36 patients.

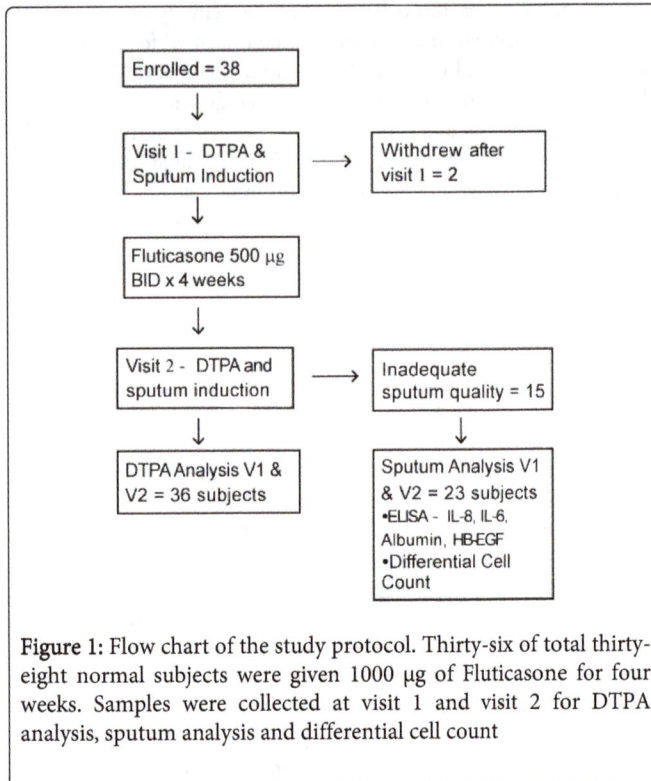

Figure 1: Flow chart of the study protocol. Thirty-six of total thirty-eight normal subjects were given 1000 µg of Fluticasone for four weeks. Samples were collected at visit 1 and visit 2 for DTPA analysis, sputum analysis and differential cell count

Epithelial cell shedding

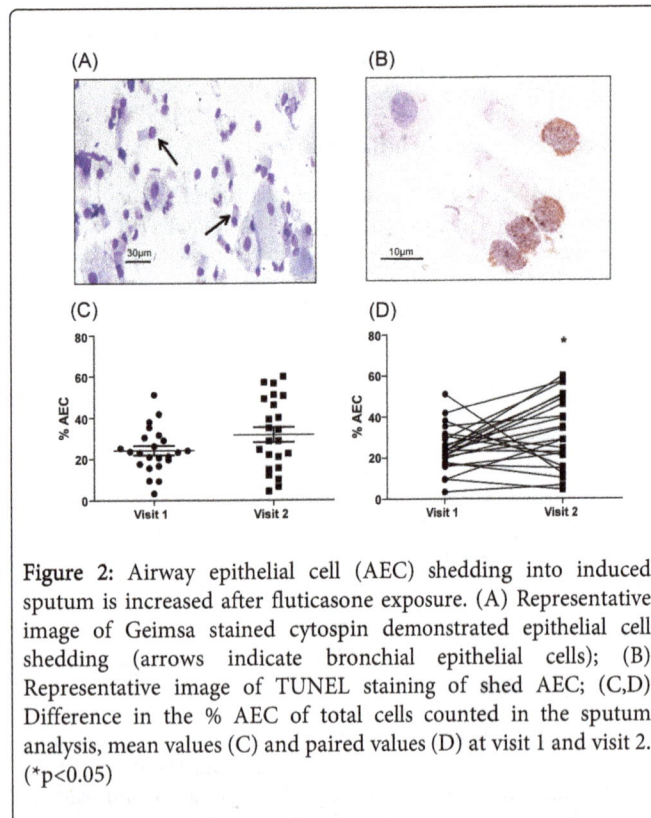

Figure 2: Airway epithelial cell (AEC) shedding into induced sputum is increased after fluticasone exposure. (A) Representative image of Geimsa stained cytospin demonstrated epithelial cell shedding (arrows indicate bronchial epithelial cells); (B) Representative image of TUNEL staining of shed AEC; (C,D) Difference in the % AEC of total cells counted in the sputum analysis, mean values (C) and paired values (D) at visit 1 and visit 2. (*p<0.05)

Sputum induction was of insufficient quality (poor viability or squamous cell contamination) at one or both visits for 13 of 36 patients,

thus data for epithelial cell shedding, airway inflammation and albumin influx are presented for 23 subjects (Figure 1).

The percentage of AEC in induced sputum increased from 24.2 (SEM ±2.3) to 31.8 (SEM ±3.6) following fluticasone treatment. There was no significant difference in the means (p=0.08) (Figure 2C) however the difference by paired analysis was significant at p<0.05 (Figure 2D). All of the shed AECs in our study were apoptotic, as determined by terminal deoxynucleotidyl transferase dUTP nick end labeling (TUNEL) staining (Figure 2A and 2B).

DTPA clearance

The mean (SEM) half-life of DTPA in the lungs increased from 90.1 (4.3) seconds to 106 (5.4) seconds following 28 days of inhaled fluticasone. The difference between the means was significant at p<0.05 (Figure 3A), and paired analysis showed a significant increase in T½ between visit 1 and visit 2 at p<0.02 (Figure 3B).

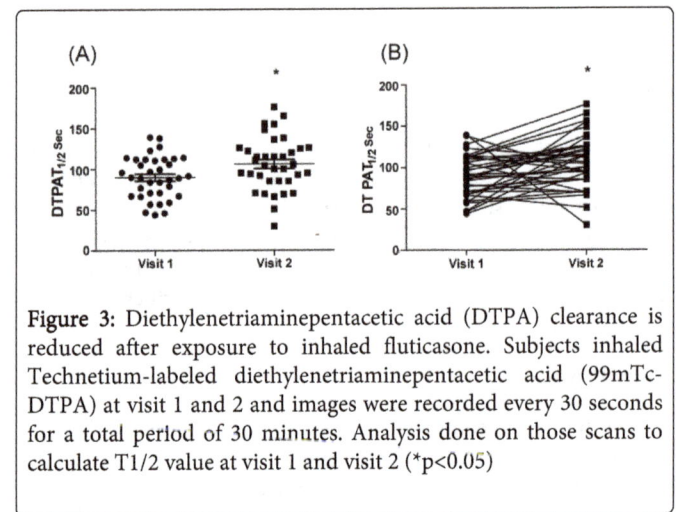

Figure 3: Diethylenetriaminepentacetic acid (DTPA) clearance is reduced after exposure to inhaled fluticasone. Subjects inhaled Technetium-labeled diethylenetriaminepentacetic acid (99mTc-DTPA) at visit 1 and 2 and images were recorded every 30 seconds for a total period of 30 minutes. Analysis done on those scans to calculate T1/2 value at visit 1 and visit 2 (*p<0.05)

Albumin influx

Albumin levels in induced sputum decreased from 761 (SEM ±72) µg/ml to 618 (SEM ±64) µg/ml following 4 weeks of inhaled fluticasone.

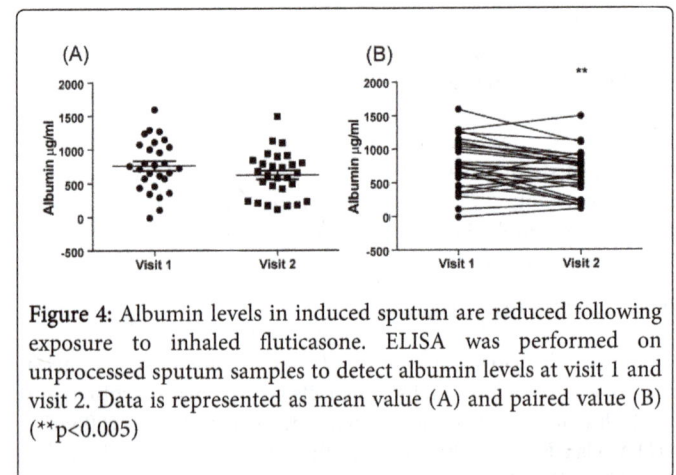

Figure 4: Albumin levels in induced sputum are reduced following exposure to inhaled fluticasone. ELISA was performed on unprocessed sputum samples to detect albumin levels at visit 1 and visit 2. Data is represented as mean value (A) and paired value (B) (**p<0.005)

There was no significant difference between the means p=0.14 (Figure 4A) however paired analysis showed a highly significant reduction in albumin levels following fluticasone treatment at p<0.005 (Figure 4B).

Airway inflammation

There was no significant difference in the levels of pro- inflammatory cytokines IL-6 and IL-8 following fluticasone treatment (Table 1). HB-EGF levels were similarly unchanged. There was no difference in the inflammatory differential cell counts in the induced sputum following fluticasone exposure (data not shown).

Concentration (pg/ml)	Visit 1	Visit 2	P- value
IL-6	113.9 (139.4)	79.7 (85.9)	0.27
IL-8	755.3 (906.1)	611.8 (757.2)	0.72
HB-EGF	609.6 (298.1)	679.8 (457.2)	0.54

Table 1: Concentrations of inflammatory mediators (IL-6, IL-8 and HB-EGF) in induced sputum

Cell free supernatants from induced sputum were analyzed for IL-6, IL-8 and HB-EGF by ELISA (as described in Material and Methods). No change was observed for IL-6, IL-8 and HB-EGF after fluticasone exposure. Data are mean (SEM). P- Value refers to paired t-test.

Discussion

The airway epithelium is constantly exposed to inhaled agents that injure the epithelium, and maintains homeostasis through an efficient and highly regulated cycle of injury, inflammation and repair [34]. Our results demonstrate that subjects taking regular inhaled fluticasone for four weeks manifest a degree of airway epithelial injury reflected by a significant increase in the number of shed apoptotic AECs. Epithelial injury occurred in the absence of measurable inflammatory response, and was associated with a reduction in airway permeability and increased barrier function, likely representing an active repair response.

Epithelial shedding and desquamation is considered by many to be a hallmark of asthma, based on post-mortem and biopsy studies [7,9,35,36], along with findings of increased numbers of epithelial cells in sputum [37] and bronchoalveolar lavage fluid [38]. Epithelial loss is largely confined to the columnar epithelial cells [39], and is accompanied by phenotypic changes in the epithelium consistent with the repair process. Persistent repair mechanisms are also implicated in airway remodeling [40,41]. These include upregulation of cyclin- dependent kinase inhibitor, p21 (waf) [42], EGFR [43] and CD-44 [44,45]. In asthma, epithelial shedding is largely attributed to the induction of apoptosis in AECs by infiltrating T cells and eosinophils along with increased pro-inflammatory cytokines including IFN- gamma and TNF-alpha [46]. While cell-mediated inflammation is reduced by corticosteroids, our study was performed in normal individuals without baseline airway inflammation and we observed no changes in the inflammatory indices in induced sputum following corticosteroid therapy. Therefore the epithelial shedding observed in this study likely represents direct apoptotic effect of corticosteroids on AECs as previously demonstrated in vitro and in animal studies by ours [23-25,30] and other groups [47].

The potential significance of this corticosteroid induced AEC shedding in asthma is unclear. It might be expected that in asthma, any direct cytopathic effects of corticosteroid would be offset by the ben-

eficial anti-inflammatory effects. We have previously shown however that pre-treatment with corticosteroid reduced allergen- induced inflammation but did not reduce epithelial shedding in an animal model of allergic asthma [23]. Direct corticosteroid-induced AEC injury may be a factor in airway remodeling and explain at least in part the failure of steroid therapy to impact on this process. However, the response of asthmatic epithelial cells to corticosteroids may be different to that of phenotypically normal cells. Vignola and colleagues previously demonstrated increased levels of the anti- apoptotic molecule Bcl-2 in asthmatic subjects compared to controls and there was no difference in the number of apoptotic epithelial cells between corticosteroid-treated and -untreated asthmatic subjects in their study of bronchial biopsies [40]. It would be important therefore to define these effects in subjects with asthma.

The airway mucosa exhibits properties of a selective and tightly regulated permeability barrier that is direction dependent [48], properties which have been used experimentally to assess the presence of airway damage in response to various epithelial insults. Clearance of inhaled labeled-DTPA is considered to be an accurate measurement of lung epithelial permeability, as movement of this molecule into the circulation is limited by the epithelium rather than the endothelium [31]. DTPA is a small hydrophilic molecule that is believed to be cleared from the airway in an apical to basolateral direction via paracellular diffusion; this diffusion is increased following exposure to an allergen or other inflammatory insult [12,49-51] and is thought to be mediated by alterations in cellular contacts such as tight junctions and adherents junctions [12,49]. In addition to DTPA clearance, the presence of serum proteins such as albumin in the airway and measured in induced sputum may reflect altered barrier function in the basolateral-to-apical direction. Plasma extravasation into the sub- epithelial tissue occurs rapidly in response to inhaled allergen reflecting an acute vascular response, but extravasation into the epithelium is not observed [52]. The sustained transepithelial exudation of plasma seen in chronic airway inflammation reflects epithelial injury and repair [53], as almost all (92%) of resistance to albumin flux across the epithelial-capillary barrier occurs in the epithelium [54]. Passive bulk flow of plasma through a "leaky" epithelium is regulated by cellular junctions [48,55], or via diffusive vesicular transport across cells [54].

Intuitively one might expect that epithelial shedding would result in increased permeability and loss of barrier function. However, the complex structure and repair characteristics of the airway epithelium are such that this is not the case. In vivo experiments in guinea-pig trachea demonstrate that epithelial shedding is immediately followed by repair responses directed towards covering of the basement membrane and epithelial restitution [52,53,56]. The microcirculation exudes a plasma-rich fibrin-fibronectin gel rich in inflammatory cells, while the cells neighboring the denuded area dedifferentiate, flatten and migrate over the membrane to fill the gap. Columnar cells are likely more easily shed than basal cells [57], and the residual basal cells undergo extensive flattening and develop interdigitating cytoplasmic protrusions observed by electron microscopy [34]. The large flattened cells again have less junctional area than the shed columnar cells, with less potential for paracellular transit of proteins. Thus, in the setting of normal repair, desquamative processes may be accompanied by the apparent paradox of reduced permeability, as a mechanism to reduce further injury [48]. The observation of reduced clearance of DTPA and decreased luminal albumin in the context of epithelial shedding in our normal subjects likely represents initiation of a normal injury repair response.

Corticosteroids have long been known to reduce endothelial permeability, particularly at the blood brain barrier, where they are used therapeutically to reduce cerebral edema [58]. The mechanisms of improved barrier function are not fully understood, but include glucocorticoid mediated induction of junctional proteins including occludin, ZO-1 and claudin [59-61]. Evidence from lung epithelium is less abundant, but suggests similar effects. In a co-culture model of immortalized lung epithelial cell lines in monolayer with primary human pulmonary microvascular endothelial cells, dexamethasone treatment resulted in increased membrane staining of E-Cadherin and ZO-1 in the NCI H441 epithelial cells which was associated with increased transepithelial resistance (TER), a surrogate of reduced permeability [62]. While it is difficult to extrapolate these results to the polarized pseudo-stratified airway epithelium in vivo, it is possible that modulation of junctional proteins contributes to the observed reduction in permeability.

Some studies of epithelial permeability have failed to demonstrate a significant difference between normal subjects and mild stable asthmatics [63-65]. Lemarchand et al. [66] however showed increased DTPA clearance in asthmatics during acute exacerbations, which decreased within 4 weeks of the acute attack but still remained increased compared to the control group. Ilowite et al. [67] adjusted their results for mucociliary clearance, which was reduced in the asthmatics, and found that while total clearance was the same between asthmatics and controls, airway permeability was in fact increased in the asthmatics [50]. Another recent study of chronic persistent asthma, which excluded the component of mucociliary transport by careful exclusion of the hilar regions, found increased permeability in asthma compared to control and the degree of permeability was correlated with severity of asthma [68]. It would appear therefore that epithelial damage in asthma, at least during acute attacks, is associated with loss of barrier function.

This study was performed in normal subjects in order to isolate the cytopathic effects of corticosteroids on the epithelium from the anti-inflammatory effects. One limitation of this approach is in then extrapolating the results to the asthmatic airway, which by definition will have differences in the injury and repair responses. Asthma is characterized by a cycle of chronic injury and dysregulated repair [69,70]. Recent studies demonstrate that airway epithelial cells from asthmatic children express significantly less fibronectin compared to non-asthmatic controls, resulting in reduced reparative capacity [71]. Thus, while corticosteroid induced cytopathology and epithelial injury may be inconsequential in the context of normal repair mechanisms which quickly restore and even improve barrier function, where these responses are inadequate or abnormal, permeability may increase. The first studies of inhaled corticosteroids and permeability in asthma used low daily doses (200 μg and 400 μg Beclomethasone) for short duration (1 week), and found no difference in DTPA clearance rates [72,73]. However, in the only other human study of the effect of chronic inhaled corticosteroids on airway permeability, treatment with corticosteroids (budesonide) in atopic asthmatic children did in fact result in increased permeability as measured by DTPA clearance [74].

Evidence from both biopsy and differentiated culture studies indicate that expression and assembly of tight junctions is abnormal in asthma [75,76]. This may contribute to the epithelial "fragility" in asthma, while failure to upregulate tight junctions in response to corticosteroid may contribute to an altered permeability response in the context of epithelial shedding. It is unclear whether the direct cytopathic effects of corticosteroids observed in this study are glucocorticoid receptor-mediated and would occur in the population of steroid resistant asthmatics. Certainly these effects in the absence of the beneficial anti-inflammatory effects could be potentially catastrophic with regard to airways remodeling. This further underlines the importance of early identification of these patients and avoiding the use of both systemic and inhaled corticosteroids.

The Flovent inhaler used in this study consists of 99.66 - 99.91% 1,1,1,2-tetrafluoroethane propellant (carrier) and 0.09 - 0.34% fluticasone propionate powder. 1,1,1,2-tetrafluoroethane (also known as the Glaxo compound HFA134a) was developed in the early 1990s as an alternative propellant to chlorofluorocarbons as it has a far lower ozone-depleting potential. Inhaled radiolabelled HFA134a is rapidly removed from the body by ventilation and does not accumulate significantly in any specific region of the body [77]. Multiple other safety studies have demonstrated that HFA134a has no negative impact on various respiratory and systemic health indices in healthy volunteers [78,79] and in patients with mild-moderate asthma [80-82]. Even whole body exposure to increasing concentrations of HFA234a did not trigger any adverse effects, including upper respiratory tract irritation [83]. There has been a single case of extrinsic allergic alveolitis with eosinophil infiltration triggered by 1,1,1,2- tetrafluoroethane inhalation [84], but the vast majority of individuals do not show any adverse health effects. There is little evidence to suggest that the effects we observed in patients using the Flovent inhaler were caused by the propellant.

Conclusions

In summary, our results demonstrate that normal subjects taking inhaled fluticasone at clinically relevant doses for 4 weeks show evidence of epithelial damage in the absence of airway inflammation. This is associated with reduced airway permeability and albumin extravasation, reflecting repair. The airway epithelium in asthma is held in a cycle of chronic injury, inflammation and dysregulated repair. Inhaled corticosteroids in asthma may contribute to epithelial injury, while at the same time reducing the accompanying inflammatory response. Failure of appropriate repair mechanisms may result in increased permeability and increased susceptibility to inhalational injury. We have no reason to believe that the observed results are unique to the particular steroid used in this study; however further studies using other inhaled steroid preparations and carrier only placebo controls would be of interest.

While the beneficial effects of corticosteroids on cell-mediated immunopathology in asthma are manifold, our study suggests that the direct toxic effects on the epithelium may not be inconsequential, particularly in the context of inappropriate repair, and could in fact contribute to airway remodeling. Care should be taken in extrapolating our findings to asthmatic subjects recognizing the potential differences in apoptotic susceptibility, inflammation and repair. Given the widespread use of inhaled corticosteroids and their failure to prevent airway remodeling, further careful investigation of these effects in asthmatic subjects is warranted.

Acknowledgement

This study was supported by operating grants from National Institutes of Health (NIH) HL60531, HL66026 and the Canadian

Institutes of Health Research, the Canadian/British Columbia Lung Associations, and AllerGen-NCE and personal support awards from the Michael Smith Foundation for Health Research (D.R.D. and R.M.), and the Canadian Institutes of Health Research (D.R.D.).

References

1. Becker A, Lemière C, Bérubé D, Boulet LP, Ducharme FM, et al. (2005) Summary of recommendations from the Canadian Asthma Consensus guidelines, 2003. CMAJ 173: S3-11.

2. Cohn L, Elias JA, Chupp GL (2004) Asthma: mechanisms of disease persistence and progression. Annu Rev Immunol 22: 789-815.

3. Fahy JV (2001) Remodeling of the airway epithelium in asthma. Am J Respir Crit Care Med 164: S46-51.

4. Murphy DM, O'Byrne PM (2010) Recent advances in the pathophysiology of asthma. Chest 137: 1417-1426.

5. Holgate ST, Roberts G, Arshad HS, Howarth PH, Davies DE (2009) The role of the airway epithelium and its interaction with environmental factors in asthma pathogenesis. Proc Am Thorac Soc 6: 655-659.

6. Swindle EJ, Collins JE, Davies DE (2009) Breakdown in epithelial barrier function in patients with asthma: identification of novel therapeutic approaches. J Allergy Clin Immunol 124: 23-34.

7. Jeffery PK, Wardlaw AJ, Nelson FC, Collins JV, Kay AB (1989) Bronchial biopsies in asthma. An ultrastructural, quantitative study and correlation with hyperreactivity. Am Rev Respir Dis 140: 1745-1753.

8. Vignola AM, Chanez P, Campbell AM, Souques F, Lebel B, et al. (1998) Airway inflammation in mild intermittent and in persistent asthma. Am J Respir Crit Care Med 157: 403-409.

9. Laitinen LA, Heino M, Laitinen A, Kava T, Haahtela T (1985) Damage of the airway epithelium and bronchial reactivity in patients with asthma. Am Rev Respir Dis 131: 599-606.

10. Barbato A, Turato G, Baraldo S, Bazzan E, Calabrese F, et al. (2006) Epithelial damage and angiogenesis in the airways of children with asthma. Am J Respir Crit Care Med 174: 975-981.

11. Erjefält JS (2010) The airway epithelium as regulator of inflammation patterns in asthma. ClinRespir J 4 Suppl 1: 9-14.

12. Holgate ST (2008) Pathogenesis of asthma. Clin Exp Allergy 38: 872-897.

13. Bateman ED, Hurd SS, Barnes PJ, Bousquet J, Drazen JM, et al. (2008) Global strategy for asthma management and prevention: GINA executive summary. Eur Respir J 31: 143-178.

14. Barnes PJ (2000) Molecular basis for corticosteroid action in asthma. Chem Immunol 78: 72-80.

15. LeVan TD, Babin EA, Yamamura HI, Bloom JW (1999) Pharmacological characterization of glucocorticoid receptors in primary human bronchial epithelial cells. Biochem Pharmacol 57: 1003-1009.

16. Stellato C (2007) Glucocorticoid actions on airway epithelial responses in immunity: functional outcomes and molecular targets. J Allergy Clin Immunol 120: 1247-1263.

17. Barnes N (1998) Relative safety and efficacy of inhaled corticosteroids. J Allergy Clin Immunol 101: S460-464.

18. Calverley PM (2004) Effect of corticosteroids on exacerbations of asthma and chronic obstructive pulmonary disease. Proc Am Thorac Soc 1: 161-166.

19. Murray CS (2008) Can inhaled corticosteroids influence the natural history of asthma? Curr Opin Allergy Clin Immunol 8: 77-81.

20. Bisgaard H, Bønnelykke K (2010) Long-term studies of the natural history of asthma in childhood. J Allergy Clin Immunol 126: 187-197.

21. Goleva E, Hauk PJ, Boguniewicz J, Martin RJ, Leung DY (2007) Airway remodeling and lack of bronchodilator response in steroid-resistant asthma. J Allergy Clin Immunol 120: 1065-1072.

22. Sumi Y, Hamid Q (2007) Airway remodeling in asthma. Allergol Int 56: 341-348.

23. Dorscheid DR, Low E, Conforti A, Shifrin S, Sperling AI, et al. (2003) Corticosteroid-induced apoptosis in mouse airway epithelium: effect in normal airways and after allergen-induced airway inflammation. J Allergy Clin Immunol 111: 360-366.

24. Dorscheid DR, Patchell BJ, Estrada O, Marroquin B, Tse R, et al. (2006) Effects of corticosteroid-induced apoptosis on airway epithelial wound closure in vitro. Am J Physiol Lung Cell Mol Physiol 291: L794-801.

25. Dorscheid DR, Wojcik KR, Sun S, Marroquin B, White SR (2001) Apoptosis of airway epithelial cells induced by corticosteroids. Am J Respir Crit Care Med 164: 1939-1947.

26. MacRedmond RE, Greene CM, Dorscheid DR, McElvaney NG, O'Neill SJ (2007) Epithelial expression of TLR4 is modulated in COPD and by steroids, salmeterol and cigarette smoke. Respir Res 8: 84.

27. Singhera GK, Chan TS, Cheng JY, Vitalis TZ, Hamann KJ, et al. (2006) Apoptosis of viral-infected airway epithelial cells limit viral production and is altered by corticosteroid exposure. Respir Res 7: 78.

28. Tse R, Marroquin BA, Dorscheid DR, White SR (2003) Beta-adrenergic agonists inhibit corticosteroid-induced apoptosis of airway epithelial cells. Am J Physiol Lung Cell MolPhysiol 285: L393-404.

29. Undevia NS, Dorscheid DR, Marroquin BA, Gugliotta WL, Tse R, et al. (2004) Smad and p38-MAPK signaling mediates apoptotic effects of transforming growth factor-beta1 in human airway epithelial cells. Am J Physiol Lung Cell Mol Physiol 287: L515-524.

30. White SR, Dorscheid DR (2002) Corticosteroid-induced apoptosis of airway epithelium: a potential mechanism for chronic airway epithelial damage in asthma. Chest 122: 278S-284S.

31. Effros RM, Mason GR (1983) Measurements of pulmonary epithelial permeability in vivo. Am Rev Respir Dis 127: S59-65.

32. Levin S (1984) Statistical methods, Textbook of Nuclear Medicine (2nd Edn), Philadelphia: Lea &Fehinger: 70-91.

33. Allahverdian S, Harada N, Singhera GK, Knight DA, Dorscheid DR (2008) Secretion of IL-13 by airway epithelial cells enhances epithelial repair via HB-EGF. Am J Respir Cell Mol Biol 38: 153-160.

34. Erjefält JS, Sundler F, Persson CG (1997) Epithelial barrier formation by airway basal cells. Thorax 52: 213-217.

35. Dunnil MS (1960) The pathology of asthma, with special reference to changes in the bronchial mucosa. J Clin Pathol 13: 27-33.

36. Houston JC, De Navasquez S, and Trounce JR (1953) A clinical and pathological study of fatal cases of status asthmaticus. Thorax 8: 207-213.

37. Naylor B (1962) The shedding of the mucosa of the bronchial tree in asthma. Thorax 17: 69-72.

38. Wardlaw AJ, Dunnette S, Gleich GJ, Collins JV, Kay AB (1988) Eosinophils and mast cells in bronchoalveolar lavage in subjects with mild asthma. Relationship to bronchial hyperreactivity. Am Rev Respir Dis 137: 62-69.

39. Beasley R, Roche WR, Roberts JA, Holgate ST (1989) Cellular events in the bronchi in mild asthma and after bronchial provocation. Am Rev Respir Dis 139: 806-817.

40. Vignola AM, Chiappara G, Siena L, Bruno A, Gagliardo R, et al. (2001) Proliferation and activation of bronchial epithelial cells in corticosteroid-dependent asthma. J Allergy Clin Immunol 108: 738-746.

41. Cohen L, E X, Tarsi J, Ramkumar T, Horiuchi TK, et al. (2007) Epithelial cell proliferation contributes to airway remodeling in severe asthma. Am J RespirCrit Care Med 176: 138-145.

42. Puddicombe SM, Torres-Lozano C, Richter A, Bucchieri F, Lordan JL, et al. (2003) Increased expression of p21(waf) cyclin-dependent kinase inhibitor in asthmatic bronchial epithelium. Am J Respir Cell Mol Biol 28: 61-68.

43. Puddicombe SM, Polosa R, Richter A, Krishna MT, Howarth PH, et al. (2000) Involvement of the epidermal growth factor receptor in epithelial repair in asthma. FASEB J 14: 1362-1374.

44. Lackie PM, Baker JE, Günthert U, Holgate ST (1997) Expression of CD44 isoforms is increased in the airway epithelium of asthmatic subjects. Am J Respir Cell Mol Biol 16: 14-22.

45. Peroni DG, DjukanoviÄ‡ R, Bradding P, Feather IH, Montefort S, et al. (1996) Expression of CD44 and integrins in bronchial mucosa of normal and mildly asthmatic subjects. Eur Respir J 9: 2236-2242.

46. Trautmann A, Kruger K, Akdis M, Muller-Wening D, Akkaya A, et al. (2005) Apoptosis and loss of adhesion of bronchial epithelial cells in asthma. Int Arch Allergy Immunol 138: 142-150.

47. Andersson K, Shebani EB, Makeeva N, Roomans GM, Servetnyk Z (2010) Corticosteroids and montelukast: effects on airway epithelial and human umbilical vein endothelial cells. Lung 188: 209-216.

48. Persson CG, Andersson M, Greiff L, Svensson C, Erjefält JS, et al. (1995) Airway permeability. Clin Exp Allergy 25: 807-814.

49. Knight D (2002) Increased permeability of asthmatic epithelial cells to pollutants. Does this mean that they are intrinsically abnormal? Clin Exp Allergy 32: 1263-1265.

50. Ilowite JS, Bennett WD, Sheetz MS, Groth ML, Nierman DM (1989) Permeability of the bronchial mucosa to 99mTc-DTPA in asthma. Am Rev Respir Dis 139: 1139-1143.

51. Kennedy SM, Elwood RK, Wiggs BJ, Paré PD, Hogg JC (1984) Increased airway mucosal permeability of smokers. Relationship to airway reactivity. Am Rev Respir Dis 129: 143-148.

52. Erjefält JS, Andersson P, Gustafsson B, Korsgren M, Sonmark B, et al. (1998) Allergen challenge-induced extravasation of plasma in mouse airways. Clin Exp Allergy 28: 1013-1020.

53. Erjefält JS, Sundler F, Persson CG (1996) Eosinophils, neutrophils, and venular gaps in the airway mucosa at epithelial removal-restitution. Am J Respir Crit Care Med 153: 1666-1674.

54. Gorin AB, Stewart PA (1979) Differential permeability of endothelial and epithelial barriers to albumin flux. J Appl Physiol Respir Environ Exerc Physiol 47: 1315-1324.

55. Persson CG (1990) Plasma exudation in tracheobronchial and nasal airways: a mucosal defence mechanism becomes pathogenic in asthma and rhinitis. Eur Respir J Suppl 12: 652s-656s.

56. Erjefält I, Greiff L, Persson CG (1993) Exudation versus absorption across the airway epithelium. Pharmacol Toxicol 72 Suppl 3: 14-16.

57. Montefort S, Roberts JA, Beasley R, Holgate ST, Roche WR (1992) The site of disruption of the bronchial epithelium in asthmatic and non-asthmatic subjects. Thorax 47: 499-503.

58. Rabinstein AA (2006) Treatment of cerebral edema. Neurologist 12: 59-73.

59. Förster C, Waschke J, Burek M, Leers J, Drenckhahn D (2006) Glucocorticoid effects on mouse microvascular endothelial barrier permeability are brain specific. J Physiol 573: 413-425.

60. Romero IA, Radewicz K, Jubin E, Michel CC, Greenwood J, et al. (2003) Changes in cytoskeletal and tight junctional proteins correlate with decreased permeability induced by dexamethasone in cultured rat brain endothelial cells. Neurosci Lett 344: 112-116.

61. Kröll S, El-Gindi J, Thanabalasundaram G, Panpumthong P, Schrot S, et al. (2009) Control of the blood-brain barrier by glucocorticoids and the cells of the neurovascular unit. Ann N Y Acad Sci 1165: 228-239.

62. Hermanns MI, Unger RE, Kehe K, Peters K, Kirkpatrick CJ (2004) Lung epithelial cell lines in coculture with human pulmonary microvascular endothelial cells: development of an alveolo-capillary barrier in vitro. Lab Invest 84: 736-752.

63. Del Donno M, Chetta A, Foresi A, Gavaruzzi G, Ugolotti G, et al. (1997) Lung epithelial permeability and bronchial responsiveness in subjects with stable asthma. Chest 111: 1255-1260.

64. Elwood RK, Kennedy S, Belzberg A, Hogg JC, Paré PD (1983) Respiratory mucosal permeability in asthma. Am Rev Respir Dis 128: 523-527.

65. O'Byrne PM, Dolovich M, Dirks R, Roberts RS, Newhouse MT (1984) Lung epithelial permeability: relation to nonspecific airway responsiveness. J Appl Physiol Respir Environ Exerc Physiol 57: 77-84.

66. Lemarchand P, Chinet T, Collignon MA, Urzua G, Barritault L, et al. (1992) Bronchial clearance of DTPA is increased in acute asthma but not in chronic asthma. Am Rev Respir Dis 145: 147-152.

67. Bennett WD, Ilowite JS (1989) Dual pathway clearance of 99mTc-DTPA from the bronchial mucosa. Am Rev Respir Dis 139: 1132-1138.

68. Bhure UN, Bhure SU, Bhatt BM, Mistry S, Pednekar SJ, et al. (2009) Lung epithelial permeability and inhaled furosemide: added dimensions in asthmatics. Ann Nucl Med 23: 549-557.

69. Bucchieri F, Puddicombe SM, Lordan JL, Richter A, Buchanan D, et al. (2002) Asthmatic bronchial epithelium is more susceptible to oxidant-induced apoptosis. Am J Respir Cell Mol Biol 27: 179-185.

70. Holgate ST (2008) The airway epithelium is central to the pathogenesis of asthma. AllergolInt 57: 1-10.

71. Kicic A, Hallstrand TS, Sutanto EN, Stevens PT, Kobor MS, et al. (2010) Decreased fibronectin production significantly contributes to dysregulated repair of asthmatic epithelium. Am J Respir Crit Care Med 181: 889-898.

72. Wang SJ, Kao CH, Lin WY, Hsu CY, Chang CP, et al. (1995) Effects of inhalation of steroids on lung permeability in patients with asthma. Clin Nucl Med 20: 494-496.

73. Tsai SC, Kao CH, Wang SJ, Lan JL, ChangLai SP (1995) Effects of corticosteroid inhalation therapy on lung ventilation and alveolar permeability in asthma using TC-99M DTPA radioaerosol inhalation lung scintigraphy. Gaoxiong Yi Xue Ke Xue ZaZhi 11: 436-442.

74. Yuksel H, Yuksel D, Demir E, Tanaç R (2001) Influence of inhaled steroids on pulmonary epithelial permeability to Tc99m-dTPA in atopic asthmatic children. J Investig Allergol Clin Immunol 11: 188-192.

75. de Boer WI, Sharma HS, Baelemans SM, Hoogsteden HC, Lambrecht BN, et al. (2008) Altered expression of epithelial junctional proteins in atopic asthma: possible role in inflammation. Can J Physiol Pharmacol 86: 105-112.

76. Wan H, Winton HL, Soeller C, Gruenert DC, Thompson PJ, et al. (2000) Quantitative structural and biochemical analyses of tight junction dynamics following exposure of epithelial cells to house dust mite allergen Der p 1. Clin Exp Allergy 30: 685-698.

77. Pike VW, Aigbirhio FI, Freemantle CA, Page BC, Rhodes CG, et al. (1995) Disposition of inhaled 1,1,1,2-tetrafluoroethane (HFA134A) in healthy subjects and in patients with chronic airflow limitation. Measurement by 18F-labeling and whole-body gamma-counting. Drug Metab Dispos 23: 832-839.

78. Donnell D, Harrison LI, Ward S, Klinger NM, Ekholm BP, et al. (1995) Acute safety of the CFC-free propellant HFA-134a from a pressurized metered dose inhaler. Eur J Clin Pharmacol 48: 473-477.

79. Kirby SM, Smith J, Ventresca GP (1995) Salmeterol inhaler using a non-chlorinated propellant, HFA134a: systemic pharmacodynamic activity in healthy volunteers. Thorax 50: 679-681.

80. Jenkins M (1995) Clinical evaluation of CFC-free metered dose inhalers. J Aerosol Med 8 Suppl 1: S41-47.

81. Ramsdell JW, Colice GL, Ekholm BP, Klinger NM (1998) Cumulative dose response study comparing HFA-134a albuterol sulfate and conventional CFC albuterol in patients with asthma. Ann Allergy Asthma Immunol 81: 593-599.

82. Nelson HS, Kane RE, Petillo J, Banerji D (2000) Long-term safety of a non-chlorofluorocarbon-containing triamcinolone acetonide inhalation aerosol in patients with asthma. Azmacort HFA Study Group. J Asthma 37: 145-152.

83. Emmen HH, Hoogendijk EM, Klöpping-Ketelaars WA, Muijser H, Duistermaat E, et al. (2000) Human safety and pharmacokinetics of the CFC alternative propellants HFC 134a (1,1,1,2-tetrafluoroethane) and HFC 227 (1,1,1,2,3,3,3-heptafluoropropane) following whole-body exposure. Regul Toxicol Pharmacol 32: 22-35.

84. Ishiguro T, Yasui M, Nakade Y, Kimura H, Katayama N, et al. (2007) Extrinsic allergic alveolitis with eosinophil infiltration induced by 1,1,1,2-tetrafluoroethane (HFC-134a): a case report. Intern Med 46: 1455-1457.

27

Obesity, Circulating Androgens and their Precursors

Michaela Dušková, Hana Pospíšilová, Martin Hill and Luboslav Stárka*

Institute of Endocrinology, Prague, Czech Republic

Abstract

Objective: The association of obesity with a lower circulating testosterone level in men is well documented. However, reports on possible changes in the androgen spectrum in obesity are rare.

Methods: To investigate this phenomenon, serum sex hormone–binding globulin (SHBG), testosterone, dihydrotestosterone, androstenedione, dehydroepiandrosterone and its sulphate, 17α-hydroxypregnenolone, 17α-hydroxyprogesterone and gonadotrophins LH and FSH concentrations were measured in fasting blood samples of 224 men divided into three groups – normal (BMI=18-25, n=109, overweight (BMI 25.10-30, n=78) and obese (BMI=30.1-39, n=37).

Results: A significant decrease in testosterone, dihydrotestosterone, 17α-hydroxypregnenolone, 17α-hydroxyprogesterone and SHBG with increasing body mass index was observed, whereas insignificant changes for dehydroepiandrosterone and its sulphate, androstenedione and gonadotrophins LH and FSH, were found. The ratios of corresponding pairs of steroids were in agreement with the concept that in obesity splitting of the side chain of C_{21}-steroids, and 17β-hydroxysteroid dehydrogenase-reducing activity are decreased. No changes for steroid 5α-reductase or 3β-hydroxysteroid dehydrogenase (HSD3B2) were found.

Conclusion: The findings demonstrate that, in men with increasing body mass index, the formation of C_{19} steroids decreases from their C_{21} precursors and lower 17β-hydroxysteroid dehydrogenase further confines the production of testosterone and dihydrotestosterone.

Keywords: Obesity; Testosterone; Dihydrotestosterone; Androgens; 17α-hydroxyprogesterone; 17α-hydroxypregnenolone

Introduction

Reduced testosterone levels, well into the hypogonadal range, are common in male obesity [1-5]. The mechanism of circulating total testosterone concentration decrease is explained by a high expression of aromatase, the enzyme that converts testosterone to estradiol, in adipose tissue and by the resulting elevated estradiol. Together with the increased leptin and adipokines from fat tissue, this triggers inhibition of the hypothalamic-pituitary-gonadal axis [6, 7]. This results in hypogonadotrophic hypogonadism, which is observed in a large percentage of obese men.

Whereas a handful of publications deal with the relation of testosterone, dihydrotestosterone or estradiol levels to obesity, less attention has been paid to the influence of obesity on androgen metabolism. Some important data were acquired by measuring the intra-adipose metabolism of androgens [8-10]. The activity of enzymes involved in androgen metabolism varies in the different parts of fat tissue and, together with local glucocorticoid activity, constitutes an important factor for fat distribution.

Data concerning circulating androgens and their precursors in obese men, with the exception of that on testosterone or dihydrotestosterone [11], are scarce [12-15]. This short study aims to determine the impact of obesity on the pattern of circulating androgens and to show whether all changes in the concentration of androgens and their precursors 17α-hydroxypregnenolone and 17α-hydroxyprogesterone are proportional to the reduced level of testosterone and if this decline also applies to androgens of mainly adrenal origin.

Materials and Methods

Subjects

A group of 224 healthy (except for their obesity and associated symptoms) men aged 20 to 78 with a broad range of body mass index (BMI) 18 to 39 was enrolled in this study. Anthropometric parameters (i.e. weight, height, BMI) were measured. Blood withdrawal was carried out in fasting subjects in the morning between 7:30 and 8:30 a.m. from the forearm vein. Serum was stored at -80°C until it was processed in the laboratory.

The Ethical Committee approved the study and all patients signed informed consent forms before taking part in the study.

Anthropometric data

Anthropometric data were obtained in a fasting state. Body weight and height were measured in all participants in order to calculate body mass index (BMI). Weight (to the nearest 0.1 kg) and height (to the nearest cm) were measured. Body mass index was calculated as the weight (kg) divided by height squared (m^2).

The group of 224 healthy men was divided into three subgroups according to BMI. The first subgroup consisted of 109 men with BMI between 18 and 25. The second group included 78 men with BMI between 25 and 30. The third subgroup had 37 men with BMI 30 to 39.

Steroid analysis

Laboratory analyses of sex hormone binding globulin (SHBG),

***Corresponding author:** Luboslav Stárka, Institute of Endocrinology, Narodni 8, 116 94 Prague 10, Czech Republic, E-mail: lstarka@endo.cz

LH, FSH and steroid hormones: dihydrotestosterone, testosterone, 17α-hydroxyprogesterone, dehydroepiandrosterone (DHEA), dehydroepiandrosterone sulfate (DHEAS), 4-androstene-3,17-dione (androstenedione), and 17α-hydroxypregnenolone were carried out.

Serum testosterone was determined by standard radioimmunoassay (RIA) using antiserum anti-testosterone-3-carboxymethyloxim: BSA and testosterone-3-carboxymethyloxim-tyrosylmethyl-ester-[^{125}I] as a tracer. Intra-assay and inter-assay coefficient variants were 7.2% and

10%, respectively, and sensitivity was 0.21 nmol/l. Androstenedione was determined by standard RIA with antiserum anti-androstenedione-6-carboxy-methyloxim: BSA and [^{3}H] androstenedione as tracer. Intra-assay and inter-assay coefficient variants were 8.1% and 10.2% and sensitivity was 0.39 nmol/l. Sexual hormones binding globulin was assayed using an IRMA kit (Orion, Espoo, Finland). Commercial kits (Immunotech, Marseilles, France) were used for the determination of LH, FSH (IRMA kit), 17α-hydroxyprogesterone, dehydroepiandrosterone (DHEA) and dehydroepiandrosterone

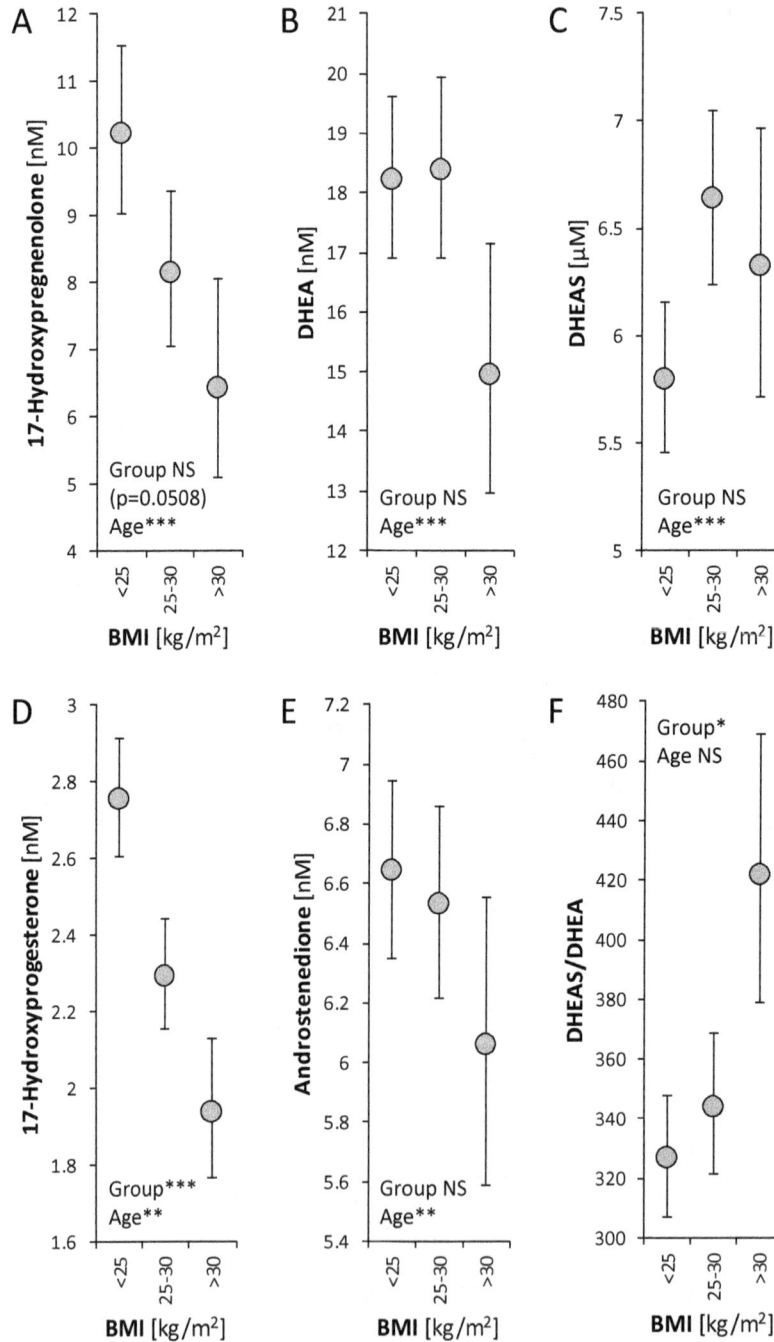

Figure 1: Relationships between steroid levels, DHEAS/DHEA ratio and BMI as evaluated using ANCOVA with BMI group as a main factor and age of the subject as a covariate (for details see statistical data analysis). The circles with error bars represent the group means with their 95% confidence intervals as computed for least significant difference (LSD) multiple comparisons (p=0.05). The confidence values, which do not overlap, represent statistical significant difference between the corresponding groups. Statistical significance: NS=not significant, *p<0.05, **p<0.01, ***p<0.001.

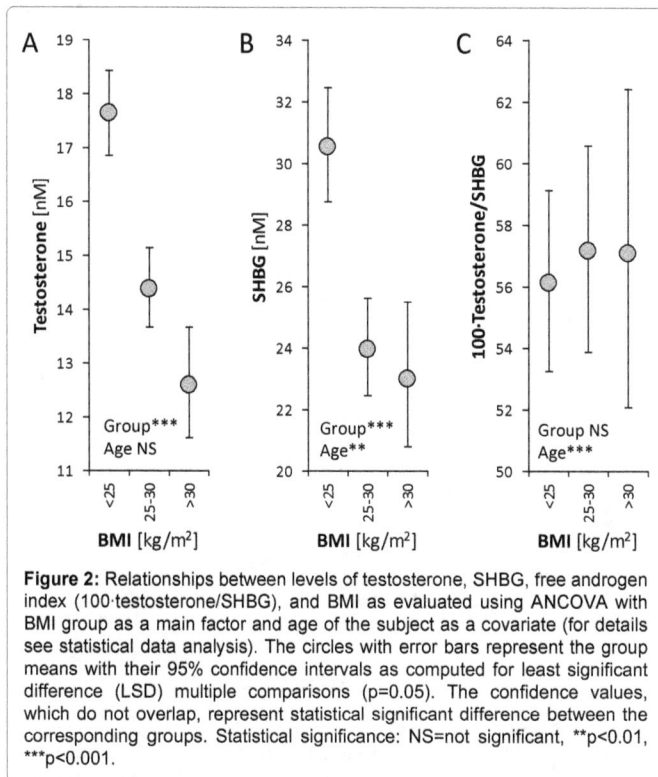

Figure 2: Relationships between levels of testosterone, SHBG, free androgen index (100·testosterone/SHBG), and BMI as evaluated using ANCOVA with BMI group as a main factor and age of the subject as a covariate (for details see statistical data analysis). The circles with error bars represent the group means with their 95% confidence intervals as computed for least significant difference (LSD) multiple comparisons (p=0.05). The confidence values, which do not overlap, represent statistical significant difference between the corresponding groups. Statistical significance: NS=not significant, **p<0.01, ***p<0.001.

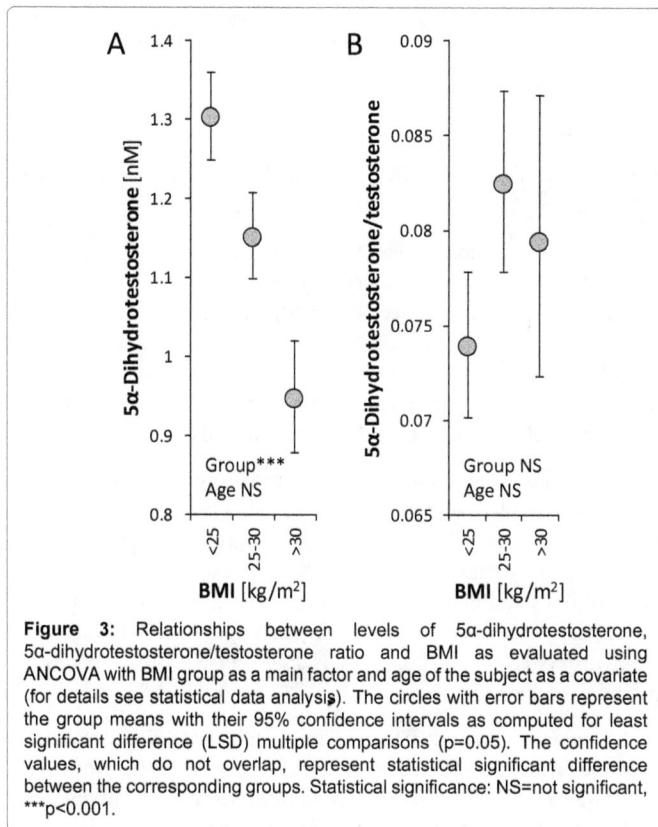

Figure 3: Relationships between levels of 5α-dihydrotestosterone, 5α-dihydrotestosterone/testosterone ratio and BMI as evaluated using ANCOVA with BMI group as a main factor and age of the subject as a covariate (for details see statistical data analysis). The circles with error bars represent the group means with their 95% confidence intervals as computed for least significant difference (LSD) multiple comparisons (p=0.05). The confidence values, which do not overlap, represent statistical significant difference between the corresponding groups. Statistical significance: NS=not significant, ***p<0.001.

sulfate (DHEAS) (RIA kit). Dihydrotestosterone was determined by an original methodology [16,17]. 17α-Hydroxypregnenolone was determined by an in-house RIA method.

Statistical data analysis

To evaluate the relationships between dependent variables, we used the ANCOVA model with BMI group as a main factor and age of the subject as a covariate (age–adjusted ANOVA) followed by least significant difference (LSD) multiple comparisons. The original dependent variables and the covariate were transformed by power transformations to attain a constant variance and symmetric distribution of the data and residuals [18]. Statistical software Statgraphic Centurion version XVI (Herndon, VA, USA) was used for the calculations. The homogeneity of the data and residual were checked as described elsewhere [19].

Results

The comparison of men with normal body mass index, overweight and obese men showed that a significant continuous decrease of parameters for testosterone (Figure 2A), dihydrotestosterone (Figure 3A) and SHBG (Figure 2B) correlates with increasing body mass. Also the circulating both C_{21} androgen precursors, 17α-hydroxyprogesterone and 17α-hydroxypregnenolone, decrease with increasing BMI (Figures 1A and 1D), whereas the changes in androstenedione, DHEA, and DHEAS levels as well as in gonadotrophins do not reach statistical significance (Figures 1B, 1C and 1E). Since the decrease of SHBG (Figure 2B) parallels the decrease of testosterone level (Figure 2A), thus compensating the loss of free testosterone, no change was observed in the free androgen index (Figure 2C).

The dihydrotestosterone : testosterone ratio does not correlate with the degree of obesity (Figure 3B), to the 17α-hydroxyprogesterone : 17α-hydroxpregnenolone ratio or

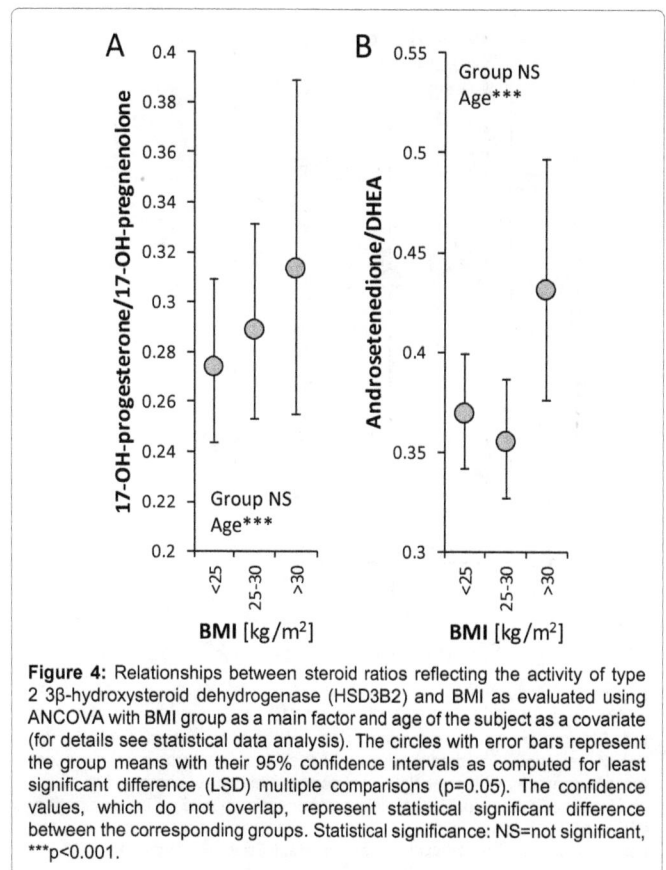

Figure 4: Relationships between steroid ratios reflecting the activity of type 2 3β-hydroxysteroid dehydrogenase (HSD3B2) and BMI as evaluated using ANCOVA with BMI group as a main factor and age of the subject as a covariate (for details see statistical data analysis). The circles with error bars represent the group means with their 95% confidence intervals as computed for least significant difference (LSD) multiple comparisons (p=0.05). The confidence values, which do not overlap, represent statistical significant difference between the corresponding groups. Statistical significance: NS=not significant, ***p<0.001.

androstenedione : dehydroepiandrosterone ratio (Figures 4A and 4B), which demonstrates the undisturbed activity of 3β-hydroxysteroid dehydrogenase type 2 (HSD3B2). On the contrary, it is evident from the DHEA : 17α-hydroxypregnenolone and androstenedione : 17α-hydroxprogesterone ratios (Figure 5A) that the activity of C_{17}, C_{20}-lyase (CYP17A1) decreases with the degree of obesity, especially for the Δ^4 pathway (Figure 5B).

The testosterone: androstenedione ratio (Figure 6) decreases significantly, which is in agreement with the decreased activity of 17β-hydroxysteroid dehydrogenase type 3 (HSD17B3).

Multivariate statistical analysis showed that age was a significant factor for the correlation of BMI and the levels of 17α-hydroxypregnenolone, 17α-hydroxyprogesterone, androstenedione, dehydroepiandrosterone and its sulfate and SHBG. The decrease of testosterone and dihydrotestosterone with increasing BMI was independent of age.

Discussion

We can derive from the data that testosterone biosynthesis in overweight and obese men is inhibited already in the step of splitting the side chain of C_{21} steroids and further by the decrease of 17β-hydroxysteroid dehydrogenase type 3 (HSD17B3) reducing activity. The changed ratio of dehydroepiandrosterone sulfate to DHEA, which might be a consequence of decreased sulfatase or increased sulfotransferase or increased secretion of DHEA sulfate from the adrenals, is of interest.

No changes with increasing BMI were observed with regards to

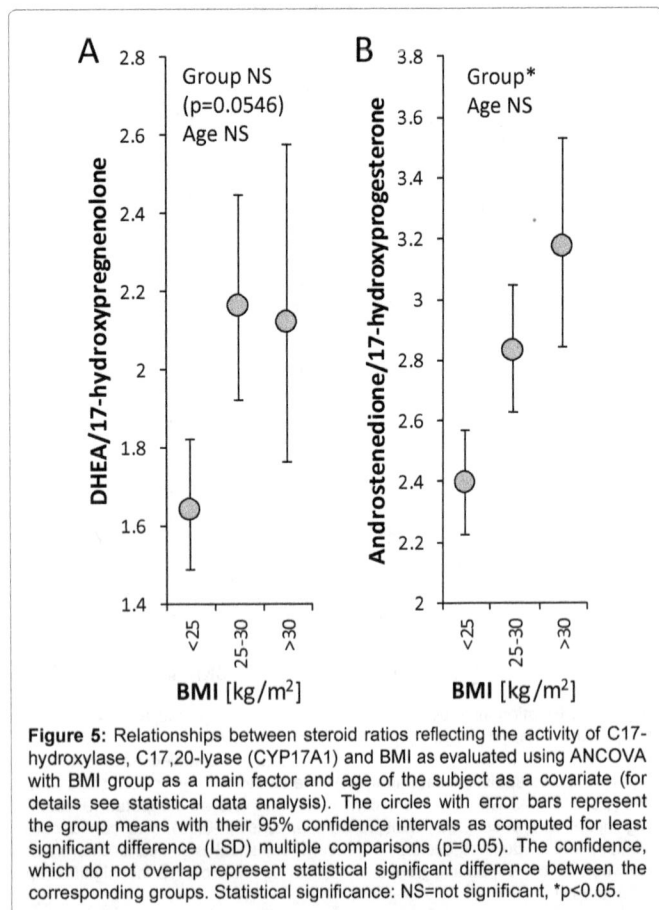

Figure 6: Relationships between steroid ratios reflecting the activity of type 3 17-hydroxysteroid dehydrogenase (HSD17B3) and BMI as evaluated using ANCOVA with BMI group as a main factor and age of the subject as a covariate (for details see statistical data analysis). The circles with error bars represent the group means with their 95% confidence intervals as computed for least significant difference (LSD) multiple comparisons (p=0.05). The confidence, which do not overlap represent statistical significant difference between the corresponding groups. Statistical significance: NS=not significant, *p<0.05, **p<0.01, *p<0.001.

steroid 5α-reducatse (SRD5A1) or 3β-hydroxysteroid dehydrogenase (HSD3B2).

These findings concur with the studies on in vitro metabolism of testosterone in the fat tissue of various localisations. In a study of intra-adipose sex steroid metabolism [9], generalized obesity (BMI) was associated with increased aromatase mRNA and 5α-reductase type 1 levels did not did not predict fat amount or its distribution. This supported the hypothesis that intra-adipose sex steroid metabolism is a determinant of gynoid vs. android patterns of body fat [9].

Modified androgen metabolism pathway influences fat tissue, as androgens modulate adipocyte function and affect the size of adipose tissue compartments in humans. For instance, aldo-keto reductase 1C (AKR1C) enzymes, especially AKR1C2 and AKR1C3, through local synthesis and inactivation of androgens, may be involved in the fine regulation of androgen availability in adipose tissue [10]. Type 3 17β-hydroxysteroid dehydrogenase is co-expressed with aromatase in the abdominal preadipocytes [8].

It could be concluded that in men with increasing body mass index the formation of C_{19} steroids decreases from their C_{21} precursors, and lower 17β-hydroxysteroid dehydrogenase further confines the production of testosterone and dihydrotestosterone.

Acknowledgement

The project was supported by the grant No. NT 13542-3 of the Internal Grant Agency of the Ministry of Health IGA MZ, Czech Republic and grant GAUK No. 367511 of the Grant Agency of Charles University.

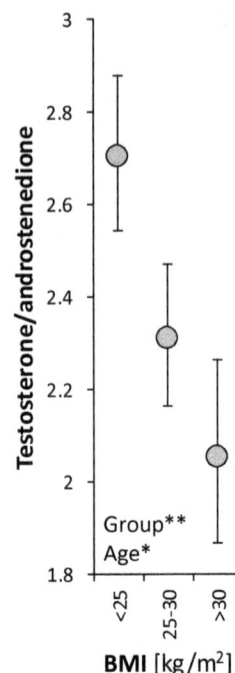

Figure 5: Relationships between steroid ratios reflecting the activity of C17-hydroxylase, C17,20-lyase (CYP17A1) and BMI as evaluated using ANCOVA with BMI group as a main factor and age of the subject as a covariate (for details see statistical data analysis). The circles with error bars represent the group means with their 95% confidence intervals as computed for least significant difference (LSD) multiple comparisons (p=0.05). The confidence, which do not overlap represent statistical significant difference between the corresponding groups. Statistical significance: NS=not significant, *p<0.05.

References

1. Hofstra J, Loves S, van Wageningen B, Ruinemans-Koerts J, Jansen I, et al. (2008) High prevalence of hypogonadotropic hypogonadism in men referred for obesity treatment. Neth J Med 66: 103-109.

2. De Maddalena C, Vodo S, Petroni A, Aloisi AM (2012) Impact of testosterone on body fat composition. J Cell Physiol 227 : 3744-3748.

3. Dandona P, Dhindsa S (2011) Update: Hypogonadotropic hypogonadism in type 2 diabetes and obesity. J Clin Endocrinol Metab 96: 2643-2651.

4. Allan CA, McLachlan RI (2010) Androgens and obesity. Curr Opin Endocrinol Diabetes Obes 17: 224-232.

5. Wang C, Jackson G, Jones TH, Matsumoto AM, Nehra A, et al. (2011) Low testosterone associated with obesity and the metabolic syndrome contributes to sexual dysfunction and cardiovascular disease risk in men with type 2 diabetes. Diabetes Care 34: 1669-1675.

6. Glass AR (1989) Endocrine aspects of obesity. Med Clin North Am 73: 139-160.

7. Cohen PG (1999) The hypogonadal-obesity cycle: role of aromatase in modulating the testosterone-estradiol shunt - a major factor in the genesis of morbid obesity. Med Hypotheses 52: 49-51.

8. Corbould AM, Bawden MJ, Lavranos TC, Rodgers RJ, Judd SJ (2002) The effect of obesity on the ratio of type 3 17β-hydroxysteroid dehydrogenase mRNA to cytochrome P450 aromatase mRNA in subcutaneous abdominal and intra-abdominal adipose tissue of women. Int J Obes Relat Metab Disord 26: 165-175.

9. Wake DJ, Strand M, Rask E, Westerbacka J, Livingstone DE, et al. (2007) Intra-adipose sex steroid metabolism and body fat distribution in idiopathic human obesity. Clin Endocrinol (Oxf) 66: 440-446.

10. Blouin K, Veilleux A, Luu-The V, Tchernof A (2009) Androgen metabolism in adipose tissue: recent advances. Mol Cell Endocrinol 301: 97-103.

11. Côté JA, Lessard J, Mailloux J, Laberge P, Rhéaume C, et al. (2012) Circulating 5α-dihydrotestosterone, abdominal obesity and adipocyte characteristics in women. Horm Mol Biol Clin Invest 12: 391-400.

12. De Pergola G, Triggiani V, Giorgino F, Cospite MR, Garruti G, et al. (1994) The free testosterone to dehydroepiandrosterone sulphate molar ratio as a marker of visceral fat accumulation in premenopausal obese women. Int J Obes Relat Metab Disord 18: 659-664.

13. Labrie F, Bélanger A, Cusan L, Gomez JL, Candas B (1997) Marked decline in serum concentrations of adrenal C19 sex steroid precursors and conjugated androgen metabolites during aging. J Clin Endocrinol Metab 82: 2396-2402.

14. Tchernof A, Labrie F (2004) Dehydroepiandrosterone, obesity and cardiovascular disease risk: a review of human studies. Eur J Endocrinol 151: 1-14.

15. Barrett-Connor E, Ferrara A (1996) Dehydroepiandrosterone, dehydroepiandrosterone sulfate, obesity, waist-hip ratio, and noninsulin-dependent diabetes in postmenopausal women: the Rancho Bernardo Study. J Clin Endocrinol Metab 81: 59-64.

16. Sedláčková B, Dušátková L, Zamrazilová H, Matucha P, Bičíková M, et al. (2012) 7-oxygenated derivatives of dehydroepiandrosterone and obesity. Prague Med Rep 113 : 147-155.

17. Hampl R, Putz Z, Stárka L (1990) Radioimmunolaogical determination of dihydrotestosterone and its importance for laboratory diagnostic. Biochemia Clin bohemoslov 19: 157-163.

18. Meloun M, Hill M, Militky J, Kupka K (2000) Transformation in the PC-aided biochemical data analysis. Clin Chem Lab Med 38: 553-559.

19. Meloun M, Militky J, Hill M, Brereton RG (2002) Crucial problems in regression modelling and their solutions. Analyst 127: 433-450.

28

Progesterone and Melanoma Cells: An Old Story Suspended between Life and Death

Gabriella Moroni, Roberta Gaziano, Cristina Buè, Massimiliano Agostini, Carlo-Federico Perno, Paola Sinibaldi-Vallebona and Francesca Pica*

Department of Experimental Medicine and Surgery, University of Rome Tor Vergata, Rome, Italy

Abstract

Melanoma is a widespread cancer with poor prognosis. Female hormones are known to be capable of influencing melanoma progression but clinical data related to pregnancy, oral contraception and hormone replacement therapy are controversial. A few reports show that *in vitro* progesterone (PG) affects melanoma growth in nuclear progesterone receptor (nPR)-positive and nPR-negative cells, but the experimental protocols used are quite different and the results are not univocal. Further research on this topic is thus needed especially in view of the widespread use of PG in clinical practice. In this study, we used human melanoma cells (A-375), which were cultured *in vitro* in the presence or absence of a wide range of PG concentrations (from 0.01 to 1000 µM) in single treatment. Daily cell count, cell cycle analysis and apoptosis assay were performed. Our results show that the low PG concentrations (from 0.01 to 1.0 µM) promote a significant increase of melanoma cell proliferation but this growth-stimulatory effect is not observed at 10 µM PG and the higher PG concentrations (i.e. 100 and 1000 µM) induce a cell density reduction which is the result of both cell cycle arrest and apoptosis. These findings confirm and extend previous observations reported in the international literature. A higher caution in the clinical use of progesterone is thus mandatory, since PG concentrations capable of stimulating melanoma cell proliferation are very close to those commonly used in a wide spectrum of physio-pathological conditions.

Keywords: Progesterone; Cancer; Human melanoma; Steroid hormones; Cell proliferation; Cell-cycle; Apoptosis

Introduction

Steroid hormones regulate cell proliferation, survival and development and have been involved in the origin and/or progression of cancer [1-6]. In the last decades, many epidemiological and experimental studies have suggested that steroid hormones may be etiologic factors in tumor generation, but whereas for some tumors, the link between hormones and cancer is well established, in other cases the relationship is not fully defined or even contradictory [1, 7-9].

Many human cancers, especially those of reproductive tissues, depend on progesterone (PG) [9]. PG is known to participate in the regulation of several physiological and pathological processes in mammals, such as ovarian function, growth and differentiation of the uterine endometrium and mammary gland [10]. However, PG also participates in non-reproductive processes, such as neural excitability, learning and memory, and in pathological processes like cancer [10-12]. In literature, however, data exploring the relationship between progesterone and cancer are controversial. One of the main problems lies in the fact that depending on the cell type, hormonal environment, growth conditions, and developmental stage, progesterone can either stimulate or inhibit cell proliferation or promote cell differentiation [13]. It has been reported that the lifetime exposure to reproductive hormones, in particular progesterone and/or estrogens, affects the risk of breast cancer and melanoma [12]. Melanoma is a widespread skin cancer with very poor prognosis. It is an old story, however still debated, that the outcome of established melanoma is influenced by endocrine status although the acquisition of melanoma does not seem to be influenced by female sex hormones [14, 15]. Early studies showed that female patients with malignant melanoma had some survival advantage [16], which in some studies was observed in pre- as opposed to post-menopausal women [17-19]. Others larger multi-variate analyses, however, demonstrated that it was equally strong in

pre- as well as in post-menopausal groups [20]. Parallely, the literature concerning melanoma progression in pregnancy is also controversial [21-24], although several recent reports demonstrate that pregnancy-associated melanomas have poorer outcomes than other melanomas [25-29].

In vitro progesterone influences melanoma growth [30-33], but several melanoma cell lines have been studied and very different experimental protocols have been used, so that the results actually available in literature are not univocal. Further research on this topic is thus needed, especially in view of the widespread use of PG in clinical practice. In this study, we report the results obtained by testing *in vitro* the effects of a wide range of concentrations of PG on the growth and viability of human melanoma cells.

Materials and methods

Cell Culture and Treatments

The human melanoma A-375 cell line was purchased from the American Type Culture Collection (ATCC, Rockville, MD) and grown in DMEM supplemented with 10% (v/v) heat-inactivated fetal calf serum (FCS) (Euroclone, Milan, Italy), 2 mM L-glutamine, 100 IU/ml penicillin and 100 g/ml streptomycin at 37 °C in a humidified 5% $CO2$ atmosphere. Cells were passaged two or three times a week after detachment from culture flasks with 0.05% trypsin and 0.02% EDTA solution in PBS. Progesterone Water-soluble was purchased from Sigma-Aldrich Chemical Company, St. Louis, MO, USA.

Corresponding author: Francesca Pica, Department of Experimental Medicine and Surgery University of Rome Tor Vergata, Via Montpellier, 1 00133 Rome, Italy, E-mail: pica@uniroma2.it

For dose-response curve experiments, exponentially growing A-375 were seeded into 6-well plates at a density of 1.5×10^5 cells/well in complete culture medium (CM). After an over-night of adherence, fresh medium containing various PG concentrations (i.e. 0,01 μM, 0,1 μM, 1 μM, 10 μM, 100 μM and 1000 μM) or control diluent was added to the wells and cell cultures were incubated at 37°C for additional 72 hours. Cell count and viability were evaluated daily in PG-treated and control cultures by light microscope after trypan blue vital-dye staining.

Cell cycle kinetics and apoptosis

Twenty-four, 48 and 72 hours post-treatment, A-375 cells were harvested and cell cycle analysis and quantification of apoptosis were performed by flow cytometry using a FACScan flow cytometer (Becton Dickinson Immunocytometry Systems, San Jose, CA, USA) equipped with an argon-ion laser (488 nm). The assay of cell cycle kinetics was carried out as described previously [34]. Cell cycle analysis was performed using ModFit software. Two different approaches were used to study apoptosis. The appearance of a Hypo diploid DNA peak (sub-G1 fraction) indicates the presence of an apoptotic cell population [35]. Induction of nuclear fragmentation characteristic of apoptosis was also determined by the DAPI staining of treated and untreated cells according to the standard technique [36].

Statistics

All experimental points were carried out in duplicate. Average of the duplicate samples was taken as mean value and standard error was calculated. Each experimental point was expressed as Mean ± SEM. Each experiment was repeated at least three times. Significance of differences between PG-treated and -untreated control cells was assessed by using the Student's t test and p values ≤ 0.05 were considered significant.

Results

Effect of PG addition on human melanoma A-375 cell density

Dose and time course experiments were carried out using different PG concentrations (from 0.01 to 1000 μM) addition to human melanoma A-375 cells. As shown in Figure 1, low PG concentrations, i.e. 0.01, 0.1 and 1.0 μM, induce a clear-cut elevation of the A-375 cell growth above the control values ($p < 0.05$ vs untreated controls, for each concentration at each time point tested, except than 0.01 μM at 24h p=0,126). This effect is not observed in A-375 cells exposed to 10 μM PG, whose growth curves appear to be overlapping those of the untreated controls. Conversely, higher PG concentrations induced a dramatic reduction of cell density, which was evident at PG 100 μM ($p < 0.05$ vs untreated controls at each time point tested, except than 100 μM at 72h p=0.0009) and reached its maximum of inhibition at the dose PG 1000 μM ($p < 0.001$ vs untreated controls at each time point tested). The block of cell proliferation induced by 100 μM PG shows a recovery trend at 72 hours post-treatment, whereas 1000 μM PG produce a more dramatic and prolonged effect (Figures 1 and 2). Although A-375 cells exposed to the highest PG dose were found to be suppressed up to 72 hours post-treatment, they showed a normal pattern of cell growth after being seeded in fresh medium without PG (data not shown). No macroscopic change in cell shape or spreading was observed in A-375 cells exposed to the lower doses PG (from 0.01 to 1.0 μM) when compared to the untreated control cells (data not shown). By contrast, evidence of reduced cell density was found in A-375 cells treated with the highest doses of PG, as assessed by means of microscope examination (Figure 2).

Effect of PG addition on human melanoma A-375 cell cycle kinetics and apoptosis

The effect observed on cell density in the dose-response curve experiments led us to investigate whether PG could affect cell cycle and/ or cell viability. Thus, flow-cytometry analysis was performed on A-375 cells treated or not with different PG concentrations, as shown in (Figure 3) (left panel), no significant change in the percentage of cells found in the various phases of the cell cycle was observed in cells treated with PG from 0.01 to 10.0 μM, throughout the whole period of observation. By contrast, cells exposed to 100 μM and 1000 μM PG showed an alteration of the cell cycle. In particular, we observed an increase in the percentage of the cells in S-phase with a concomitant reduction of the cells in G1-phase. No significant changes in G2/M-phase were observed. Moreover, a slight increase in the percentages of sub-G1 fraction, consistent with cell death, was observed in A-375 cells exposed at the highest doses of PG, starting from 48 hours post-treatment and increasing further in the following days. This finding was confirmed by the detection of characteristic aspects of nuclear fragmentation, which were observed at microscopic examination (Figure 3). All together these results indicate that high PG concentrations induce cell cycle arrest,which appears to be most likely associated with a reduction in S-G2/M transition, rather than cell death.

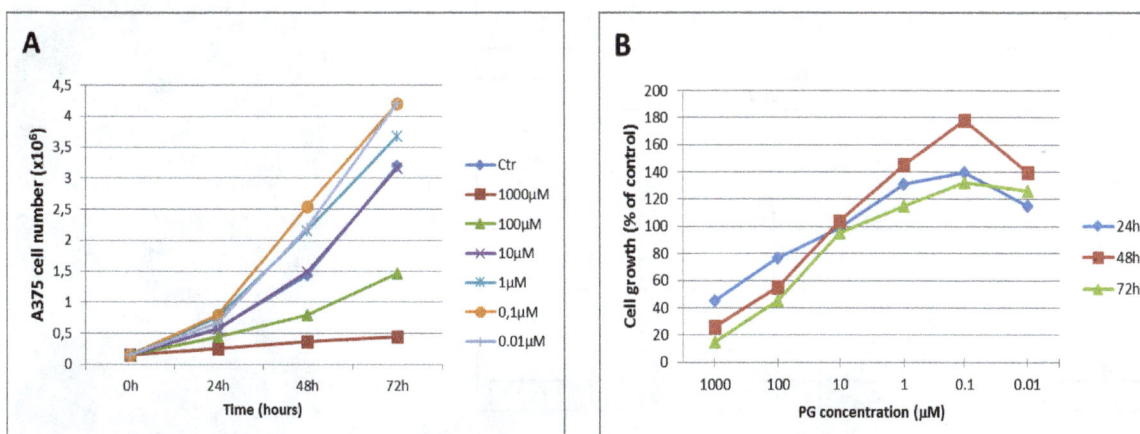

Figure 1: Effects of Progesterone on human melanoma A-375 cells.

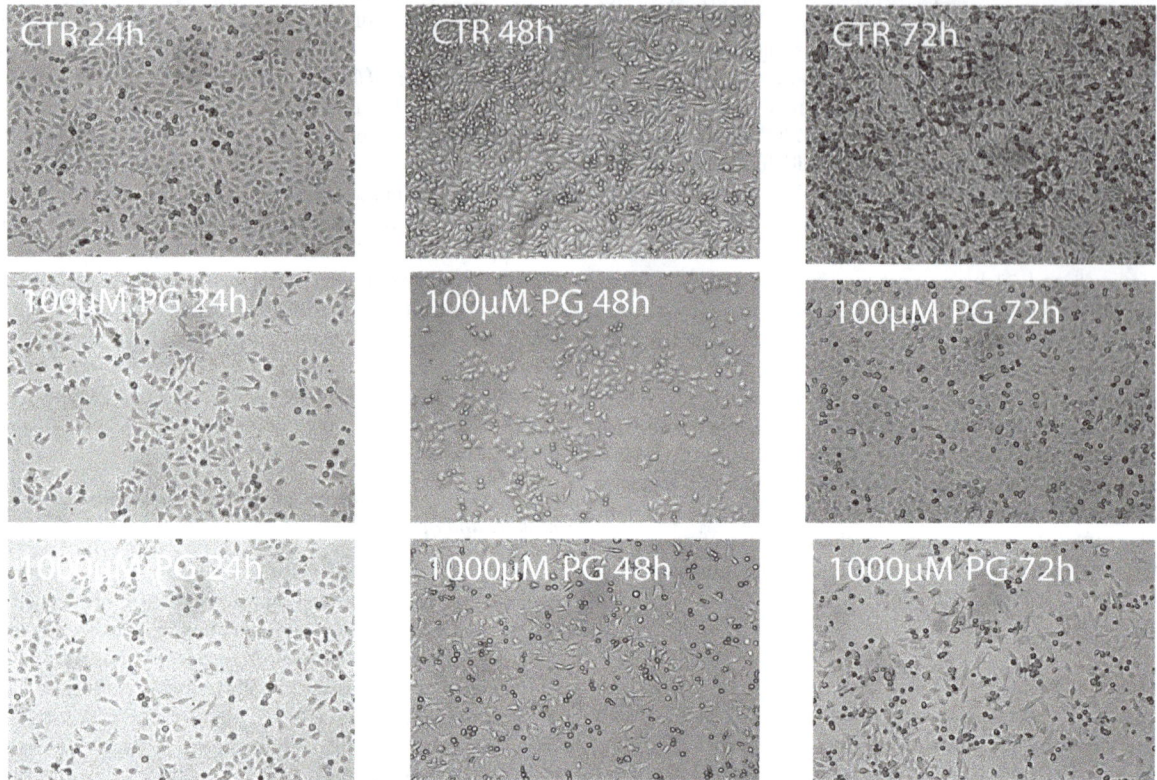

Figure 2: Effects of high-dose Progesterone on human melanoma A-375 cells.

PG (µM)	Time (hrs)	G_0/G_1 (%)	S (%)	G_2/M (%)	Sub-G_1
0	24	47.4	32.4	19.6	0.4
0.01	"	48.5	33,6	17.9	0.3
0.1	"	48,9	32.7	18.4	0.3
1.0	"	48.3	32.9	18.8	0.2
10	"	48.3	33.6	18	0.2
100	"	46	34.1	19.9	0.56
1000	"	24,6	65.8	9.7	3,7
PG (µM)	Time (hrs)	G_0/G_1 (%)	S (%)	G_2/M (%)	Sub-G_1
0	48	59.4	26.9	13.7	0.3
0.01	"	61.9	26.7	11.4	0.3
0.1	"	63	23.4	11.7	0.2
1.0	"	63.1	25.1	11.8	0.2
10	"	64.1	25.1	10.8	0.4
100	"	58,6	30.8	10.7	1.6
1000	"	42.7	43.5	13.9	8.4
PG (µM)	Time (hrs)	G_0/G_1 (%)	S (%)	G_2/M (%)	Sub-G_1
0	72	78.3	14.2	7.5	0.7
0.01	"	79.8	12.7	7.5	0.6
0.1	"	80.5	13.3	6.2	0.6
1.0	"	79.0	13.5	7.5	0.5
10	"	78.6	13.7	7.7	0.6
100	"	65.4	27.6	7.2	2
1000	"	48	42.7	9.3	10.7

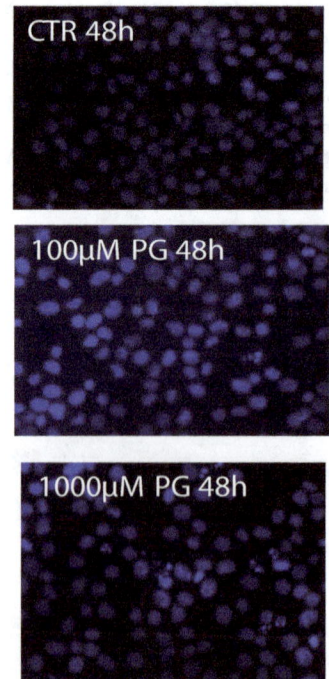

Figure 3: Effects of Progesterone on human melanoma A-375 cell cycle kinetic and apoptosis.

Discussion

The results of our experiments show that progesterone affects the human melanoma A-375 cell growth and viability in a complex and opposite direction depending on the dose employed. Indeed, low PG concentrations (from 0.01 to 1.0 μM) induce a significant increase of cell proliferation, but the effect seems to vanish at 10 μM PG and higher PG concentrations (100 and 1000 μM PG) induce both cell cycle arrest and a slight increase in cell death.

A similar result was reported previously by Fang and coll. in a paper where PG treatments were carried out after an overnight of serum deprivation and the effects on the melanoma cells viability were evaluated by MTT assay exclusively 24 hours post-treatment [31]. In this regard, two considerations prompted us to repeat the experiments using a different protocol. First, previous evidence had been reported that human melanoma cells *in vitro* undergo a transition *versus* a more malignant phenotype associated with increased proliferation when exposed to stress conditions such as serum deprivation [37] and this fact could represent a potential bias for the observed PG effects. Second, the several limitations of the the MTT- and MTS-based assays have been discussed recently as well as the importance of careful evaluation of the methods used for the *in vitro* assessment of cell viability and proliferation[38]. Indeed, not even the cell-cycle kinetic studies appear to be reliable in this sense, as demonstrated by us in this report, since only microscopic cell counts after vital staining allowed us to check the stimulation of cell growth induced by low-dose PG. These seemingly trivial considerations, actually make us realize how important are the experimental conditions employed in the evaluation of the hormones' effects *in vitro* with consistent reliability, and then explain why data in the literature are often conflicting. Moreover, what is new respect to previous work, we show that both the growth-stimulatory and the growth-inhibitory effects of PG, which were obtained by means of the treatment with a single dose of low-PG (≤1μM) or high PG (≥100 μM), lasted for at least 72 hours after PG addition, i.e. for the whole period of observation. Further experiments showed that the seeding of A-375 cells, which had been exposed or not to the different PG concentrations, in fresh medium without PG, produced normal cell growth patterns; conversely, the daily administration of PG to the cultures increased the hormone- induced effects, especially those induced by high-dose PG (data not shown). Other *in vitro* studies on different melanoma cell lines have failed to demonstrate the cell growth stimulatory effect induced by low-dose PG, although confirming that high-dose PG inhibit melanoma cell growth and viability by means of different mechanisms such as the induction of marked apoptosis and/or autophagy [32]. In our hands, the cell density reduction induced by high-dose PG was primarily the result of cell cycle arrest. However, a small contribution of cell death on cell number has been observed in our experimental setting.

The exact mechanisms underlying the effects of PG on A-375 cell growth and viability have been not completely elucidated. It is known that PG exerts its actions through various mechanisms that are classified as classical and non-classical [10]. The classical mechanisms are mediated by n-PR and induce modifications of gene expression, whereas the non-classical ones rapidly proceed and are mediated by different pathways including the interaction with membrane receptors (mPR), ionic channels, growth factors and their receptors coupled to G proteins. These last interactions are associated with increased cAMP production, phosphoinositide turnover and protein kinase C and MAP kinase activation [10]. The A-375 melanoma cell line used in our experiments is negative for the presence of the n-PR, but has not been characterized for the presence of mPR [31]. Also, the possibility

that, depending on the dose employed, PG can use different cellular receptors which are present on melanoma cells, i.e. various growth factor receptors, which mediate different signal transduction pathways, cannot be ruled out [10].Finally, it is worth mentioning that melanomas are, in addition to teratocarcinomas and human breast cancer, the third tumor type with enhanced expression of HERV-K [39], and A-375 melanoma cells have been found to be positive for HERV-K encoded proteins in different studies [37, 39, 40]. Interestingly, a study performed almost thirty years ago by Ono and coll. on the human breast cancer cell line T47D, which possess different steroid receptors and is positive for HERV-K, showed that the combination of estradiol and progesterone was capable of stimulating the HERV-K genome expression [41]. Recent studies also point to activation of HERV-K expression as one of the key elements contributing to both morphological and functional modifications during melanoma progression.

In conclusion, the mechanisms by which hormones induce cell proliferation *in vivo* are poorly understood. Further studies are needed for a better comprehension of the many and complex effects of progesterone and other steroid hormones on melanoma and other cancers. This need is made urgent especially when considering that progesterone and its synthetic progestin analogs are clinically employed as methods of contraception and in hormone replacement therapies [42-47], in the treatment of recurrent miscarriage and during assisted reproductive technologies [48]. A higher caution in the clinical use of progesterone is thus mandatory, since PG concentrations capable of stimulating melanoma cell proliferation are very close to the pharmacological doses of PG commonly used in a wide spectrum of physio-pathological conditions.

Acknowledgements

The study was supported by a grant from MIUR to CFP (Project grant: PRIN 2010PHT9NF)

References

1. Madhunapantula SV, Mosca P, Robertson GP (2010) Steroid hormones drive cancer development. Cancer Biol Ther 10: 765-766.

2. Driscoll MS, Grant-Kels JM (2007) Hormones, nevi, and melanoma: an approach to the patient. J Am Acad Dermatol 57: 919-931.

3. Lens M, Bataille V (2008) Melanoma in relation to reproductive and hormonalfactors in women: current review on controversial issues. Cancer Causes Control 19: 437-442.

4. Kim JJ, Chapman-Davis E (2010) Role of progesterone in endometrial cancer. Semin Reprod Med 28: 81-90.

5. Villa E. (2008) Role of estrogen in liver cancer. Womens Health (Lond Engl) 4: 41-50.

6. Keely NO, Meegan MJ (2009) Targeting tumors using estrogen receptor ligand conjugates. Curr Cancer Drug Targets 9: 370-380.

7. Freedman RA, Winer EP (2010) Adjuvant therapy for postmenopausal women with endocrine-sensitive breast cancer. Breast 19: 69-75.

8. Yager JD, Davidson NE (2006) Estrogen carcinogenesis in breast cancer. N Engl J Med 354: 270-282.

9. Spicer DV, Pike MC (1994) Sex steroids and breast cancer prevention. J Natl Cancer Inst Monogr 16: 139-147.

10. Hernández-Hernández OT, Camacho-Arroyo I (2013) Regulation of gene expression by progesterone in cancer cells: effects on cyclin D1, EGFR and VEGF. Mini Rev Med Chem 13: 635-642.

11. Cabrera-Muñoz E, Hernández-Hernández OT, Camacho-Arroyo I (2011) Role of progesterone in human astrocytomas growth. Curr Top Med Chem 11: 1663-1667.

12. Conneely OM, Jericevic BM, Lydon JP (2003) Progesterone receptors in

mammary gland development and tumorigenesis. J Mammary Gland Biol Neoplasia 8: 205-214.

13. Edwards DP (2005) Regulation of signal transduction pathways by estrogen and progesterone. Annu Rev Physiol 67: 335-376.

14. Richardson B, Price A, Wagner M, Williams V, Lorigan P, et al. (1999) Investigation of female survival benefit in metastatic melanoma. Br J Cancer 12: 2025-2033.

15. Gefeller O, Hassan K, Wille L (1998) Cutaneous malignant melanoma in women and the role of oral contraceptives. Br J Dermatol 138: 122-124.

16. Miller JG, Mac Neil S (1997) Gender and cutaneous melanoma. Br J Dermatol 136: 657-665.

17. Shaw HM, McGovern VJ, Milton GW, Farago GA, McCarthy WH (1980) Malignant melanoma: influence of site of lesion and age of patient in the female superiority in survival. Cancer 46: 2731-2735.

18. Karjalainen S, Hakulinen T (1988) Survival and prognostic factors of patients with skin melanoma. A regression-model analysis based on nationwide cancer registry data. Cancer 62: 2274-2280.

19. Cocconi G, Bella M, Calabresi F, Tonato M, Canaletti R, et al. (1992) Treatment of metastatic malignant melanoma with dacarbazine plus tamoxifen. N Engl J Med 327: 516-523.

20. Stidham KR, Johnson JL, Seigler HF (1994) Survival superiority of females with melanoma. A multivariate analysis of 6383 patients exploring the significance of gender in prognostic outcome. Arch Surg 129: 316-324.

21. MacKie RM, Bufalino R, Morabito A, Sutherland C, Cascinelli N (1991) Lack of effect of pregnancy on outcome of melanoma. For The World Health Organisation Melanoma Programme. Lancet 337: 653-655.

22. Slingluff CL Jr, Seigler HF (1992) Malignant melanoma and pregnancy. Ann Plast Surg 28: 95-99.

23. Shaw HM, Milton GW, Farago G, McCarthy WH (1978) Endocrine influences on survival from malignant melanoma. Cancer 42: 669-677.

24. Travers RL, Sober AJ, Berwick M, Mihm MC Jr, Barnhill RL, et al. (1995) Increased thickness of pregnancy-associated melanoma. Br J Dermatol 132: 876-883.

25. Byrom L, Olsen C, Knight L, Khosrotehrani K, Green AC (2015) Increased mortality for pregnancy-associated melanoma: systematic review and meta-analysis. J Eur Acad Dermatol Venereol 29: 1457-1466.

26. Janik ME, Bełkot K, Przybyło M (2014) Is oestrogen an important player in melanoma progression? Contemp Oncol (Pozn) 18: 302-306.

27. Cardonick E (2014) Pregnancy-associated breast cancer: optimal treatment options. Int J Womens Health 6: 935-943.

28. Enninga EA, Holtan SG, Creedon DJ, Dronca RS, Nevala WK, et al. (2014) Immunomodulatory effects of sex hormones: requirements for pregnancy and relevance in melanoma. Mayo Clin Proc 89: 520-535.

29. Jhaveri MB, Driscoll MS, Grant-Kels JM (2011) Melanoma in pregnancy. Clin Obstet Gynecol 54: 537-545.

30. Mordoh J, Tapia IJ, Barrio MM (2013) A word of caution: do not wake sleeping dogs; micrometastases of melanoma suddenly grew after progesterone treatment. BMC Cancer 13: 132.

31. Fang X, Zhang X, Zhou M, Li J (2010) Effects of progesterone on the growth regulation in classical progesterone receptor-negative malignant melanoma cells. J Huazhong Univ Sci Technolog Med Sci 30: 231-234.

32. Ramaraj P, Cox JL (2014) In vitro effect of progesterone on human melanoma (BLM) cell growth. Int J Clin Exp Med 7: 3941-3953 eCollection 2014.

33. Kanda N, Watanabe S (2011) 17beta-estradiol, progesterone, and dihydrotestosterone suppress the growth of human melanoma by inhibiting interleukin-8 production. J Invest Dermatol 117: 274-283.

34. Tucci P, Porta G, Agostini M, Dinsdale D, Iavicoli I, et al. (2013) Metabolic effects of TiO2 nanoparticles, a common component of sunscreens and cosmetics, on human keratinocytes. Cell Death Dis Mar 21;4:e549.

35. Kajstura M, Halicka HD, Pryjma J, Darzynkiewicz Z (2007) Discontinuous fragmentation of nuclear DNA during apoptosis revealed by discrete „sub-G1" peaks on DNA content histograms. Cytometry A 71: 125-131.

36. Kubista M, Akerman B, Nordén B (1987) Characterization of interaction between DNA and 4',6-diamidino-2-phenylindole by optical spectroscopy. Biochemistry 26: 4545-4553.

37. Serafino A, Balestrieri E, Pierimarchi P, Matteucci C, Moroni G, et al. (2009) The activation of human endogenous retrovirus K (HERV-K) is implicated in melanoma cell malignant transformation. Exp Cell Res 315: 849-862.

38. Wang P, Henning SM, Heber D (2010) Limitations of MTT and MTS-based assays for measurement of antiproliferative activity of green tea polyphenols. PLoS One 5(4): e10202.

39. Büscher K, Trefzer U, Hofmann M, Sterry W, Kurth R, et al. (2005) Expression of human endogenous retrovirus K in melanomas and melanoma cell lines. Cancer Res 65: 4172-4180.

40. Li Z, Sheng T, Wan X, Liu T, Wu H, et al. (2010) Expression of HERV-K correlates with status of MEK-ERK and 16INK4A16ICDK4 pathways in melanoma cells. Cancer Invest 28: 1031-1037.

41. Ono M, Kawakami M, Ushikubo H (1987) Stimulation of expression of the human endogenous retrovirus genome by female steroid hormones in human breast cancer cell line T47D. J Virol 61: 2059-2062.

42. Chlebowski RT, Anderson GL, Gass M, Lane DS, Aragaki AK, et al. (2010) Estrogen plus progestin and breast cancer incidence and mortality in postmenopausal women. JAMA 304: 1684-16892.

43. Tang JY, Spaunhurst KM, Chlebowski RT, Wactawski-Wende J, Keiser E, et al. (2011) Menopausal hormone therapy and risks of melanoma and nonmelanoma skin cancers: women's health initiative randomized trials. J Natl Cancer Inst 103: 1469-1475.

44. Govender Y, Avenant C, Verhoog NJ, Ray RM, Grantham NJ, et al. (2014) The injectable-only contraceptive medroxyprogesterone acetate, unlike norethisterone acetate and progesterone, regulates inflammatory genes in endocervical cells via the glucocorticoid receptor. PLoS One. May 19;9(5):e96497.

45. Hapgood JP, Ray RM, Govender Y, Avenant C, Tomasicchio M (2014) Differential glucocorticoid receptor-mediated effects on immunomodulatory gene expression by progestin contraceptives: implications for HIV-1 pathogenesis. Am J Reprod Immunol 71: 505-512.

46. Arroyo IC, Montor JM (2011) Non-reproductive effects of sex steroids: their immunoregulatory role. Curr Top Med Chem 11: 1661-1662.

47. Colditz GA, Rosner BA, Chen WY, Holmes MD, Hankinson SE (2004) Risk factors for breast cancer according to estrogen and progesterone receptor status. J Natl Cancer Inst 96: 218-228.

48. Whitley KA, Ural SH (2014) Treatment modalities in recurrent miscarriages without diagnosis. Semin Reprod Med 32: 319-322.

29

Synthetic Epoxy-Pregnan Steroids: Effects on Anxiety Behavior in Rats

Rey M[1], Ghini AA[2] and Coirini H[1,3,*]

[1]Laboratorio de Neurobiología, Instituto de Biología y Medicina Experimental (IBYME-CONICET), Vuelta de Obligado 2490, (C1428ADN), Ciudad Autónoma de Buenos Aires, Argentina.
[2]Departamento de Química Orgánica, Unidad de Microanálisis y Métodos Físicos aplicados a Química Orgánica (UMYMFOR-CONICET) Facultad de Ciencias Exactas y Naturales, Universidad de Buenos Aires (FCEN-UBA), Pabellón 2, Ciudad Universitaria, Intendente Güiraldes 2160, (C1428EHA) Ciudad Autónoma de Buenos Aires, Argentina
[3]Departamento de Bioquímica Humana, Facultad de Medicina, Universidad de Buenos Aires, Paraguay 2155, 5to Piso, (C1121ABG) Ciudad Autónoma de Buenos Aires, Argentina.

Abstract

Neurosteroids like 3α-OH-5α-pregnan-20-one (allopregnanolone) and 3α-OH-5β-pregnan-20-one (pregnanolone) modulate the γ-aminobutyric acid-A (GABAA) receptor function and produce several effects that can be considered for therapeutical pruposes like antidepressant and anxiolyticts, in a similar way to benzodiazepines. However, their rapid metabolism is a great disadvantage for medicinal treatments consideration. Synthetic steroid analogues with more bioavailability and stability arise like a solution to overcome these limitations. In previous studies, we evaluated the performance of a synthetic steroid group (Epoxies, similar to allopregnanolone and pregnanolone) throughout different assays in rat cerebral cortex and hippocampus, including neuroprotection and GABAA receptor modulation obtaining promising results. Taking into account the anxiolytic effect of allopregnanolone and pregnanolone, in this work we evaluated the effect of an intracranial administration (in dorsal hippocampus) of two synthetic steroids, Epoxy 1 and Epoxy 2, in an anxiety animal model to provide knowledge about the possible in vivo effects of these steroids. Allopregnanolone and pregnanolone produced increases in vertical and horizontal exploration behaviors, interpreted as anxiolytic-like effects. However, the two Epoxies capable to modulate GABAA receptor binding have no effect on anxiety at the dose evaluated. These features make them suitable for other therapeutical purposes where the anxiogenic behaviors are not involved.

Keywords: Neurosteroids; Synthetic analogues; Allopregnanolone; Pregnanolone; Open field

Introduction

Inside the central nervous system, the in situ synthesized steroids (neurosteroids, NS) are capable of modify the brain excitability [1,2]. Due to their chemical structure, the steroids may produce positive or negative modulations over receptors, like the γ-aminobutyric acid-A (GABAA) receptor [3,4]. Among the positive modulators of this receptor are two progesterone's metabolites: the 5α-pregnane-3α-ol-20- one (allopregnanolone, A) and its isomer 5α-pregnane-3β-ol-20-one (pregnanolone, P) [5]. In the last decades, the relevance of NS, like A and P, also has been increasing due to their multiple roles in normal and pathological behavior, ageing processes, damaged tissue regeneration and neuroprotection [6-9].

The interest on these steroids arises specifically from their potential activity as anticonvulsants, anesthetics, anxiolytic or sedative-hypnotic agents [10] useful for the treatment of several neurological and psychiatric disorders [5]. But, the main limitation for the therapeutical administration of these NS is their rapid in vivo biotransformation to other metabolites. Therefore, synthetic steroids (SS) analogues with better bioavailability and efficacy have an important therapeutic potential in brain disorders, becoming an alternative approach for different pathologies [11,12].

In the last decades, a significant increase around NS physiology and synthetic analogues development has been observed. The medicinal chemistry of neuroactive steroids (NAS) has been focused in the development of SS analogues preserving the absolute configuration of naturally occurring steroids. Structure/activity studies of the progester-

one metabolites, indicate that the 3α-hydroxyl configuration is required for binding and activity maintenance [13], while modifications in some carbon atoms do not affect their functions [14-16]. In previous works we evaluated the performance of a SS group Epoxies (similar to A and P) through different assays as well as neuroprotection and inhibition/stimulation binding of specific ligands of the GABA$_A$ receptor in rat cerebral cortex and hippocampus [17,18]. The main feature of these Epoxies is the presence of an oxygen bridge that holds the A/B angle of steroidal nucleus in a controlled way, conferring conformational restricted analogues [19]. In those studies, we demonstrated that, of all the *Epoxies* tested, the *Epoxy 1* (3α- hydroxy-2β,19-epoxy-5α-pregnan-20-one; A analogue) and the Epoxy 2 (3α-hydroxy-6,19-epoxypregn-4-ene-20-one; P analogue) produced the most similar effects to A and P [17,18].

On the other hand, severe psychiatric conditions like anxiety and stress-related disorders affect daily performance in tasks and represent a high cost to public health. Thus, the search of new and improve therapeutical alternatives remains currently. Also, the fact that neurosteroidogenic agents lack benzodiazepine-like side effects shows promise in the treatment of anxiety and depression [11]. Administration of A or P produces anxiolytic, ataxic, hypnotic- anesthetic and anticonvulsant effects as well as locomotor stimulation [5,20-30], being able to mimic the actions of benzodiazepines. Taking into account their effects as modulators of the GABAA receptor-ion- channel complex [5] mentioned before, the mechanism underlying their anxiolytic properties appears to be due to a potentiation of neural inhibition via this receptor

*Corresponding author: Prof. Dr. Héctor Coirini, Laboratorio de Neurobiología, Instituto de Biología y Medicina Experimental (IBYME-CONICET), Vuelta de Obligado 2490, (C1428ADN), Ciudad Autónoma de Buenos Aires, Argentina, E-mail: hcoirini@ibyme.conicet.gov.ar

[31-34]. Previous studies suggest that A increases the channel conductance of GABAA receptor-gated Cl- in hippocampal neurons, promoting anxiolytic-like effects [35-37]. This supports the hypothesis about the role that the dorsal (CA1) hippocampus area plays in emotional processes and NS modulation of anxiety and exploration. It has also been postulated that the dorsal region of this brain structure is involved in memory-related functions, whereas the ventral region mediates fear and anxiety responses[38]. In contrast to these anatomical and functional considerations, the recent results of Mòdol et al. [39] demonstrate that the dorsal (CA1) area of the hippocampus is also implicated in the modulation of anxiety- related behaviors. Their studies indicate that the hippocampal administration of A produces an anxiolytic-like profile and also increases exploratory behavior, observed trough the enhancement of the number of entries into the open arms in the elevated plus-maze device. This suggests that CA1 region together with other brain structures (such as the amygdala or the medial septum) could be an important target for explaining the NS effects on exploration, anxiety, learning and memory [39]. P administration in the dorsal hippocampus or in the lateral septum also produces dose-dependent anxiolytic-like effects in several animal models [36]. Moreover, both steroids have shown a comparable potency eliciting anxiolytic effects [24,27,31]. In addition, the ability of these and other NS to decrease anxiety-induced behavior has been demonstrated in several tests such as light/dark transition, rearing events and open-field [22,34,40]. In fact, there is evidence that the anxiolytic action of progesterone is mediated by its reduced metabolites, A and P [41,42]. Based in the previous results obtained with the Epoxies in the GABAA receptor modulation and the neuroprotective actions [17,18], and the anxiolytic-like effects mediated by A and P, the aim of this work was to evaluate the effects of two of these SS (Epoxy 1 and Epoxy 2) administration over the animal behavior. These analysis were performed in an anxiety model (open-field test), assessing horizontal and vertical exploration and the anxiolytic-like effects; comparing results between synthetic and natural steroids.

Materials and Methods

Steroids

Two natural steroids (A and P) and two synthetic analogues, 3α-hydroxy-1β,11α-epoxy-5α-pregnan-20-one (Epoxy 1, A analogue) [43] and 3α-hydroxy-6,19-epoxypregn-4-ene-20-one (Epoxy 2, P analogue) [44] were used. Steroid concentration used for microinfusion (6.7 µg/µl) was selected according to our previous results [17,18]. The solutions were prepared using cyclodextrin 30% in artificial cerebrospinal fluid (aCSF) as vehicle one hour before the administration.

Experimental animals

Ninety day old adult male Sprague Dawley rats (400 g; n=48) were housed under standard laboratory conditions with a 12-h light-dark cycle, with food and water ad libitum on a temperature (21ºC) and humidity (40-70%) controlled vivarium. The animal surgical procedures and treatments were evaluated by the Ethics Committee of the Instituto de Biología y Medicina Experimental (IBYME), CABA, Argentine, and approved according to the described on the protocol CE 040-Jun/2014, in accordance with guidelines defined by the European Community Council Directive (86/609/EEC) and the National Institutes of Health Guide for the Care and Use of Laboratory Animals.

Male rats were anesthetized with ketamine-xylazine (40:4 mg/Kg i.p.; Holliday, Richmond, Argentina) and placed in a stereotaxic apparatus (David Kopf Instruments, Tujunga CA, USA). Handmade 23-gauge stainless steel cannulae with 30-gauge removable inserts (dummy cannulae) were unilaterally implanted on the dorsal hippocampus using flat skull coordinates (anteroposterior, -2.3 mm; mediolateral, ± 1.6 mm; dorsoventral, 2.8 mm; from Bregma) according to the atlas Paxinos and Watson [45]. Three stainless steel screws and dental cement were used to fix the cannulae to the skull surface. After the surgery, animals were subcutaneously injected with a nonsteroidal anti-inflammatory (Meloxican 2 mg/Kg body weight, Boehringer Ingelheim, Argentina). A painkiller (Tramadol chlorhydrate 0.15 g/L; Finadiet SACIFI, Argentina) and an antibiotic (Enrofloxaxine 5 mg/L; Afford SA, Argentina) were administered in the drinking water for the next 3 days.

Bilateral implants in some brain areas have been widely used to explore the anxiolytic and/or antidepressant like-effects [46-48]. Although, the choice of unilateral cannulation (with left/right alternations) performed in this work, was based in previous reports that described anxiolytic and antidepressant effects with unilateral microinjections of A [49] or progesterone [50], without behavioral differences between brain sides.

Microinfusion procedure

Animals were allowed to recover for 10 days before performing the behavioral trials. Vehicle (cyclodextrin 30% in aCSF) or steroids (A, P, Epoxy 1 and Epoxy 2; 2 µg) were administered in 0.3 µl using a 30-gauge injection needle connected by PC-40 tubing (Rivero SA, Argentina) to a 10 µl glass syringe (Hamilton, Reno NV, USA; 0.1 µl/ min). After the 3 minutes of microinfusion, the injection needle was kept in place for 1 additional minute to allow diffusion away from the cannula tip before the dummy cannula reposition. According to the condition, 5 groups of animals (n=8) were established: Vehicle (cyclodextrin 30% in aCSF treatment), A (A treatment), P (P treatment), Epoxy 1 (Epoxy 1 treatment) and Epoxy 2 (Epoxy 2 treatment). Animals were hand restrained during all microinfusion procedure.

Behavioral testing

The open-field task [51,52] was used in accordance with the methods described by McCarthy et al. [53]. Behavioral testing occurred between 10:00 and 15:00h. The open-field device (housed in a dimly lit room with controlled temperature 21ºC and humidity 40-70%) consisted of 75 cm side squared box divided in 25 quadrants, with 30 cm height walls and an open roof. All animals were allowed to explore the device for 15 minutes (precondition test) one day before steroids microinfusion. At the next day, one minute after the dummy cannula relocation, animals were placed in the center of the device and were allowed to explore it for 300 seconds. The animal activity was videotaped with a digital camera suspended above the test apparatus. The behavioral parameters evaluated were: Freezing (duration of the animal in a completely stationary state), Active time (determined as total time test minus Freezing time), Line Crossing (number of grid lines crossed with all four paws), the frequency and duration of Grooming (when the animal licks and/or scratches itself while it stays still) and Rearing (when the animal stands up on its hind legs). After each trial, the apparatus was thoroughly cleaned with damp and dry towels to prevent olfactory cues. Behavioral videos were scored by two observers who were blind to the rat's treatment condition.

Histology

At the end of the behavioral testing period, animals were rendered unconscious by CO_2 and killed by decapitation. The brains were removed, frozen and stored at -80ºC. Coronal sections (40 μm thick) obtained with a cryostat were mounted on subbed slides and stained with cresyl violet [54] for microscopic visualization of cannulae placements. The results from animals with accurately placed cannulae were used for the statistical analyses.

Statistical analysis

Statistical analyses were performed with commercial softwares GraphPad Prism (Graphpad Software Inc., v.4) and Statview (SAS Institute Inc. v5.0.1). The effects of intracranial microinfusions on the behavioral parameters were analyzed by a one-way ANOVA and comparisons between each steroid and vehicle were made by Newman-Keuls post hoc test. Differences were considered significant when $p < 0.05$.

Results

Histological analysis

Cannulae tip localizations in the brain from those animals used for statistical analyses are schematically represented in Figure 1a. They were mainly placed on the dorsal (CA1) area of the hippocampus throughout the rostral-caudal extent. Cresyl violet staining was used for the visualization (Figure 1b). Cannulae distribution was more frequently positioned in -2.40 mm anteroposterior; 1.3 and 2.4 mm mediolateral (left or right sides) and 2.6 mm dorsoventral from Bregma (Figure 1c; Paxinos and Watson [45]). Animals with bad placed cannulae (n=8) were discarded for statistical analyses.

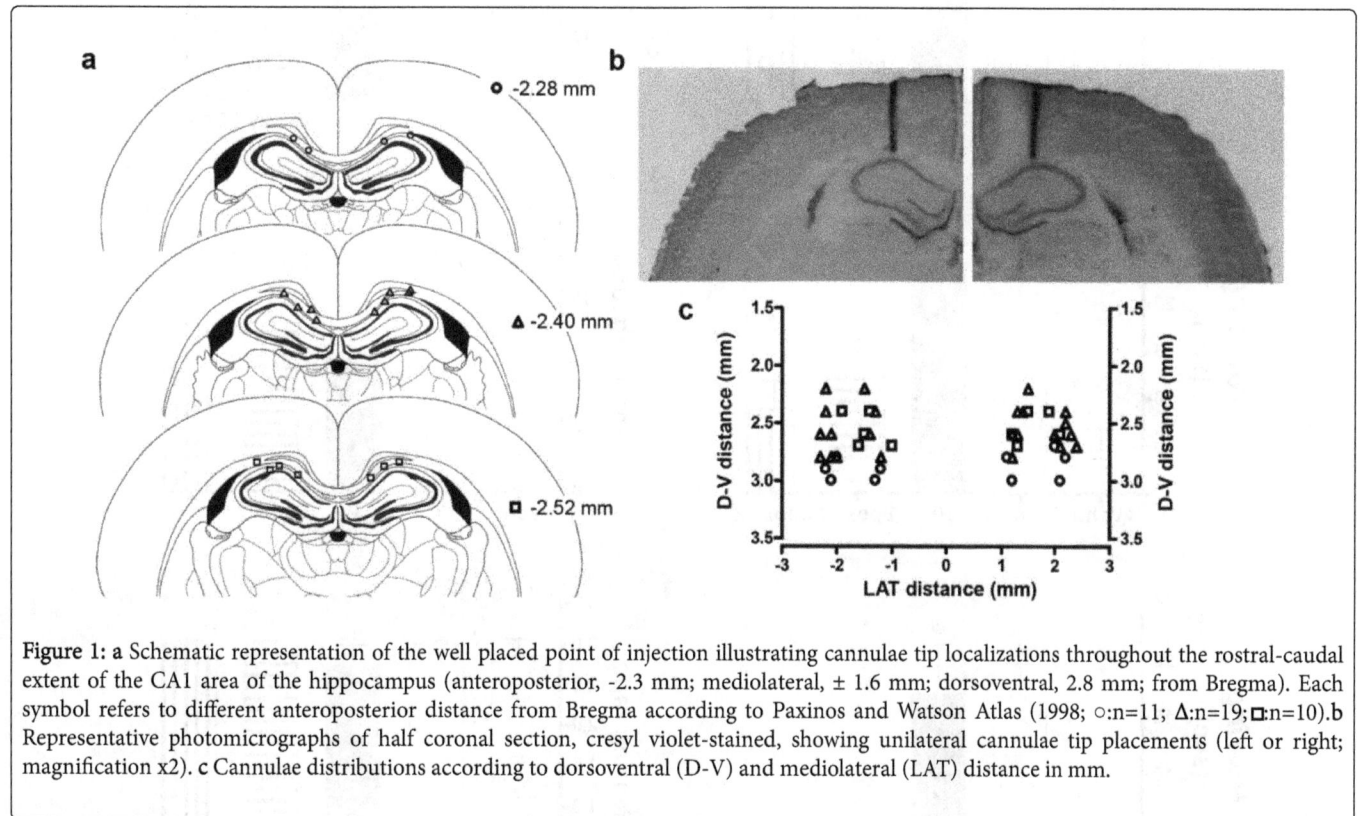

Figure 1: a Schematic representation of the well placed point of injection illustrating cannulae tip localizations throughout the rostral-caudal extent of the CA1 area of the hippocampus (anteroposterior, -2.3 mm; mediolateral, ± 1.6 mm; dorsoventral, 2.8 mm; from Bregma). Each symbol refers to different anteroposterior distance from Bregma according to Paxinos and Watson Atlas (1998; ○:n=11; △:n=19;□:n=10).b Representative photomicrographs of half coronal section, cresyl violet-stained, showing unilateral cannulae tip placements (left or right; magnification x2). c Cannulae distributions according to dorsoventral (D-V) and mediolateral (LAT) distance in mm.

Active time

The amount of time in which animals were in activity was determined as the total time of the test (300 sec) minus the Freezing time (when the animals remain completely immobile). A significant increase on Active time was observed with A and P treatments compared to control (143% and 147% respectively; p<0.05). These increases can be translated as an augmentation in total locomotor activity and horizontal and vertical explorations (Figure 2a). Although, no effects were observed with Epoxy 1 and Epoxy 2 treatments.

Line crossing

Ambulation was quantified as the number of grid lines crossed with all four paws within the 300 sec of testing. A and P administrations produced significant increases of this parameter compared to vehicle (114% and 136% respectively; p<0.05; Figure 2b). That can be interpret-

ed as an increase in horizontal exploration activity, although no effects were observed with Epoxy 1 and Epoxy 2 administrations.

Grooming and grooming ratio

The frequency and duration of each occurrence (when the animal licks and scratches itself) was measured throughout the 300 sec of testing. A significant increase in Grooming duration was observed only with P microinfusion (428% compared to control; p<0.05; Figure 2c). However, no significant effects were observed on the duration of each Grooming event indicated by the "Grooming ratio" (defined like Grooming duration/Grooming frequency; Figure 2d). No effects were observed with the other three steroids in any of both variables.

Rearing and rearing ratio

The frequency and duration of each occurrence (when the animal stands up on its hind legs) was measured in the 300 sec of testing. Significant increases in total Rearing duration were observed with A and P treatments compared to vehicle (265% and 271% respectively; p<0.05; Figure 2e). The increase of this parameter can be interpreted as an augmentation of vertical exploration activity, although no effects were observed on the duration of each Rearing event indicated by the "Rearing ratio" (defined like Rearing duration/Rearing frequency; Figure 2f). No effects were observed with Epoxy 1 and Epoxy 2 administrations in any of both parameters.

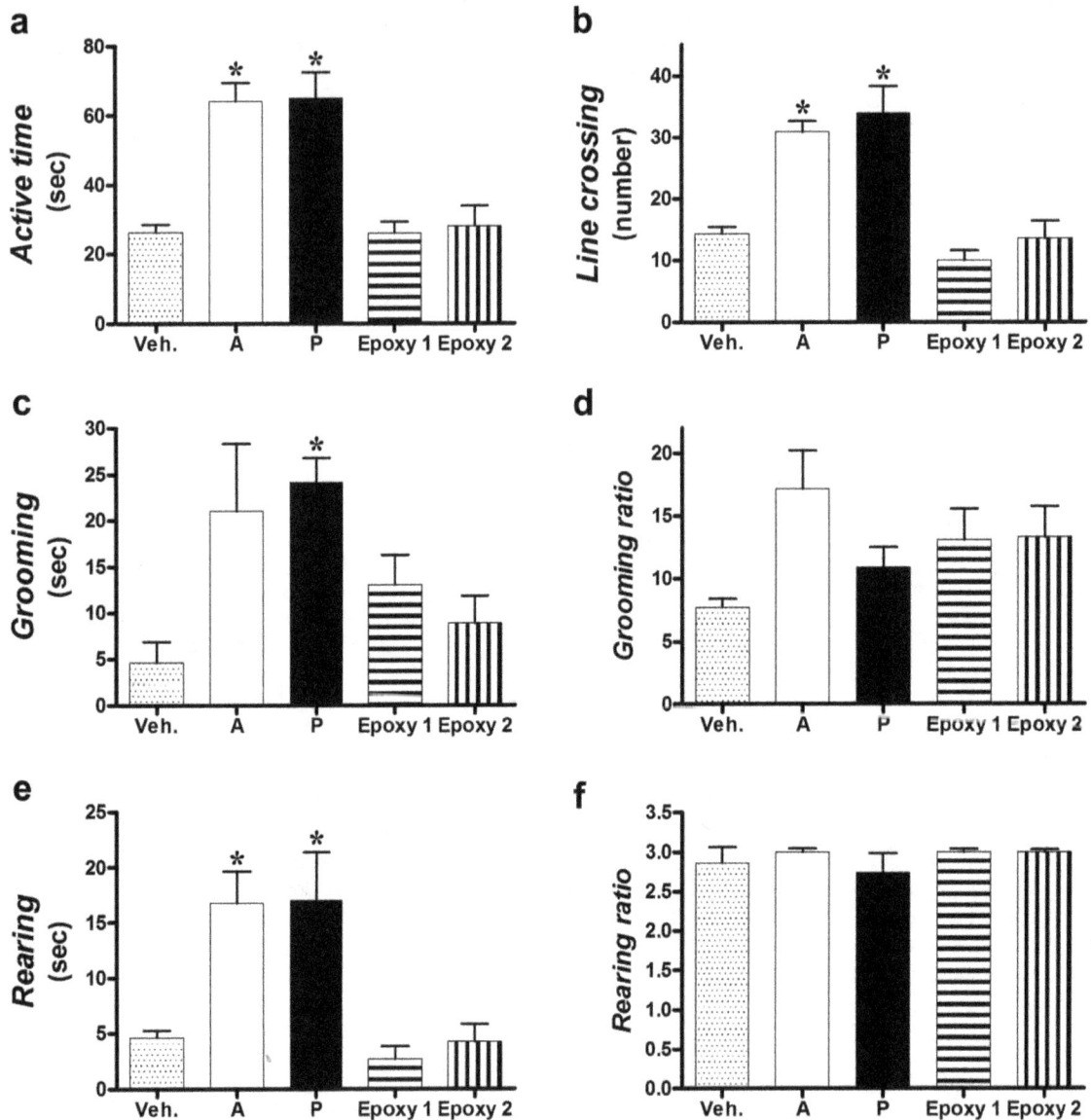

Figure 2: Unilateral microinfusion (0.3 μl) on dorsal hippocampus of vehicle (Veh., cylcodextrin 30% in aCSF) or steroid (A, P, *Epoxy 1* and *Epoxy 2*, 2 μg) and changes in open-field behavioral parameters: **a** *Active time* (difference between total time test and freezing in sec) **b** *Line crossing* (number of grid lines crossed with all four paws), **c** *Grooming* (when the animal licks or scratches itself while stays still in sec) and **d** ratio (duration/frequency) and **e** *Rearing* (when the animal stands up on its hind legs in sec), and f ratio (duration/frequency). Significant effect was determined by one-way ANOVA: $F_{Active\ time}(4,35)=15.3$; $p<0.001$, $F_{Line\ crossing}(4,35)=18.2$; $p<0.001$, $F_{Grooming}(4,35)=2.8$; $p<0.05$, $F_{Grooming\ ratio}(4,24)=1.1$; $p=0.12$, $F_{Rearing}(4,35)=13.3$; $p<0.001$ and $F_{Rearing\ ratio}(4,28)=0.5$; $p=0.75$, sub index in each F indicates the variable analysed. *$p<0.05$ Newman-Keuls post hoc test.

Correlation between Active time and Line crossing

Analysis of Line crossing variable based on Active time, showed a positive correlation factor of 0.74, when all the treatments were considered toghether (Figure 3 C). When this correlation was performed for each treatment, significant effects of P and its analogue, Epoxy 2 (r2=0.77 and r2=0.69 respectively; Figure 3 P and Figure 3 Epoxy

2) were observed, but with lower Active time for the Epoxy 2 than P. On the other hand, the Epoxy 1 showed similar pattern than its

natural analogue A and vehicle, with no significant ANOVA p values (Figure 3).

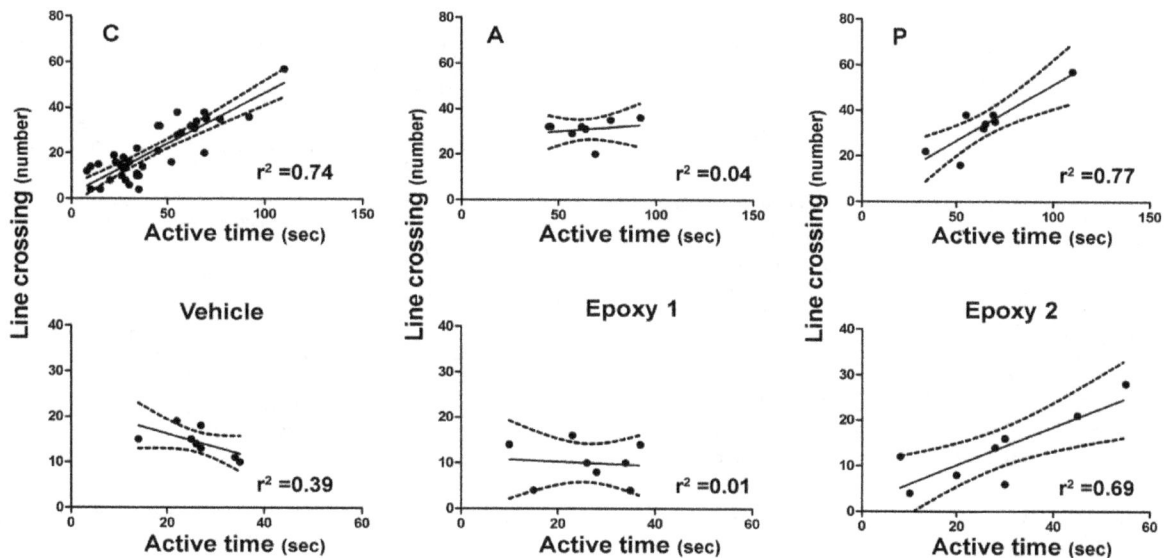

Figure 3: Correlation between *Line crossing* and *Active time* behavioral parameters, under all conditions together (C) or for each microinfusion treatment (Vehicle, **A:** allopregnanolone, **P:** pregnanolone, *Epoxy 1* and *Epoxy 2*). Each point represents a value corresponding to an individual animal test. Correlation coefficients are showed in each panel. Significant effects were determined by one-way ANOVA: $F_C(1,40)=108.2$; $p<0.0001$, $F_{Vehicle}(1,6)=3.9$; $p=0.09$, $F_A(1,6)=0.3$; $p=0.62$, $F_P(1,6)=20.5$; $p=0.004$, $F_{Epoxy\ 1}(1,6)=0.1$; $p=0.82$ and $F_{Epoxy\ 2}(1,6)=19.6$; $p=0.01$, sub index in each F indicates the treatment analyzed. Dotted lines indicate the 95% confidence intervals.

Discussion

Anxiety is an unpleasant nervous state of inner restlessness. Although benzodiazepines and barbiturates are among the treatments of choice for this kind of pathologies, they may induce various side effects [55]. Their actions may be mediated by the GABAA receptor located within the hippocampal formation, which mediates postsynaptic inhibition [56].

Progesterone and its reduced metabolites, A and P, were found to produce anxiolytic-like effects similar to benzodiazepines [36,57,58]. In the brain, in situ synthetized NS are capable of modulating neuronal excitability by rapid non-genomic actions [59] acting as potent modulators of GABAA receptor-mediated neurotransmission [5]. They can locally influence neuronal activity through their effects as paracrine messengers [60]. Thus, NS may have important effects on the regulation of the behavior in humans and in different murine models.

On the other hand, the hippocampal formation is important for the acquisition of short-term memory [61] and it has been also related to anxiety behaviors. Recently, reports described an association between dorsal hippocampus and the modulation of anxiety behavior [39]. Moreover, other studies have shown a significant correlation between low-anxiety or increased exploratory behaviors and A concentration in the hippocampus [52]. Several studies developed in rodents show that

A and P reduce stress and anxiety-like behavior [1,36,62-67]. In fact, the blockade of progesterone's conversion to its metabolites impairs social behavior and induces anxiety-related behavior in rats [68].

The SS arise as a promising solution to the poor bioavailability and rapid metabolism of natural NS administration [12], but it is necessary to compare their biological effects in similar targets and doses of the NS.

In this work, an anxiety model developed to identify the pharmacological mechanisms and potential clinical effects of synthetic and natural steroids was used. Usually, this kind of model based on conflict situations can generate opposite motivational states induced by approach-avoidance situations, however it does not attempt to replicate all features and symptoms of a specific anxiety disorder. Rather, it tries to generate a state of anxiety that could be related to these disorders. Another important methodological consideration that needs to be taken into account is our choice to cannulate animals in a unilateral way (with left/right alternations). Although bilateral cannulae have been widely used to explore the anxiolytic and antidepressant-like effects [46-48], we relied in reports that have not found behavioral differences describing these effects between the brain sides with unilateral progesterone or A microinfusions [49,50]. In agreement with this information, we do not observe lateral influence on the horizontal and vertical exploratory activities either.

Here, we evaluated the anxiolytic properties of an equal dose of A, P or two synthetic steroid analogues (Epoxy 1 and Epoxy 2) by microinfusions in dorsal hippocampus on the open-field test, quantifying horizontal and vertical exploration. The changes observed on the behavioral parameters by A and P can be interpreted as anxiolytic-like effects. Both natural NS enhanced the exploratory activity observed trough the Line crossing, Grooming and Rearing increases and Freezing decrease. However, in some cases P treatment produced the most potent anxiolytic-like effects. Although anxiolytic effects of A are widely described in literature [69-72], only few reports have shown that P administration is able to produce similar effects [28,36,57] with an improved efficacy in some cases [27].

Therefore, the results described in this work support these last findings and add more evidence to this topic. Moreover, none of the treatment affected the duration of Grooming and Rearing events observed through the absence of significant differences in their ratios.

Although A and P treatments produce a significant increase in the Active time and Line crossing, correlations analyses of Line crossing based Active time were not equal. Only a positive correlation of these parameters was observed with microinfusions of P or its analogue Epoxy 2. These differences may probably due to the molecular features of each steroid. These analyses allow to describe similar behavioral effects for steroids with similar A/B rings conformations and suggest that the SS and probably A doses should be administered in higher concentrations to probably produce anxiolytic-like effects. Although, these SS had a limited solubility in aqueous medium.

Previously, we described similar responses to A and P with these SS administrations in a variety of assays, including binding modulation of specific ligands to the GABAA receptor, the 3β-hydroxysteroid dehydrogenase activity alteration and neuroprotection in cerebral cortex and hippocampus cultures against a hypoxic event [17,18]. However, no effects were observed in these behavioral assays, we do not discard these SS for further in vivo evaluations that include another doses and more behavioral assays.

Summarizing, in this work we evaluated, in an open-field test, the in vivo anxiolytic-like effects of two synthetic analogues of A and P with a decreased molecular flexibility (that confers a favorable spatial arrangement for the steroid binding site). Only an increase in animal exploratory activities interpreted as anxiolytic-like effects were observed with A and P microinfusions. The lack of anxiolytic-like effect at the dose evaluated, and the previously reported modulation on the GABAA receptor [17,18] may these SS suitable for therapeutical treatments in other mood disorders where the GABAergic function is involved like early chronic psychosocial stress or depression. Nevertheless the action of these Epoxies should be further evaluated for these conditions.

Acknowledgment

This work was supported by grants from ANPCYT PICT-2006-727; CONICET PIP-860, PIP-243 and partially supported by UBACYT. M R was supported by a fellowship from CONICET.

References

1. Lambert JJ, Belelli D, Peden DR, Vardy AW, Peters JA (2003) Neurosteroid modulation of GABAA receptors. Prog Neurobiol 71: 67-80.

2. Akk G, Covey DF, Evers AS, Steinbach JH, Zorumski CF, et al. (2009) The influence of the membrane on neurosteroid actions at GABA(A) receptors. Psychoneuroendocrinology 34 Suppl 1: S59-66.

3. Majewska MD (1992) Neurosteroids: endogenous bimodal modulators of the GABAA receptor. Mechanism of action and physiological significance. Prog Neurobiol 38: 379-395.

4. Reddy DS (2003) Is there a physiological role for the neurosteroid THDOC in stress-sensitive conditions? Trends Pharmacol Sci 24: 103-106.

5. Gasior M, Carter RB, Witkin JM (1999) Neuroactive steroids: potential therapeutic use in neurological and psychiatric disorders. Trends Pharmacol Sci 20: 107-112.

6. Rupprecht R, di Michele F, Hermann B, Ströhle A, Lancel M, et al. (2001) Neuroactive steroids: molecular mechanisms of action and implications for neuropsychopharmacology. Brain Res Brain Res Rev 37: 59-67.

7. Mellon SH (2004) Synthesis, enzyme localization, and regulation of neurosteroids. In: Smith SS Editor. Neurosteroid effects in the central nervous system: the role of the GABAA receptor. Boca Raton: CRC Press 1-46.

8. Dubrovsky BO (2005) Steroids, neuroactive steroids and neurosteroids in psychopathology. Prog Neuropsychopharmacol Biol Psychiatry 29: 169-192.

9. Hirst JJ, Kelleher MA, Walker DW, Palliser HK (2014) Neuroactive steroids in pregnancy: key regulatory and protective roles in the foetal brain. J Steroid Biochem Mol Biol 139: 144-153.

10. Akk G, Covey DF, Evers AS, Steinbach JH, Zorumski CF, et al. (2007) Mechanisms of neurosteroid interactions with GABA(A) receptors. Pharmacol Ther 116: 35-57.

11. Reddy DS (2010) Neurosteroids: endogenous role in the human brain and therapeutic potentials. Prog Brain Res 186: 113-137.

12. Rey M, Coirini H (2015) Synthetic neurosteroids on brain protection. Neural Regen Res 10: 17-21.

13. Purdy RH, Morrow AL, Blinn JR, Paul SM (1990) Synthesis, metabolism, and pharmacological activity of 3a-hydroxy steroids which potentiate GABA-receptor-mediated chloride ion uptake in rat cerebral cortical synaptoneurosomes. J Med Chem 33: 1572-1581.

14. Souli C, Avlonitis N, Calogeropoulou T, Tsotinis A, Maksay G, et al. (2005) Novel 17beta-substituted conformationally constrained neurosteroids that modulate GABAA receptors. J Med Chem 48: 5203-5214.

15. Scaglione JB, Manion BD, Benz A, Taylor A, DeKoster GT, et al. (2006) Neurosteroid analogues. 11. Alternative ring system scaffolds: gamma- aminobutyric acid receptor modulation and anesthetic actions of benz[f]indenes. J Med Chem 49: 4595-4605.

16. Suñol C, García DA, Bujons J, Kristofíková Z, Matyás L, et al. (2006) Activity of B-nor analogues of neurosteroids on the GABA(A) receptor in primary neuronal cultures. J Med Chem 49: 3225-3234.

17. Rey M, Kruse MS, Alvarez LD, Ghini AA, Veleiro AS, et al. (2013) Neuroprotective action of synthetic steroids with oxygen bridge. Activity on GABAA receptor. Exp Neurol 249: 49-58.

18. Rey M, Veleiro AS, Ghini AA, Kruse MS, Burton G, et al. (2015) Effect of synthetic steroids on GABAA receptor binding in rat brain. Neuroscience 290: 138-146.

19. Veleiro AS, Burton G (2009) Structure-activity relationships of neuroactive steroids acting on the GABAA receptor. Curr Med Chem 16: 455-472.

20. Norberg L, Wahlström G, Bäckström T (1987) The anaesthetic potency of 3 alpha-hydroxy-5 alpha-pregnan-20-one and 3 alpha-hydroxy-5 beta- pregnan-20-one determined with an intravenous EEG-threshold method in male rats. Pharmacol Toxicol 61: 42-47.

21. Belelli D, Lan NC, Gee KW (1990) Anticonvulsant steroids and the GABA/benzodiazepine receptor-chloride ionophore complex. Neurosci Biobehav Rev 14: 315-322.

22. Wieland S, Lan NC, Mirasedeghi S, Gee KW (1991) Anxiolytic activity of the progesterone metabolite 5 alpha-pregnan-3 alpha-o1-20-one. Brain Res 565: 263-268.

23. Devaud LL, Purdy RH, Morrow AL (1995) The neurosteroid, 3 alpha- hydroxy-5 alpha-pregnan-20-one, protects against bicuculline-induced seizures during ethanol withdrawal in rats. Alcohol Clin Exp Res 19: 350-355.

24. Picazo O, Fernández-Guasti A (1995) Anti-anxiety effects of progesterone and some of its reduced metabolites: an evaluation using the burying behavior test. Brain Res 680: 135-141.

25. Wang MD, Wahlström G, Gee KW, Bäckström T (1995) Potency of lipid and protein formulation of 5 alpha-pregnanolone at induction of anaesthesia and the corresponding regional brain distribution. Br J Anaesth 74: 553-557.

26. Weiland NG, Orchinik M (1995) Specific subunit mRNAs of the GABAA receptor are regulated by progesterone in subfields of the hippocampus. Brain Res Mol Brain Res 32: 271-278.

27. Wieland S, Belluzzi JD, Stein L, Lan NC (1995) Comparative behavioral characterization of the neuroactive steroids 3 alpha-OH,5 alpha- pregnan-20-one and 3 alpha-OH,5 beta-pregnan-20-one in rodents. Psychopharmacology (Berl) 118: 65-71.

28. Carboni E, Wieland S, Lan NC, Gee KW (1996) Anxiolytic properties of endogenously occurring pregnanediols in two rodent models of anxiety. Psychopharmacology (Berl) 126: 173-178.

29. Finn DA, Roberts AJ, Lotrich F, Gallaher EJ (1997) Genetic differences in behavioral sensitivity to a neuroactive steroid. J Pharmacol Exp Ther 280: 820-828.

30. Palmer AA, Miller MN, McKinnon CS, Phillips TJ (2002) Sensitivity to the locomotor stimulant effects of ethanol and allopregnanolone is influenced by common genes. Behav Neurosci 116: 126-137.

31. Bitran D, Hilvers RJ, Kellogg CK (1991) Anxiolytic effects of 3 alpha- hydroxy-5 alpha[beta]-pregnan-20-one: endogenous metabolites of progesterone that are active at the GABAA receptor. Brain Res 561: 157-161.

32. Bitran D, Purdy RH, Kellogg CK (1993) Anxiolytic effect of progesterone is associated with increases in cortical allopregnanolone and GABAA receptor function. Pharmacol Biochem Behav 45: 423-428.

33. Fernández-Guasti A, Picazo O (1995) Flumazenil blocks the anxiolytic action of allopregnanolone. Eur J Pharmacol 281: 113-115.

34. Brot MD, Akwa Y, Purdy RH, Koob GF, Britton KT (1997) The anxiolytic- like effects of the neurosteroid allopregnanolone: interactions with GABA(A) receptors. Eur J Pharmacol 325: 1-7.

35. Reddy DS, Kulkarni SK (1997) Differential anxiolytic effects of neurosteroids in the mirrored chamber behavior test in mice. Brain Res 752: 61-71.

36. Bitran D, Dugan M, Renda P, Ellis R, Foley M (1999) Anxiolytic effects of the neuroactive steroid pregnanolone (3 alpha-OH-5 beta-pregnan-20- one) after microinjection in the dorsal hippocampus and lateral septum. Brain Res 850: 217-224.

37. Rupprecht R (2003) Neuroactive steroids: mechanisms of action and neuropsychopharmacological properties. Psychoneuroendocrinology 28: 139-168.

38. Bannerman DM, Rawlins JN, McHugh SB, Deacon RM, Yee BK, et al. (2004) Regional dissociations within the hippocampus--memory and anxiety. Neurosci Biobehav Rev 28: 273-283.

39. Mòdol L, Darbra S, Pallarès M (2011) Neurosteroids infusion into the CA1 hippocampal region on exploration, anxiety-like behaviour and aversive learning. Behav Brain Res 222: 223-229.

40. Pick CG, Peter Y, Terkel J, Gavish M, Weizman R (1996) Effect of the neuroactive steroid alpha-THDOC on staircase test behavior in mice. Psychopharmacology (Berl) 128: 61-66.

41. Mok WM, Krieger NR (1990) Evidence that 5 alpha-pregnan-3 alpha- ol-20-one is the metabolite responsible for progesterone anesthesia. Brain Res 533: 42-45.

42. Bitran D, Mc Leod M, Schiekh M (1995) Blockade of the bioconversion of progesterone to allopregnanolone prevents the anxiolytic effects and potentiation of cortical GABAA receptor function observed in progesterone treated ovariectomized rats. Soc Neurosci Abstr 19: 373-379

43. Eduardo SL, Ghini AA, Burton G (2003) Oxido-bridged neurosteroid analogues Synthesis of 2,19-oxido-allopregnanolone. ARKIVOC X: 468-476.

44. Veleiro AS, Rosenstein RE, Jaliffa CO, Grilli ML, Speroni F, et al. (2003) Synthesis and GABA(A) receptor activity of a 6,19-oxido analogue of pregnanolone. Bioorg Med Chem Lett 13: 343-346.

45. Paxinos G, Watson C (1998) The rat brain in stereotaxic coordinates (4thedn) Academic Press, San Diego California.

46. Engin E, Treit D (2007) The anxiolytic-like effects of allopregnanolone vary as a function of intracerebral microinfusion site: the amygdala, medial prefrontal cortex, or hippocampus. Behav Pharmacol 18: 461-470.

47. Frye CA, Paris JJ, Rhodes ME (2008) Estrogen is necessary for 5alpha- pregnan-3alpha-ol-20-one (3alpha,5alpha-THP) infusion to the ventral tegmental area to facilitate sexual and social, but neither exploratory nor affective behavior of ovariectomized rats. Pharmacol Biochem Behav 91: 261-270.

48. Nin MS, Salles FB, Azeredo LA, Frazon AP, Gomez R, et al. (2008) Antidepressant effect and changes of GABAA receptor gamma2 subunit mRNA after hippocampal administration of allopregnanolone in rats. J Psychopharmacol 22: 477-485.

49. Rodríguez-Landa JF, Contreras CM, Bautista-Martínez FE, Saavedra M, Bernal-Morales B, et al. (2005) Antidepressant-like effect of a microinjection of allopregnanolone in the dorsal hippocampus and lateral septal nucleus in the rat; involvement of GABAA receptor. Behav Pharmacol 16: S45.

50. Estrada-Camarena E, Contreras CM, Saavedra M, Luna-Baltazar I, López-Rubalcava C (2002) Participation of the lateral septal nuclei (LSN) in the antidepressant-like actions of progesterone in the forced swimming test (FST). Behav Brain Res 134: 175-183.

51. Blizard DA, Lippman HR, Chen JJ (1975) Sex differences in open-field behavior in the rat: the inductive and activational role of gonadal hormones. Physiol Behav 14: 601-608.

52. Frye CA, Petralia SM, Rhodes ME (2000) Estrous cycle and sex differences in performance on anxiety tasks coincide with increases in hippocampal progesterone and 3alpha,5alpha-THP. Pharmacol Biochem Behav 67: 587-596.

53. McCarthy MM, Felzenberg E, Robbins A, Pfaff DW, Schwartz-Giblin S (1995) Infusions of diazepam and allopregnanolone into the midbrain central gray facilitate open-field behavior and sexual receptivity in female rats. Horm Behav 29: 279-295.

54. Schumacher M, Coirini H, Pfaff DW, McEwen BS (1990) Behavioral effects of progesterone associated with rapid modulation of oxytocin receptors. Science 250: 691-694.

55. Woods JH, Katz JL, Winger G (1992) Benzodiazepines: use, abuse, and consequences. Pharmacol Rev 44: 151-347.

56. Sperk G, Schwarzer C, Tsunashima K, Fuchs K, Sieghart W (1997) GABA(A) receptor subunits in the rat hippocampus I: immunocytochemical distribution of 13 subunits. Neuroscience 80: 987-1000.

57. Gomez C, Saldivar-Gonzalez A, Delgado G, Rodriguez R (2002) Rapid anxiolytic activity of progesterone and pregnanolone in male rats. Pharmacol Biochem Behav 72: 543-550.

58. Schüle C, Eser D, Baghai TC, Nothdurfter C, Kessler JS, et al. (2011) Neuroactive steroids in affective disorders: target for novel antidepressant or anxiolytic drugs? Neuroscience 191: 55-77.

59. Zheng P (2009) Neuroactive steroid regulation of neurotransmitter release in the CNS: action, mechanism and possible significance. Prog Neurobiol 89: 134-152.

60. Gago N, El-Etr M, Sananès N, Cadepond F, Samuel D, et al. (2004) 3alpha,5alpha-Tetrahydroprogesterone (allopregnanolone) and gamma- aminobutyric acid: autocrine/paracrine interactions in the control of

neonatal PSA-NCAM+ progenitor proliferation. J Neurosci Res 78: 770-783.

61. Harrison NL, Simmonds MA (1984) Modulation of the GABA receptor complex by a steroid anaesthetic. Brain Res 323: 287-292.

62. Majewska MD, Harrison NL, Schwartz RD, Barker JL, Paul SM (1986) Steroid hormone metabolites are barbiturate-like modulators of the GABA receptor. Science 232: 1004-1007.

63. Belelli D, Peden DR, Rosahl TW, Wafford KA, Lambert JJ (2005) Extrasynaptic GABAA receptors of thalamocortical neurons: a molecular target for hypnotics. J Neurosci 25: 11513-11520.

64. Martín-García E, Pallarès M (2005) Intrahippocampal nicotine and neurosteroids effects on the anxiety-like behaviour in voluntary and chronic alcohol-drinking rats. Behav Brain Res 164: 117-127.

65. Frye CA, Rhodes ME (2006) Infusions of 5alpha-pregnan-3alpha-ol-20- one (3alpha,5alpha-THP) to the ventral tegmental area, but not the substantia nigra, enhance exploratory, anti-anxiety, social and sexual behaviours and concomitantly increase 3alpha,5alpha-THP concentrations in the hippocampus, diencephalon and cortex of ovariectomised oestrogen-primed rats. J Neuroendocrinol 18: 960-975.

66.

Darbra S, Pallarès M (2010) Alterations in neonatal neurosteroids affect exploration during adolescence and prepulse inhibition in adulthood. Psychoneuroendocrinology 35: 525-535.

67. Frye CA, Paris JJ (2011) Progesterone turnover to its 5l±-reduced metabolites in the ventral tegmental area of the midbrain is essential for initiating social and affective behavior and progesterone metabolism in female rats. J Endocrinol Invest 34: e188-199.

68. Finn DA, Roberts AJ, Long S, Tanchuck M, Phillips TJ (2003) Neurosteroid consumption has anxiolytic effects in mice. Pharmacol Biochem Behav 76: 451-462.

69. Bäckström T, Bixo M, Johansson M, Nyberg S, Ossewaarde L, et al. (2014) Allopregnanolone and mood disorders. Prog Neurobiol 113: 88-94.

70. Bali A, Jaggi AS (2014) Multifunctional aspects of allopregnanolone in stress and related disorders. Prog Neuropsychopharmacol Biol Psychiatry 48: 64-78.

71. Melcangi RC, Panzica GC (2014) Allopregnanolone: state of the art. Prog Neurobiol 113: 1-5.

72. Schüle C, Nothdurfter C, Rupprecht R (2014) The role of allopregnanolone in depression and anxiety. Prog Neurobiol 113: 79-87.

Permissions

List of Contributors

Mancini A, Raimondo S, Di Segni C, Persano M, Cammarano M and Pontecorvi A
Department of Medical Sciences, Division of Endocrinology, The Catholic University School of Medicine, Rome, Italy

Festa R
Department of Clinical and Molecular Sciences, Polytechnic University of Marche, Ancona, Italy

Tiano L
Institute of Biochemistry, Polytechnic University of the Marche, Ancona, Italy

Silvestrini A and Meucci E
Institute of Biochemistry and Clinical Biochemistry, Catholic University of the Sacred Heart, Rome, Italy

Toru Sanai, Takako Hirakawa, Toru Mizumasa and Hideyuki Koga
Department of Internal Medicine and Clinical Research Institute, National Kyushu Medical Center, 1-8-1 Jigyohama, Chuo-ku, Fukuoka-city, 810-8563 Fukuoka, Japan

Basma K Ramadan
Department of Physiology, Faculty of Medicine for Girls (Cairo), Al-Azhar University, Egypt

Mona F Schaalan
Department of Clinical Pharmacy, Faculty of Pharmacy, Misr International University, Cairo, Egypt

Eman S Mahmoud
Department of Histology, Faculty of Medicine for Girls (Cairo), Al-Azhar, University, Egypt

Mohammad S Abdallah
Critical Care Clinical Pharmacist at King Saud Medical City Riyadh, Saudi Arabia

Ahmad F Madi and Muhammad A Rana
ICU consultant at King Saud Medical City Riyadh, Saudi Arabia

Christine Carlsson-Skwirut, Konstantin V Svechnikov and Olle Söder
Department of Woman and Child Health, Paediatric Endocrinology Unit, Astrid Lindgren Children's Hospital, Karolinska Institute and University Hospital, SE 17176 Stockholm, Sweden

Eugenia Colón
Department of Woman and Child Health, Paediatric Endocrinology Unit, Astrid Lindgren Children's Hospital, Karolinska Institute and University Hospital, SE 17176 Stockholm, Sweden
Department of Pathology and Cytology, Sodersjukhuset, Karolinska Institute and University Hospital, SE 11883 Stockholm, Sweden

Roxane Paulin and Sébastien Bonnet
Department of Medicine, Laval University, Centre de Recherche du CHUQ, Hôtel-Dieu de Québec, Québec City, QC, Canada

Graham MR
Sport and Exercise Science, Institute of Health, Medical Science and Society Science, Glyndwr University, Wrexham, Wales, UK, LL11 2AW

Davies B
Health and Exercise Science, University of Glamorgan, Pontypridd, Wales, UK, CF83 1DL

Grace FM and Baker JS
Exercise Science, University of the West of Scotland, Hamilton, Scotland, ML3 OJB

Evans PJ
Department of Endocrinology, Royal Gwent Hospital, Newport, Wales, UK, NP20 2UB

D. Somjen
Institute of Endocrinology, Metabolism and Hypertension, Tel-Aviv Sourasky Medical Center; Tel-Aviv 64239, and the Sackler Faculty of Medicine, Tel-Aviv University, Tel-Aviv, Israel

S. Katzburg, S. Tamir and and Y. Vaya
Laboratory of Human Health and Nutrition Sciences, MIGAL-Galilee Technology Center, Kiryat- Shmona 11016

O. Sharon and D. Hendel
Department of Orthopedic Surgery, Shaarei- Zedek Medical Center, Jerusalem, Israel

Somchit Eiam-Ong and Kittisak Sinphitukkul
Department of Physiology, Faculty of Medicine, Chulalongkorn University, Bangkok, Thailand

Krissanapong Manotham
Department of Medicine, Lerdsin General Hospital, Bangkok, Thailand

Somchai Eiam-Ong
Deparment of Medicine (Division of Nephrology), Faculty of Medicine, Chulalongkorn University, Bangkok, Thailand

Ahmed SI and Attia GA
Department of Anatomy, Faculty of Medicine, Najran University, Saudi Arabia

Ali TO
Faculty of Graduate Studies & Scientific Research, National Ribat University, Sudan

Elsheikh AS
Department of Applied Medical Sciences, Community faculty Najran, Saudi Arabia

Abdalla AM
Department of Anatomy, Faculty of Medicine, King Khalid University, Saudi Arabia

Mohamed MH
Department of Anatomy, Faculty of Medicine, Jazan University, Saudi Arabia

Wendell SG and Edward JP
Department of Chemistry and Biochemistry, College of Science and Mathematics, Auburn University, Auburn, Alabama 36849-5319, USA

Medras M
Department of Endocrinology, Diabetology and Isotope Treatment, Wroclaw Medical University, ul. Pasteura 4, 50-367 Wroclaw, Poland
Department of Sports Medicine, University School of Physical Education, ul, Paderewskiego 35, 51-612 Wroclaw, Poland

Jozkow P
Department of Sports Medicine, University School of Physical Education, ul, Paderewskiego 35, 51-612 Wroclaw, Poland

Terpilowski L
Department of Emergency Medical Services, Wroclaw Medical University, ul. Pasteura 4, 50-367 Wroclaw, Poland

Zagocka E
Laboratory of Male Infertility, ul. Kosciuszki 108A/18, 50-441 Wroclaw, Poland

Monika Modrzejewska, Ewelina Lachowicz, Joanna Kot D, Wojciech Lubiński and Anna Modrzejewska
Department of Ophthalmology, Pomeranian Medical University, Powst, Wlkp. Str. 72, 70 111 Szczecin, Poland

Jacek Rudnicki
Department of Neonatal Pathology, Pomeranian Medical University, Powst, Wlkp. Str. 72, 70 111 Szczecin, Poland

Beata Czeszyńska
Departament of Neonatology Pomeranian Medical University, Siedlecka Str. 2, Police, Poland

Jacek Patalan
Department of Neonatal Intensive Care Sp SZOZ-Zdroje, Mączna Str. 4, Szczecin, Poland

Ikki Sakuma, Jun Saito, Yoko Matsuzawa, Masao Omura and Tetsuo Nishikawa
Endocrinology and Diabetes Center, Yokohama Rosai Hospital, Yokohama, Japan

Seiji Matsui
Department of Radiology, Yokohama Rosai Hospital, Yokohama, Japan

Koshiro Nishimoto
Departments of Urology, School of Medicine, Keio University, Tokyo, Japan
Department of Urology, Tachikawa Hospital, Tokyo, Japan

Kuniaki Mukai
Department of Biochemistry, School of Medicine, Keio University, Tokyo, Japan

Asami Kato, Shimpei Higo and Fusako Sakai
Department of Biophysics and Life Sciences, Graduate School of Arts and Sciences, The University of Tokyo, 3-8-1 Komaba, Meguro, Tokyo 153-8902, Japan, 9 The University of Tokyo, Japan

Yasushi Hojo and Suguru Kawato
Department of Biophysics and Life Sciences, Graduate School of Arts and Sciences, The University of Tokyo, 3-8-1 Komaba, Meguro, Tokyo 153-8902, Japan, 9 The University of Tokyo, Japan
Bioinformatics Project of Japan Science and Technology Agency, The University of Tokyo, Japan

Masahiro Okamoto
Department of Biophysics and Life Sciences, Graduate School of Arts and Sciences, The University of Tokyo, 3-8-1 Komaba, Meguro, Tokyo 153-8902, Japan, 9 The University of Tokyo, Japan
Research Fellow of the Japan Society for the Promotion of Science, Japan

Hideaki Soya
Laboratory of Exercise Biochemistry and Neuroendocrinology, Institute for Health & Sports Sciences, University of Tsukuba, Tsukuba, Ibaraki, Japan

Takeshi Yamazaki
Laboratory of Molecular Brain Science, Graduate School of Integrated Arts and Sciences, Hiroshima University, Higashi-Hiroshima, Japan

Mohanty BK
School of MVM, 1417 Baramunda Colony, Bhubaneswar-751003, Orissa, India

Neelima P. Sidharthan and Addicam Jagannadha Rao
Department of Biochemistry, Indian Institute of Science, Bangalore, India

Bánhegyi RJ, Laczó I and Pikó B
Oncology Centre, Pandy Kalman Bekes County Hospital, Hungary

Fülöp F and Mellár E
Department of Radiology, Pandy Kalman Bekes County Hospital, Hungary

Pooja Shree
Department of Biotechnology, SSIET-Anna University, Chennai, India

Renan Pozzi, Leandro Fernandes, Bruno FA Calegare and Vânia D'Almeida
Department of Psychobiology, Universidade Federal de São Paulo, UNIFESP, São Paulo, Brazil

Satué K
Department of Animal Medicine and Surgery, Cardenal Herrera University, Spain

Gardón JC
Department of Experimental Sciences and Mathematics, Catholic University of Valencia "San Vicente Mártir", Spain

Rabih Darwiche and Roger Schneiter
University of Fribourg, Department of Biology, 1700 Fribourg, Switzerland

Mansur A Sandhu, Muhammad S Anjum, Nasir Mukhtar and Riaz Hussain
Department of Veterinary Biomedical Sciences, PMAS-Arid Agriculture University Rawalpindi, 46300, Shamasabad square, Pakistan

Imtiaz A Khan
Department of Veterinary Pathobiology, PMAS-Arid Agriculture University Rawalpindi, 46300, Shamasabad square, Pakistan

Robert S Bowen
Science and Mathematics Division, Truett-McConnell College, Cleveland, GA 30528, USA
Department of Kinesiology, University of North Carolina Charlotte, Charlotte, NC 28223, USA

David P Ferguson and J Timothy Lightfoot
Department of Kinesiology, University of North Carolina Charlotte, Charlotte, NC 28223, USA
Department of Health and Kinesiology, Texas A&M University, College Station, TX 77845, USA

Aguilar-Díaz H and Cerbón-Cervantes MA
Facultad de Química, Departamento de Biología, Universidad Nacional Autónoma de México, México

Nava-Castro KE
Departamento de Ciencias Ambientales, Centro de Ciencias de la Atmósfera, Universidad Nacional Autónoma de México, México

Meneses-Ruiz DM and Morales-Montor J
Departamento de Inmunología, Instituto de Investigaciones Biomédicas, Universidad Nacional Autónoma de México, México

Ponce-Regalado MD
Universidad de Guadalajara, Centro Universitario de los Altos-Departamento de clínicas, México

Ruth E. MacRedmond, Gurpreet K. Singhera, Samuel J. Wadsworth, Susan Attridge, Mohammed Bahzad, Kristy Williams, Harvey O. Coxson and Delbert R. Dorscheid
Centre for Heart Lung Innovation, St. Paul's Hospital, University of British Columbia, Vancouver, Canada

Steven R. White
Department of Medicine, University of Chicago, Chicago, Illinois, USA

Michaela Dušková, Hana Pospíšilová, Martin Hill and Luboslav Stárka
Institute of Endocrinology, Prague, Czech Republic

Gabriella Moroni, Roberta Gaziano, Cristina Buè, Massimiliano Agostini, Carlo-Federico Perno, Paola Sinibaldi-Vallebona and Francesca Pica
Department of Experimental Medicine and Surgery, University of Rome Tor Vergata, Rome, Italy

Rey M
Laboratorio de Neurobiología, Instituto de Biología y Medicina Experimental (IBYME-CONICET), Vuelta de Obligado 2490, (C1428ADN), Ciudad Autónoma de Buenos Aires, Argentina

Coirini H
Laboratorio de Neurobiología, Instituto de Biología y Medicina Experimental (IBYME-CONICET), Vuelta de Obligado 2490, (C1428ADN), Ciudad Autónoma de Buenos Aires, Argentina

Departamento de Bioquímica Humana, Facultad de Medicina, Universidad de Buenos Aires, Paraguay 2155, 5to Piso, (C1121ABG) Ciudad Autónoma de Buenos Aires, Argentina

Ghini AA
Departamento de Química Orgánica, Unidad de Microanálisis y Métodos Físicos aplicados a Química Orgánica (UMYMFOR-CONICET) Facultad de Ciencias Exactas y Naturales, Universidad de Buenos Aires (FCEN-UBA), Pabellón 2, Ciudad Universitaria, Intendente Güiraldes 2160, (C1428EHA) Ciudad Autónoma de Buenos Aires, Argentina

Index

www.ingramcontent.com/pod-product-compliance
Lightning Source LLC
Chambersburg PA
CBHW070155240326
41458CB00126B/5211